Vaccine Science and Immunization Guideline

Pamela G. Rockwell

Editor

Vaccine Science and Immunization Guideline

A Practical Guide for Primary Care

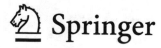 Springer

Editor
Pamela G. Rockwell, DO
Department of Family Medicine
University of Michigan Medical School
Ann Arbor, MI, USA

ISBN 978-3-319-86869-1   ISBN 978-3-319-60471-8   (eBook)
DOI 10.1007/978-3-319-60471-8

Printed on acid-free paper

This Springer imprint is published by Springer Nature
The registered company is Springer International Publishing AG
The registered company address is: Gewerbestrasse 11, 6330 Cham, Switzerland

Preface

Memories from Medical School

It was 1989. I was in my fourth year of medical school, taking care of a patient in Riverside Hospital's 6-bed ICU. Riverside was a small community hospital in Trenton, Michigan, a mostly blue-collar Detroit suburb bordering the Detroit River, surrounded by steel mills and car manufacturing plants. Practicing medicine was different then. There was less technology to aid disease diagnosis and there were fewer treatment options available. *Evidence-based medicine* was not yet a familiar term in medical education. Hospital computers were not common, electronic medical records were an innovation not yet materialized, and paper charts and books in print served as records and resources. Smoking was allowed in patient rooms which were equipped with hospital-supplied ashtrays on bedside stands. Pseudomonas was an infection commonly encountered on the wards and its *new-mown hay* smell tipped off medical staff to its existence before confirmatory cultures were complete. The Advisory Committee on Immunization Practices (ACIP) routinely recommended only four vaccines for children and one for adolescents. However, the practice of medicine in 1989 and today is similar in one important way: there were vaccine recommendations for the prevention of certain diseases for those who do not have a spleen both then and now.

David was a 26-year-old asplenic patient in ICU bed #3. He had fallen ill with a fever the day before. There was only a thin curtain partition separating David from me and my patient in bed #2 and I could hear David's doctor and family crying, inconsolable with despair. From the nursing staff I learned that David's spleen had been surgically removed after a motorcycle accident 4 years prior and he had not received the [then] two ACIP recommended postsplenectomy vaccines against pneumococcal and meningococcal infections.(1) Those gathered around his bed witnessed overwhelming postsplenectomy sepsis, a well-characterized phenomenon typically caused by encapsulated bacteria, such as *Streptococcus pneumoniae*, *Neisseria meningitides,* and *Haemophilus influenzae* type b, overwhelm his immune system and shut down his organs. Everyone knew the cocktail of antibiotics he was receiving could not help him. Sepsis took his life swiftly.

It profoundly struck me that a young, previously healthy person lying in bed a few feet from me had likely died from a vaccine-preventable disease! David's death plagued me with many "what-ifs": *What if* he had received his recommended vaccines? Would he still be alive? *What if* this fatal outcome was his doctor's fault? Had she failed to recommend the vaccines? *What if* he had been offered the vaccines but then refused them? Or, *what if* he received the vaccinations but the vaccines failed to offer protection?

The seeds of this book took root.

My hope is that this book gives the reader a broad understanding of vaccines. It chronicles vaccines from their beginnings in society, how they were developed through scientific study, and their value in preventing disease and saving lives. This book describes how a vaccine begins with an idea to prevent disease and how it is then developed in the laboratory through years of research and study and ultimately results in a recommendation put out by the Centers for Disease Control and Prevention Advisory Committee on Immunization Practices. The first chapter of this book in no way claims to cover all of the infectious disease and vaccine history or cite and acknowledge all those who were responsible to bring vaccine medical advances to where they are today. It is a collection of historical facts and interesting stories that illustrate this author's view of the development of vaccines in society. Other chapters of this book provide an understanding of vaccine science and immunology and a thorough review of routine immunizations given in the United States today and in years past, with their indications for reference. Sources and resources to determine immunization needs for patients are identified. Myths regarding vaccines are discussed and busted. Barriers to improving vaccination rates are identified and Chapters 7 and 8 detail ways to overcome those barriers, offering both evidence-based recommendations and expert opinion on how to improve immunization rates for patients. Practical as well as theoretical discussions and advice on healthcare systems, implementation science, and models of communication are presented. I hope that through this book, I can enlighten the reader on vaccines and vaccine science in new ways.

Acknowledgments

For the advancement of vaccine science, knowledge, and preventive health.

With appreciation for my smart, thoughtful, like-minded co-authors who believe in the power of vaccines.

For all my mentors, patients, family, and friends who encouraged me to undertake this book.

With special appreciation and thanks for my family who supported me with love and tolerance.

And a special thanks to my daughter Christina, who spent many hours helping edit the non-scientific portions of the text.

Contents

Contributors

Heidi L. Diez, PharmD, BCACP University of Michigan, College of Pharmacy, Ann Arbor, MI, USA

Family Medicine and Pharmacy Innovations and Partnerships, Michigan Medicine, Ann Arbor, MI, USA

Jennifer L. Hamilton, MD, PhD Department of Family, Community, and Preventive Health, Drexel University College of Medicine, Philadelphia, PA, USA

Alexandra Hayward, MPH Infection Prevention and Epidemiology, Michigan Medicine, Ann Arbor, MI, USA

Paul Hunter, MD Department of Family Medicine and Community Health, School of Medicine and Public Health, University of Wisconsin, Madison, WI, USA

City of Milwaukee Health Department, Milwaukee, WI, USA

Donald B. Middleton, MD University of Pittsburgh School of Medicine, UPMC St. Margaret, Department of Family Medicine, Pittsburgh, PA, USA

Jeffrey L. Moore, MD Department of Family Medicine, University of Wisconsin School of Medicine and Public Health, Marshfield Clinic, Merrill Center, Merrill, WI, USA

Jonathan M. Raviotta, MPH Department of Family Medicine and Clinical Epidemiology, University of Pittsburgh School of Medicine, Pittsburgh, PA, USA

Pamela G. Rockwell, DO Department of Family Medicine, University of Michigan Medical School, Ann Arbor, MI, USA

Margot Latrese Savoy, MD, MPH, FAAFP, FABC, CPE, CMQ Christiana Care Health System, Department of Family & Community Medicine, Wilmington, DE, USA

Kristi VanDerKolk, MD Western Michigan University, Homer Stryker MD School of Medicine, Department of Family and Community Medicine, Kalamazoo, MI, USA

Richard K. Zimmerman, MD, MPH University of Pittsburgh School of Medicine, Pittsburgh, PA, USA

Chapter 1
History of Infectious Diseases and Vaccines in Society: Introduction

Pamela G. Rockwell

The success or failure of any government in the final analysis must be measured by the well-being of its citizens. Nothing can be more important to a state than its public health; the state's paramount concern should be the health of its people.

Franklin Delano Roosevelt [2]

Introduction

Franklin D. Roosevelt, as governor of New York (serving from 1929 to 1932) in a report to the New York State Health Commission in 1932 [2], knew that public health was important to society as evidenced by the first line of the report quoted above. His commitment to public health and disease prevention helped incorporate vaccines into US medical practice and pave the way for eradication of polio in the United States. As the 32nd president of the United States (serving from 1933 to 1945), he founded the National Foundation for Infantile Paralysis (NFIP) in 1938, later renamed the March of Dimes. Among many other notable accomplishments, NFIP sponsored a large poliomyelitis vaccine field trial directed by Thomas Francis, Jr., MD in 1954 [3], of the University of Michigan Vaccine Evaluation Center to test the safety and efficacy of the Salk polio vaccine. It was the first wide-scale testing of a vaccine, using 65,000 children volunteered by their parents, to receive either vaccine or placebo injections [4]. Thanks to the polio trial and subsequent vaccine trials, ongoing scientific research, and scholarly activity, we can now prevent more

P.G. Rockwell, DO (✉)
Department of Family Medicine, University of Michigan Medical School, Ann Arbor, MI, USA
e-mail: prockwel@med.umich.edu

© Springer International Publishing AG 2017
P.G. Rockwell (ed.), *Vaccine Science and Immunization Guideline*,
DOI 10.1007/978-3-319-60471-8_1

infectious diseases through immunizations than ever before. In the medical communities' common goal to cure disease and treat the effects of disease as it occurs, immunizations have been hailed as one of the most effective methods of all medical and public health initiatives to save lives by way of preventing disease [5].

Infectious disease outbreaks have had devastating effects on people and populations, influencing human social and political history throughout recorded time. Hippocrates (460–377 BCE), who was among the first to record his theories on the occurrence of disease, coined the terms *endemic* and *epidemic disease*. He defined endemic diseases as diseases that were always present in a population. Conversely, epidemic diseases were not always invariably present but occurred sometimes in large numbers [6]. Civilizations and their cultures have been shaped, altered, and decimated by disease endemics and epidemics. Outbreaks of disease have been documented since 541 AD in Asia. Though the evidence for epidemics in the non-Western world and in the New World before significant contact with Europeans is scant, we can theorize that infectious diseases have been present around the world as long as man has been present [7]. Cholera, yellow fever, malaria, and plague were constant concerns in the West and in US port cities in the early twentieth century when quarantine was the principle tool of prevention [6]. Through a combination of public health initiatives including improved sanitation and introduction of vaccines, deaths declined markedly in the United States during the twentieth century. This is significantly evidenced by the sharp drop in infant and child mortality and a 29.2-year increase in life expectancy noted during that time [8]. The three leading causes of death in 1900 were pneumonia, tuberculosis (TB), diarrhea, and enteritis, which when combined with diphtheria, caused 1/3 of all deaths. Young children aged fewer than 5 years accounted for 40% of the deaths caused by the forenamed diseases and made up roughly 1/3 of all deaths from all causes. By 1997, that percentage dropped to 1.4% [9, 10] (Fig. 1.1).

The positive effects of vaccines have been documented since the late 1700s when inoculation (introduction of smallpox pustules into the skin) was practiced. Centers for Disease Control and Prevention (CDC) describes the reduction in morbidity and mortality associated with vaccine-preventable diseases in the United States as one of the ten greatest public health achievements of the first decade of the twenty-first century [11]. Despite the success of vaccination, common infectious diseases continue to confer significant societal and individual harm. For example, influenza, a common and familiar infectious disease known as "the flu," is responsible for much morbidity and mortality in the United States. CDC estimates that each year, an average of 226,000 people are hospitalized due to influenza and between 3000 and 49,000 people (mostly adults) die of influenza and its complications, depending on the year and severity of outbreaks. Other infectious diseases also result in significant morbidity and mortality: of the 32,000 cases of invasive pneumococcal disease in adults in 2012, there were approximately 3300 deaths. A total of 800,000–1.4 million people suffer from chronic hepatitis B, with complications such as liver cancer, and in the United States, human papillomavirus (HPV) causes about 17,000 cancers in women and about 9000 cancers in men each year; about 4000 women die each year from cervical cancer [12].

In addition to illness and death, cost to society from infectious diseases can be measured in terms of dollars spent in treating and preventing diseases. The economic analysis of vaccine-preventable disease (VPD) requires examination beyond

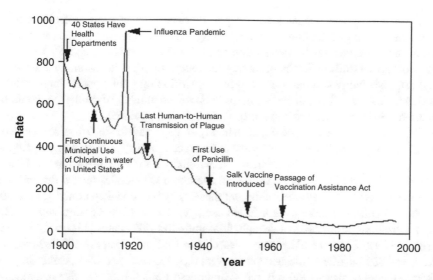

Fig. 1.1 Crude death rate (per 100,000 population per year) for infectious diseases – United States, 1900–1996 (Adapted from Armstrong et al. [8]). §American Water Works Association. Water chlorination principles and practices: AWWA manual M20. Denver, Colorado: American Water Works Association, 1973

the costs of individual illness to account for the costs of protecting society. For example, the 2004 direct cost to the public health infrastructure in Iowa containing one case of measles brought to the United States from an unvaccinated college student who had traveled to India was estimated at $142,452. This is far greater than the estimated cost of uncomplicated individual illness (fewer than $100) [13]. A 2014 report by CDC concluded that routine childhood vaccinations given to infants and young children over the previous two decades will prevent 322 million cases of disease, 21 million hospitalizations, and about 732,000 early deaths over the course of the lifetimes of children born during 1994–2013, for a net societal cost savings of $1.38 trillion which includes $295 billion in direct costs such as medical expenses [14]. Moreover, these calculations may underestimate the full impact of vaccines because only the 14 routine early childhood immunizations that are typically required for school entry were considered, leaving out flu shots and adolescent vaccines along with all the societal benefits those vaccines bestow [12].

Vaccination has led to a dramatic decline in the number of US cases of many infectious diseases. However, unvaccinated American children and adults are susceptible to diseases that are now rare stateside but may be imported into the United States from foreign travelers. Furthermore, those who are unvaccinated are susceptible to exposure to the same infectious diseases while traveling abroad as illustrated by the measles-infected college student returning from travel to India. Additionally, outbreaks of preventable diseases occur when many parents decide not to vaccinate their children, especially when living in a closed community. Pockets of unvaccinated children not only create risk for those unvaccinated children in the community, but also create risk for others outside the community unable to be vaccinated: children too young to be vaccinated and people with weakened immune systems [15].

Around the world, a much larger proportion of children are now protected against a broader range of infectious diseases through vaccinations, but there is still much room for improvement in vaccination rates. VPDs are still responsible for about 25% of the 10 million deaths occurring annually among children under 5 years of age [16]. Mortality estimates are helpful in prioritizing public health intervention, and in the case of VPDs, these estimates indicate the number of deaths that could be averted if existing vaccines were used to their fullest potential.

Take the example of measles again, a highly contagious infectious disease caused by a paramyxovirus with classic symptoms of fever, cough, coryza, conjunctivitis, Koplik spots, and rash, which in 1912 became a nationally notifiable disease in the United States. In the first decade of reporting, an average 6000 measles-related deaths were reported annually. Nearly every child got measles by the time they turned 15; an estimated 3–4 million people were infected each year in the United States, with 48,000 hospitalizations, 4000 cases of encephalitis, and ~400–500 deaths [17]. In the 4 years prior to the US licensure of the measles vaccine in 1963, an average of 503,282 measles cases and 432 measles-associated deaths were reported each year [18]. As the US public eradication of measles effort began, an ambitious Public Health Service statement in 1966 maintained that by the "effective use of [these] vaccines during the coming winter and spring should insure the eradication of measles from the United States in 1967" [19]. Though not eradicated as predicted, by 1998 measles reached a provisional record low number of 89 cases with no measles-associated deaths [20]. All cases in 1998 were either documented to be associated with international importations (69 cases) or believed to be associated with international importations [9]. Over the next decade around the globe, there was also a reduction in measles mortality from an estimated 750,000 deaths in 2000 down to 197,000 in 2007 [21, 22]. Worldwide, measles vaccination prevented an estimated 17.1 million deaths during 2000–2014 [23] (Fig. 1.2).

Infectious Disease: Its Effects on Culture and Populations

Significant Plagues, Pandemics, and Epidemics

Both in ancient times and in the modern day, infectious disease complications range from, at best, a patient forced out of commission for weeks due to illness to far more serious complications such as hearing and vision loss, disfigurement, limb paralysis, limb amputations, seizures, and death. On a much larger scale than individual complications, disease epidemics have decimated entire populations and changed cultures. It wasn't until the 1960s that historian William H. McNeill started producing scholarly writings on history in a completely novel way: he chronicled how infectious disease outbreaks have influenced history. He described how disease has molded many culture's demographics, politics, and ecological resources. His scholarly contributions are the first to correlate historical events and outcomes with disease epidemics [24].

McNeill and other historians since wrote of the Antonine Plague of 165–180 AD, the first major plague known to have influenced culture and civilization. It is reported

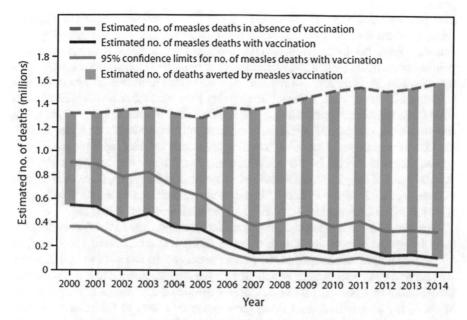

Fig. 1.2 Estimated number of measles deaths and number of averted by measles vaccination – worldwide, 2000–2014 (from citation progress toward regional measles elimination – worldwide 2000–2014 http://www.cdc.gov/mmwr/preview/mmwrhtml/mm6444a4.htm)

to have killed a quarter to a third of Rome's population [25]. Most historians agree that in 165 AD Roman soldiers returning home from war in Mesopotamia caused the plague by introducing what historians believe to be smallpox (never before seen in Europe) to Rome. Rome's two emperors Lucius Verus and Marcus Aurelius Antoninus died from the plague, giving the plague its name. Unfortunately, little record keeping of the plague disease and description of its physical and clinical effects on the sufferer exists. Though the Greek physician, Galen, recorded his observations and a description of the epidemic, his descriptions were scant and he did not give many specific details of the disease. He described the plague as "great" and of long duration and mentioned fever, diarrhea, pharyngitis, as well as a skin eruption, sometimes dry and sometimes pustular appearing on the ninth day of illness, fitting the theory that the plague was caused by smallpox (there is no actual proof of this). The majority of scholars agree that the impact of the plague was severe, affecting ancient Roman traditions and not only influencing spirituality and religion but also influencing military conscription and agricultural and urban economy and depleting the finances of the land. Artistic expression of the time depicted the renewal of spirituality and religiousness. Scholars conclude that the plague and its sequelae created the conditions for the spread of monotheistic religions, such as Mithraism and Christianity [25]. The Antonine Plague, wrote McNeill, coincided with the start of the Roman Empire's 300-year decline [24].

Several hundred years later, in 541 AD, the first of three other historically significant plague pandemics caused by the bacterium *Yersinia pestis* began, these more carefully recorded than the Antonine Plague. The *Justinian Plague* or *Bubonic Plague*, named after the sixth Byzantine Emperor Justinian I, is characterized by sudden onset fever, headache, chills, and weakness and one or more swollen, tender, and painful lymph nodes (called buboes) and is reported to have killed millions. Numerous references in art, literature, and monuments attest to the horrors and devastation that accompanied the disease. It depopulated many European cities and depressed birth rates for generations, contributing to the fall of Rome. *Yersinia pestis* infects small rodents like rats, mice, and squirrels, and it is usually transmitted to humans through the bite of an infected flea or by handling an animal infected with plague. It was spread across the world by the globalization of rats: black rats brought over from Africa as part of the grain trade to Europe. Over the next 200 years, there were several outbreaks of the Justinian Bubonic Plague which were ultimately responsible for killing over 25 million people and affecting all the Mediterranean basin [26].

The second large pandemic, rising to epidemic proportions in the fourteenth century during the Middle Ages, originated in China several hundred years later, in 1334. This plague was known as the *Black Plague*, or the *Great Plague*. The name was derived by descriptions of people ill with the plague, covered in black boils that oozed blood and pus. At that time, China was one of the busiest trading nations, allowing the plague to spread along the great trade routes to Constantinople and then to Europe where it again devastated Europe, killing nearly 50 million people, an estimated 60% of the European population. The pandemic died down in winter, when fleas went dormant, and flourished in the spring. Even after the worst of each pandemic flair was over, smaller outbreaks continued for centuries, and the disease did not disappear until the 1600s. The devastation of the Black Plague caused massive labor shortages due to high mortality rates, which in turn is credited in speeding up the development of many economic, social, and technical modernizations [27], and has been considered a factor of the onset of the Renaissance in the late fourteenth century (Fig. 1.3).

The "third great plague," the *Modern Plague*, began in the Yunnan province in China in 1855 and appeared in Hong Kong by 1894. In the following 20 years, it spread to port cities around the world via rats on steamships, causing approximately 10 million deaths. It spread from the Yunnan province to all inhabited continents, ultimately killing more than 12 million people in India and China alone [28]. The *Yersinia pestis* bacterium was originally spread by infectious flea bites from infected rats, but it then spread to local populations of ground squirrels and other small mammals. This bubonic plague was endemic in populations of infected ground rodents in central Asia and was a known cause of death among migrant and established human populations in that region for centuries. Increased globalization resulting in more heterogeneous societies led to the dissemination of bubonic plague which still exists in various parts of the world. In 2003, more than 2100 human cases and 180 deaths were recorded by the World Health Organization (WHO), nearly all of them in Africa. The last reported serious outbreak was in 2006 in the Democratic Republic of the Congo in Central Africa, when at least 50 people died. The United States, China, India, Vietnam, and Mongolia are among the other countries that have confirmed human plague cases in recent years. New research suggests Black Death is lying dormant [29].

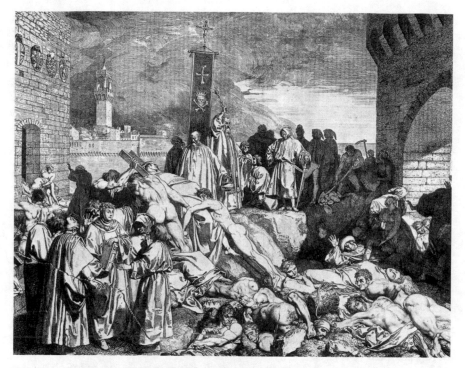

Fig. 1.3 Black plague – engraving taken from the book *Paris Through the Centuries, Tome1* (1878) (Photo courtesy of Alamy Images)

The Americas were mostly shielded by geography from the many infectious diseases endemic to Europe and Asia before the sixteenth century. Native Americans had no exposure and thus no immunity to many infectious diseases. The first large-scale contacts between Europeans and native people of the American continents brought overwhelming pandemic of measles and smallpox to the Native Americans in the sixteenth century. These diseases spread rapidly and were lethal, leading to a drastic drop in the Native American population. The Aztec and Inca civilizations in Central and South America were crippled [30], and much of Native American cultures collapsed.

The Path to Vaccine Discovery

Smallpox: From Early Recorded Man to the Twenty-First Century

To review the history of modern vaccines, one must start with a brief review of the history of smallpox, an exanthematous DNA viral disease. The deadliest form of smallpox is caused by the variola major virus and is without a known cure. It can be contracted via airborne particles or through direct contact with infected bodily fluids or contaminated objects such as bedding or clothing. There is no animal reservoir of smallpox and no human carriers – the virus has to spread continually from human to human to survive [31]. Smallpox is believed to have appeared at the time of the first agricultural settlements in northeastern Africa around 10,000 BCE. The earliest physical evidence of smallpox is the pustular rash on the mummified body of Pharaoh Ramesses V of Egypt, who died in 1157 BCE [32]. Population effects of the disease can be traced from China in 1122 BCE and on to Europe between the fifth and sixth centuries. Although epidemics of disease are described in the Bible and in Greek and Roman literature, descriptions of clinical signs are sparse [33]. One of the epidemics that can be identified with some certainty as smallpox occurred in Athens beginning in 430 BCE and was described by Thucydides, a Greek historian, born 460 BCE [31]. Later, during the fourteenth-century Middle Ages, smallpox was frequently endemic (along with other diseases like typhoid, measles, dysentery, and the plague), resulting in the fall of the Native American civilizations in the 1500s due to the introduction of smallpox by Spanish and Portuguese conquistadors to the New World.

Smallpox first appeared in England in the sixteenth century. A particularly virulent strain emerged in the early seventeenth century, and by the eighteenth century, smallpox was endemic: it killed one tenth of the population of British India, one tenth of all Swedish infants, one seventh of all Russian infants, and over 400,000 Europeans each year [34].

After several decades of endemicity, smallpox became almost wholly a disease of childhood with a high mortality rate. It resulted in a death rate of roughly 25–30% and one third of smallpox survivors were reported to have gone blind. It was common knowledge that survivors of smallpox became immune to the disease, and almost all adults were immune to smallpox, having survived the disease as children [35]. Outbreaks of variola major occurred until the end of the nineteenth century. Man's attempt to prevent smallpox initially through inoculation (also known as variolation) was the first known attempt to minimize or prevent disease.

Variolation and Inoculation: Earliest Forms of Vaccination

The terms *inoculation* from the Latin *inoculare*, meaning "to graft," and *variolation* were often used interchangeably. Variolation specifically refers to the deliberate exposure of a person to smallpox from pustules or scabs of a person with smallpox. The Chinese are generally given credit for variolation. Textual evidence such as Zhang Lu-yu's *Zhangshi Yitong* (Zhang's Medical Compendium) from 1695 offers a description of smallpox inoculation through variolation involving nasal insufflation of dried finely powdered human pox crusts taken from a patient in the recovery stages of smallpox [36]. During this same period in India, scarification procedures were invented either separately or imported from China [37]. From there, the practice of cutaneous variolation passed to the Middle East and Africa, from Turkey to Great Britain, then to the rest of Europe and elsewhere [38].

Inoculation through variolation was introduced in England in the early 1700s [39]. The smallpox virus was introduced subcutaneously via a lancet with fresh matter taken from a ripe pustule of someone suffering from smallpox. This technique carried the risk of death to the patient inoculated and also potentially infected others around the patient as the inoculated patient became infectious. However, the risk of death from inoculation was much less than the risk of death from contracting the disease outright, and vaccination through inoculation was recommended by many. Mathematically minded doctors and scientists calculated the risks of dying from inoculation – roughly 1 in 100 in the 1720s – and compared it to the risk of dying from smallpox, about 1 in 7 [40]. There were those who recommended universal inoculation like Daniel Bernoulli, a Swiss mathematician who wrote a mathematical analysis in 1760 and calculated that approximately three quarters of all living people during that time had been infected with smallpox. He argued through mathematical equations that many lives would be saved if smallpox were completely eliminated, and he encouraged universal inoculation against smallpox [35].

Edward Jenner

In 1757 a young boy by the name of Edward Jenner was inoculated with smallpox in Gloucester England and thus became immune to the disease [41]. By 1798, the young Edward Jenner had become Dr. Edward Jenner, known for developing a procedure to inoculate people with fresh cowpox lesions, conferring immunity to smallpox. Cowpox is an infectious disease caused by the cowpox virus, a zoonotic virus that can be transferred between animals and man. The transfer of the disease was observed in dairymaids who touched the udders of infected cows and who consequently developed pustules on their hands and forearms. These dairymaids were noted to have immunity to smallpox with later exposures. Jenner was the first to keep scientific records that documented that cowpox inoculation conferred immunity to those later exposed to smallpox. Through his work of inoculation with cowpox, the word *vaccination* was derived: *vacca*, Latin for cow, and *vaccina*, Latin for vaccinia virus of the genus *Orthopoxvirus* [42].

To be historically fair, prior to the work of Jenner, other country physicians and farmers in the dairy lands of eighteenth-century England and physicians and farmers in other parts of the world the previous century knew of and practiced inoculation. Recognition is due to Benjamin Jesty, a farmer in Yetminster, England, who, in an attempt to protect his family in 1774 (24 years before Jenner's experiments), used material from udders of cattle that he knew had cowpox and transferred the material with a small lancet to the arms of his wife and two young boys, ages two and three [43]. So sure of his vaccination success, Benjamin Jesty years later purposefully had one of his son's exposed to known case of smallpox, proving his son's immunity [44]. Despite his successful inoculation of his family, Jesty was said to be ridiculed by the town folk of Yetminster. Much of society at that time was not yet

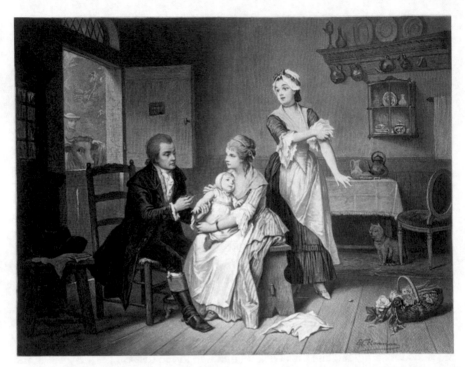

Fig. 1.4 Edward Jenner, vaccinating his young child, held by Mrs. Jenner; a maid rolls up her sleeve, a man stands outside holding a cow. Colored engraving by C. Manigaud after E Hamman. The Royal College of Surgeons of England, 35–43 Lincoln's Inn Fields, London WC2A 3PE Credit: Wellcome Library, London. *Image*: *Wellcome Images L0011550*

ready for change by way of scientific interventions. In rural areas, people were often superstitious and the last execution for witchcraft had taken place only 62 years before. Word spread of what Jesty had done to his family, and he and they became the object of their neighbors' scorn and derision. Eventually Jesty moved out of Yetminster to another part of England, and records show that he went on to successfully inoculate many others over the years [45].

However, no one before Jenner had documented or recorded any scientific investigation or study on the matter of inoculation. Jenner recorded and published his findings. Vaccines have been associated with clinical trials ever since: within 5 years of his publication, doctors in Europe and North America conducted trials both in hospitals and in communities to test the safety and efficacy of cowpox vaccine. These trials set the model for evaluations of subsequent vaccines [46]. Therefore, Jenner can be thought of as one of the first physicians to promote and practice evidenced-based medicine (Fig. 1.4).

Closer to Home: Smallpox in Eighteenth-Century Americas and the American Revolution

The early history of the United States of America is profoundly influenced by the effects of smallpox. The conflict between Great Britain and 13 of its North American colonies (self-named the United States of America) which had declared themselves independent was unduly influenced by smallpox. Outbreaks of smallpox nearly cost the Americans the Revolutionary War (1775–1783). The American Revolutionaries were fighting both the British and disease [47] as most of the British troops were immune to smallpox, either from inoculation, or from having had the disease, and the majority of the Revolutionaries were not. Furthermore, the British commanders offered voluntary inoculation to its army members not already immune to the disease, while the American commanders initially did not. Few people in North America from the 13 colonies, including the fighting troops, had been exposed to smallpox prior to the war. Quarantine was the initial American line of defense against smallpox: all incoming vessels that had smallpox on board during their voyage, or that came from a place where smallpox was known to be prevalent, were required to undergo an examination by doctors or Boston selectmen. The selectmen quarantined anyone with obvious disease or who had been known to come from an area with smallpox.

Inoculation was not new to the Americas, but it was not widely practiced. Prior to the American Revolution, sporadic inoculation had begun during a 1721 small-pox epidemic in Boston. Cotton Mather, a Puritan divine and scientist, had successfully inoculated 242 persons with good results: only four of those inoculated died from the procedure [48]. Though the risk of death due to inoculation was much less than the risk of death due to natural disease, the people of Boston did not condone inoculation for both religious and financial reasons. Many physicians and clergymen in Boston accused Mather of mocking God's will by interfering with the course of a plague. They argued that Mather subjugated a high cost to society through inoculation, determined by labor time lost to those who needed 1–2 months to recover from the effects of the inoculation. Furthermore, the risk of transmitting smallpox from those inoculated to others in the community who were not inoculated was a threat Boston society was not ready to accept. Legislative action was taken and every colony except Pennsylvania passed laws to restrict the practice of inoculation [33].

Fortunately, one very important American had been exposed to smallpox as an adolescent and survived with immunity. George Washington, the Commander in Chief of the Continental Army, who later served as the first US president (serving 1789–1797) was immune to smallpox. His immunity ultimately helped shape the course of the Revolutionary War. Washington, born in Virginia, had contracted smallpox as an adolescent during a visit to Barbados in November 1751 when he and his older brother were sent there by their parents in hopes that the warm climate would help his bother recuperate from tuberculosis – it did not.

As commander in chief during the American Revolution, Washington realized how contagious smallpox was and what a devastating effect it could have on his troops and battle outcomes. He strategically used immune troops for certain military maneuvers that resulted in close engagement with the British. Initially he declined to inoculate his troops for the same reasons many people of the American colonies professed: inoculation was dangerous with its small risk of death to those inoculated, and inoculation of large numbers of troops would render the troops ineffective for 1–2 months while they recuperated from the procedure. He instead chose to rely on quarantine measures to contain outbreaks of smallpox – until the Battle of Quebec. After the disastrous loss at Quebec in 1775–1776, reportedly largely due to smallpox infection among his troops, he changed his mind and decided to inoculate his troops. In speaking about smallpox, he stated:

> I know that it is more destructive to an army in the natural way than the sword. [47]

On February 5, 1777, Washington ordered the inoculation of all susceptible troops in the Continental camp and of every new recruit. This was the first time an American force had been immunized by command order. The Continental Army became the first in the world to have an organized program for smallpox prevention. It signaled the first of many vaccination programs US military troops would undertake. To prevent smallpox from spreading via secondary contact with inoculated troops, Washington had the procedure performed in "inoculation hospitals" and isolated the troops in vaccination huts [49]. For more than a year, the Army provided free compulsory inoculation for all soldiers [50]. Washington reportedly kept his inoculation actions secret to prevent the British from discovering the majority of his troops were temporarily incapacitated. By the end of the war, the Continental Army was virtually as immune as the British. Washington's decision to inoculate had evened the odds in the war. Some argue that had he decided to inoculate his army sooner, US land acquisition after the Revolutionary War would have been different: more of what is now Canada would belong to the United States [51].

Since the Revolutionary War, the US military has promoted vaccination of its troops and has been actively engaged in vaccine research [50]. The US Army Medical Research Institute of Infectious Diseases (USAMRIID) created in 1969 spearheads research to develop medical solutions: vaccines, drugs, diagnostics, and information to protect military service members from biological threats. USAMRIDD works alongside CDC and the World Health Organization (WHO) and collaborates with industry and federal agencies including the Department of Health and Human Services and the Department of Homeland Security, playing a critical role in the status of our country's preparedness for biological terrorism and biological warfare [52].

Smallpox Today

Before 1972, smallpox vaccination was recommended for all US children at 1 year of age, and most states required evidence of vaccination for school entry. Vaccination was also required for military recruits and tourists visiting other countries. Due to these vaccination efforts, the last natural outbreak of smallpox occurred in 1949. Routine vaccination of Americans stopped in 1972 after the disease was declared eradicated in the United States [53]. Eight years later, naturally occurring smallpox was declared eradicated from the planet thanks to a global campaign that began in 1967 under the auspices of the WHO. On May 8, 1980, the World Health Assembly announced that the world was free of smallpox and recommended that all countries cease vaccination:

"The world and all its people have won freedom from smallpox, which was the most devastating disease sweeping in epidemic form through many countries since earliest times, leaving death, blindness and disfigurement in its wake."

In 1986 the WHO proposed that all laboratories destroy their variola stocks or transfer them to one of the two WHO reference labs: the Institute of Virus Preparations in Moscow, Russia, or the CDC in Atlanta, Georgia. All countries reported compliance. Until recently, the US government provided the vaccine only to a few hundred scientists and medical professionals working with smallpox and similar viruses in a research setting. From 1983 through 2002, most service members did not get vaccinated against smallpox, but in December 2002, President George W. Bush announced that smallpox vaccination was restarted for all service members and government personnel in high-risk areas, and he set an example and received the vaccine himself on December 2, 2002. Between December 2002 and May 2014, more than 2.4 million service members received smallpox vaccinations [54].

Germ, or biological warfare, is described as the deliberate use of a microorganism or toxin as a weapon. A category "A" organism is defined as an organism/biological agent that is easy to disseminate and transmit from person to person, one that poses the highest risk to national security and public health. Smallpox was involved in what many describe as biological warfare during the 1700s. Some historians believe that roughly 20 years before the American Revolutionary War, during the French-Indian War (1754–1767), Sir Jeffrey Amherst, the commander of the British forces in North America, suggested the deliberate use of smallpox to diminish the Native Indian population hostile to the British through dissemination of pox-infested blankets to the Native Indians [55]. Today, it is reported that, beginning in 1980, the Soviet government embarked on a program to produce the smallpox virus in large quantities and adapt it for use in weapons [56]. After the anthrax terrorist attacks in September and October 2001 when powdered anthrax spores were mailed through the US postal system, preparedness for additional bioterrorist threats led the federal government to implement a smallpox vaccination program for civilian public health responders that reached nearly 40,000 workers [57]. An updated smallpox response plan was released, and the federal government has called on all states to devise comprehensive mass prophylaxis plans to ensure that civilian populations have timely access to necessary antibiotics and/or vaccines in the event of future outbreaks of infectious diseases. The government has enough vaccine stock to vaccinate every person in the United States in the event of a smallpox emergency [53]. The deliberate release of smallpox as a biological weapon today would be an international crime of unprecedented proportions – one case of smallpox would be considered an emergency.

Dryvax, the smallpox vaccine originally licensed in 1944 to Wyeth Laboratories, Inc., of Madison, N.J., was manufactured until the mid-1980s when the WHO declared that smallpox had been eradicated. Currently there is one licensed smallpox vaccine, ACAM2000, licensed on August 31, 2007, manufactured by Sanofi Pasteur Biologics Co. of Cambridge, MA, based on the same strain of virus as Dryvax. ACAM2000 is indicated for active immunization against smallpox disease for persons determined to be at high risk for smallpox infection. ACAM2000 is administered by scarification to the deltoid muscle or the posterior aspect of the arm over the triceps muscle. On May 2, 2005, the Center for Biologics Evaluation and Research (CBER), a division of the US Federal Food and Drug Administration (FDA), licensed Vaccinia Immune Globulin Intravenous (VIGIV) manufactured by Cangene Corporation of Winnipeg, Manitoba, Canada. VIGIV is used to treat rare serious complications of smallpox vaccination [58].

Development of the Germ Theory and Early Modern Vaccines

The development of the germ theory is an important step in the development of vaccines as we know them today. Louis Pasteur (1822–1895), a French scientist known for his discovery of pasteurization, developed the first laboratory vaccine and was the first to propose the "germ theory" of disease: that diseases are caused by microorganisms. He theorized that vaccination could be applied to any microbial disease. He discovered and documented methods relating to the virulence of microbes and how they could be attenuated so that live microbes could be used to make *prophylactic vaccines*. Additionally, he introduced the concept of *therapeutic vaccines* with his studies of rabies, demonstrating what we now call post-infection prophylaxis [59]. One interesting story involves Pasteur's earliest vaccine research involving chickens. Pasteur received a strain of bacteria that caused chicken cholera from Henry Toussaint, a professor of the Veterinary School of Toulouse. Pasteur learned how to grow the chicken cholera microbe in chicken broth and experimented first by feeding chickens food contaminated with a culture of chicken cholera microbes. This resulted in death for most of the chickens. Pasteur recorded his experiments: he learned that the chickens that survived were then resistant to a second exposure of the same pathogen given by an inoculation of a lethal dose of the chicken cholera microbe. He determined that those chickens had immunity against chicken cholera.

A fortuitous accident occurred when Pasteur went on vacation and his assistant forgot to continue the experiment. The bacterial inoculation cultures Pasteur meant for inoculation of the experimental chickens were left in a medium that was exposed to room air for about a month. Later, when the experiment resumed and the chickens were injected with the now unintentionally "attenuated" strains of bacteria, the chickens did not die but only contracted a mild form of the disease. When Pasteur later reinjected these chickens with lethally-dosed, fresh, purulent bacteria, they did not get ill: Pasteur had successfully vaccinated the chickens against cholera using an attenuated vaccine [60]!

Pasteur also developed another attenuated vaccine in his laboratory against anthrax. In 1881, his vaccine experiments proved vaccine-induced immunity to anthrax in animals. He gave his live, attenuated anthrax vaccine to some animals in his experiment but not all. He then proved that when later exposed to anthrax, all vaccinated animals survived while his control group died [61]. In addition, Louis Pasteur was also instrumental in documenting post-infection prophylaxis, also known as postexposure prevention (PEP), through vaccines. PEP refers to a preventive medical treatment that is started immediately after exposure to a pathogen to prevent infection and development of disease caused by the pathogen. PEP is commonly and effectively used to prevent the outbreak of rabies after a bite from or contact with a rabid animal or prevent tetanus after a potential exposure to tetanus. Pasteur first developed a vaccine against rabies in livestock in 1884, then proved its effectiveness in post-infection prophylaxis in humans in 1885 by successfully vaccinating Joseph Meister, a 9-year-old boy who was bitten several times by a rabid dog. The boy survived and did not contract rabies [62].

History of Modern Vaccines Late Nineteenth and Twentieth Centuries

Types of Vaccines

There are several different types of vaccines in use today and some currently in development.

Toxoids

When a toxin produced by a bacterial pathogen is the main cause of illness, toxoid vaccines may be effective to prevent those toxin-producing diseases. Toxoids are inactivated forms of bacterial toxins, or "detoxified" toxins, used for the purpose of immunization. They cannot cause the disease they prevent and there is no possibility of reversion to virulence [63]. When the immune system receives a vaccine containing a harmless toxoid, it learns how to fight off the natural toxin by producing antibodies that lock onto and block the toxin [41, 64]. Diphtheria and tetanus are two examples of toxoid vaccines.

Live, Attenuated Vaccines

Live, attenuated vaccines contain a version of the living microbe that has been weakened and unable to cause disease. They elicit strong cellular and antibody responses and often confer lifelong immunity with one or two doses [64]. Smallpox, yellow fever, and MMR vaccines are examples of these.

Inactivated Vaccines

Inactivated vaccines are produced by killing the disease-causing microbe with chemicals, heat, or radiation. These are more stable and safer than live vaccines; they do not require refrigeration and can be easily stored and transported in a freeze-dried form. However, these stimulate a weaker immune system response than live vaccines, often requiring booster shots [64]. Hepatitis A, rabies, and injectable polio vaccines are examples of these.

Subunit/Conjugate Vaccines

Subunit vaccines include only the antigens of a microbe that best stimulate the immune system to protect against it and do not contain live components of the pathogen. Conjugate vaccines are a special type of subunit vaccines, made to create immunity to the outer coating of polysaccharides that many bacteria have so that the immature immune systems of infants and younger children can recognize and respond to them. The hepatitis B, influenza, and Hib vaccines are examples of a subunit conjugate vaccines [64].

DNA Vaccines

DNA vaccines are still in experimental stages and developing rapidly. They involve the direct introduction into appropriate tissues of a plasmid contacting the DNA sequence encoding the antigen(s) against which an immune response is sought and relies on the in situ production of the target antigen [63–66]. The first DNA vaccines licensed for marketing are likely to use plasmid DNA derived from bacterial cells. Others may use RNA or complexes of nucleic acid molecules. Several types are currently under testing in humans including West Nile and Zika virus vaccines [64–66].

Diseases and Their Vaccines

Diphtheria toxin: diphtheria is a potentially fatal disease caused by the exotoxin produced by the bacterium *Corynebacterium diphtheriae* that primarily affects tissues of the upper respiratory tract and kills its victims slowly by suffocation. Symptoms include a thick, gray membrane covering the throat and tonsils, a sore throat, lymphadenopathy, fever, chills, and nerve damage. In 1884, German physician Edwin Klebs (1834–1913) successfully isolated the bacteria that caused diphtheria. In 1888, French physician, bacteriologist, and immunologist Emile Roux discovered the diphtheria toxin. This discovery, in conjunction with the scientific contributions of others (including Emil Von Behring and Paul Ehrlich), led to the development of the diphtheria vaccine [37].

Tetanus toxin: tetanus is an acute, often fatal disease caused by an exotoxin produced by the bacterium *Clostridium tetani*, which is characterized by generalized rigidity and convulsive spasms of skeletal muscles. The jaw is usually involved (lockjaw) and then the neck before becoming more generalized. Experiments that began in 1884 with animals injected with pus from fatal human tetanus cases eventually led to the neutralization of the toxin. During World War I (WWI), passively transferred antitoxin and passive immunization in humans were used for treatment and prophylaxis. Tetanus toxoid was developed in 1924 and used during WWII [67].

Yellow fever: yellow fever is a highly fatal hemorrhagic infection caused by a small, enveloped, single-stranded RNA virus. Symptoms include fever, chills, loss of appetite, nausea, muscle pain, and headaches. In some people symptoms worsen after 4–5 days and liver damage may occur, causing jaundice (yellow skin), bleeding risk, and kidney damage. Approximately half of those who develop severe symptoms die within 7–10 days. During the Spanish-American War of 1898, yellow fever was a serious problem for US troops. US Army physician Walter Reed headed up the Yellow Fever Commission, which traveled to Cuba and validated a theory presented by Cuban physician Carlos Finlay two decades earlier: mosquitoes were responsible for the spread of the disease. Later it was shown that the underlying cause of yellow fever is a virus that uses mosquitoes as vectors. This discovery led many scientists to work on yellow fever vaccine development until Max Theiler and other Rockefeller Foundation scientists developed a successful live attenuated vaccine for yellow fever in 1937 [68].

Tuberculosis

Tuberculosis was known as *phthisis* and *consumption* from the time of Hippocrates to the eighteenth century and known as the *white death* and the *great white plague* during the nineteenth century. It was an epidemic in Europe during the eighteenth and nineteenth centuries and caused millions of deaths [69].

Robert Koch, known as the founder of modern bacteriology, revealed in 1882 that the causative agent of tuberculosis is *Mycobacterium tuberculosis*, later known as Koch's bacillus. From there came the criteria for proof of bacterial causality. Koch's postulates state: "the organism must be present in diseased tissues; it must be isolated and grown in pure culture; and the cultured organism must induce the disease when inoculated into healthy experimental animals" [70]. Koch's discovery facilitated the development of the tuberculosis vaccine. Bacillus Calmette-Guerin (BCG), a live attenuated vaccination developed in 1924, was first used in newborns and has become the most widely administered of all vaccines in the World Health Organization (WHO) Expanded Program for Immunization. Unfortunately, it is only partially effective, providing some protection against severe forms of pediatric TB, but is not completely protective against disease in infants and is unreliable against adult pulmonary TB [71]. Nearly a century after development, this vaccine is still used today. No universal BCG vaccination policy exists. Some countries merely recommend its use and others have implemented immunization programs. It is not routinely recommended in the United States [72].

Influenza: influenza is a highly contagious disease caused by influenza viruses that infect the respiratory passages causing fever, cough (usually dry), headache, sore throat, runny nose, severe muscle and joint aches, and may result in severe illness and death. It is spread mainly via droplets, which are produced when people infected with flu cough, sneeze, or talk. Prior to 1933, the bacterium *Haemophilus influenzae* was mistakenly thought to cause the flu. The first flu vaccine was developed by Jonas Salk and Thomas Francis to protect US military forces against the flu during WWII. In 1943, a successful controlled trial of the vaccine was conducted on 12,500 men in units of the Army Specialized Training Program at universities and at medical/dental schools in different areas of the United States, proving the first effective influenza virus vaccine [73].

Note: There have been four major flu pandemics recorded throughout history. In 1918–1919 the Spanish flu pandemic was responsible for approximately 50 million deaths worldwide and for nearly 675,000 deaths in the United States. The second flu pandemic in 1957–1958 hit the United States in two waves killing 69,800 people, far fewer people than the 1918 pandemic. The elderly had the highest rates of death during these pandemics. The third pandemic occurred in 1968–1969 from a new influenza virus that originated in Hong Kong. It was the mildest of all the flu pandemics, resulting in 33,800 American deaths. Again, the elderly population was the most likely to die. The 2009–2010 H1N1 swine flu pandemic was declared a public health emergency by the US government on April 26, 2009. H1N1 was reported in mostly young people. There were approximately 60.8 million cases, 274,304 hospitalizations, and 12,469 deaths, which occurred in the United States due to H1N1 during that pandemic. Massive vaccination campaigns led to the vaccination of 80 million people during that time and a decline of flu activity. WHO declared an end to the global H1N1 flu pandemic August, 2010 [74, 75].

Poliomyelitis: polio is an acute paralytic disease caused by three poliovirus serotypes. It is an intestinal infection spread between humans through the fecal-oral route. In the 1950s Jonas Salk and Albert Sabin produced the first polio vaccines; Salk produced a killed-virus injectable vaccine (IPV) and Sabin a live-virus oral vaccine (OPV). The WHO proposed worldwide poliomyelitis eradication in 1988. Unfortunately, this goal is still not met. Sporadic cases of wildtype polio occur in various parts of the developing world in Afghanistan, India, Nigeria, and Pakistan [76, 77]. The last cases of naturally occurring paralytic polio in the United States were in 1979 when an outbreak occurred among the Amish in several Midwestern states [78]. From 1980 to date, there were 162 confirmed cases of paralytic polio reported – of those 162 cases, 8 were acquired outside the United States and imported. The last imported case caused by wild poliovirus into the United States occurred in 1993. The remaining 154 cases were vaccine-associated paralytic polio caused by live oral poliovirus vaccine. OPV has not been used in the United States since 2000 but is still used in many parts of the world. IPV is currently the only vaccine used in the United States against polio [79].

Measles, mumps, and rubella: measles, one of the most contagious infectious diseases known, is caused by an RNA virus. Until 2000, measles was still the leading cause of vaccine-preventable childhood death worldwide [80]. It is still endemic worldwide, and although declared eliminated from the United States in 2000, sporadic outbreaks still occur. Mumps, also a highly contagious viral illness, causes parotiditis and serious complications like meningitis, encephalitis, deafness, and orchitis which can lead to sterility in men. Rubella (also known as German measles) virus was isolated in the early 1960s and is associated with terrible birth defects if a pregnant woman contracts the disease. Congenital rubella syndrome (CRS) was discovered in the 1940s and is associated with cataracts, deafness, congenital heart disease, encephalitis, mental retardation, pneumonia, hepatitis, thrombocytopenia, metaphyseal defects diabetes mellitus, and thyroiditis.

The MMR vaccine is a mixture of live attenuated viruses of the three diseases. A licensed vaccine to prevent measles was first available in 1963. Live attenuated vaccines for mumps and rubella became available in 1967 and 1969, respectively [81, 82]. An attenuated combination measles-mumps-rubella vaccine was licensed in 1973 by Merck [83] in 2000; measles was declared no longer endemic in the United States in 2005; and CDC announced that rubella was no longer endemic in the United States.

MMR-Autism Hoax

The MMR vaccine is not linked in any way to autism. Perhaps one of the biggest medical hoaxes in this century is the one perpetrated by Dr. Thomas Wakefield, a British gastroenterologist [84] who described such a link in a paper published in the Lancet in 1998 [85]. His paper and the subsequent media explosion around publicizing his false theory eroded parental confidence in vaccinations, government, and public health institutions first in England and later in the United States. After 10 years of controversy and investigation and multiple studies later, Wakefield's assertion of the alleged autism-MMR link was disproved [86]. More than 20 studies found no evidence of connection between receipt of the MMR vaccine and autism disorders, and Britain's General Medical Council (GMC) determined after its hearings that Wakefield was guilty of dishonesty and serious professional misconduct with regard to his MMR-autism research and the publication of his paper [84, 87]. His paper was retracted from the Lancet and his medical license revoked. His later attempts, after moving to Texas, to sue the *British Medical Journal* for libel were dismissed in a Texas court [88]. Many believe the media has given celebrities who comment on an autism-MMR link far more attention than they deserve (Jenny McCarthy and Robert De Niro come to mind), and segments of the public have confused celebrity status with authority [89]. The GMC states that anti-vaccine groups and conspiracy proponents promoting such an association should be ignored [87].

Hepatitis A and B: hepatitis (liver inflammation) with fever, fatigue, abdominal and joint pain, loss of appetite, and jaundice is caused by several different strains of virus, and strains A and B have been isolated and differentiated since the early 1940s. Hepatitis A-inactivated vaccine was licensed in 1995. A plasma-derived hepatitis B vaccine was licensed in 1981, and in 1986 a recombinant hepatitis B vaccine was licensed. ACIP recommended routine hepatitis B vaccination for all infants in 1991. In 2001 Twinrix, a combined hepatitis A-inactivated and hepatitis B recombinant vaccine was licensed. In 2002 a vaccine combing diphtheria, tetanus, acellular pertussis, inactivated polio, and hepatitis B antigen (Pediarix) was licensed [37].

Haemophilus influenzae type b (Hib): *Haemophilus influenzae* is a bacterial infection spread person-to-person by direct contact or through respiratory droplets that mainly causes illness in babies and young children. Infections range from ear infections to pneumonia, septic arthritis, epiglottitis, meningitis, and sepsis.

Hib vaccine: in 1985 Hib vaccine was recommended routinely for children at 4 months of age and for children at 15 months of age enrolled in child care facilities. By 1988 the recommendation changed to vaccinate all children at 18 months of age. By 1990 the age for vaccine recommendation was lowered to 15 months of age for all children, and in 1991 the recommendation changed to vaccinate all children beginning at 2 months of age. In the United States between 1980 and 1990, the incidence of Hib disease was 40–100/100,000 among children under 5 years of age. Since 1990, with routine use of Hib conjugate vaccine, the incidence of invasive Hib disease has decreased to 1.3/100,000 children [90].

Pneumococcus: *Streptococcus pneumoniae* bacteria, referred to as pneumococcus, cause many types of illnesses ranging from ear/sinus infections and pneumonia to sepsis and meningitis and occur in all ages from infancy to geriatric years. Pneumonia is the most common serious form of pneumococcal disease. Two enhanced pneumococcal polysaccharide vaccines were licensed in 1983 (Pneumovax 23 and Pnu-Immune 23), covering 23 purified capsular polysaccharide antigens of *Streptococcus pneumoniae* and replacing the 1977 pneumococcal vaccine covering 14 serotypes of pneumococcal [37]. Pneumococcal 7-valent Conjugate Vaccine (Prevnar) was approved by the FDA in 2000 for immunization of infants and toddlers [91], and Pneumococcal 13-valent Conjugate Vaccine (PCV13) approved in 2010 for use in place of Prevnar expanded to broader use in all adults age 19–64 with certain underlying medical conditions and all adults over age 65 in 2014 [92].

Varicella zoster: varicella (chickenpox) and herpes zoster (shingles) are caused by the varicella zoster virus. Chickenpox, typically a relatively mild childhood illness with fever, malaise, headache, abdominal pain, and a characteristic pruritic exanthem, follows initial exposure to the virus. Shingles is a painful dermatomal rash resulting from reactivation of the dormant virus and is often followed by pain in the distribution of the rash (post-herpetic neuralgia). The varicella zoster vaccine is the first and only licensed live, attenuated herpesvirus vaccine in the world. Varivax was licensed in 1995. In 2006, VariZIG, an immune globulin product for postexposure prophylaxis of varicella, became available. Also in 2006, the FDA licensed Zostavax, approved for use in people aged 50 years of age and older to prevent shingles and ACIP recommended for those over 60 years old [37].

Rotavirus: rotavirus is the leading cause of severe acute gastroenteritis in young infants and children worldwide, transmitted primarily by the fecal-oral route, both through close person-to-person contact and through fomites. The virus is highly contagious. Millions to billions of viral particles can be present within one gram of diarrheal stool. In 2008, rotavirus caused an estimated 453,000 deaths worldwide in children younger than 5 years of age. Prior to the vaccine, almost all US infants were infected with rotavirus before their fifth birthday. The original live, oral vaccine was introduced in 1999 but was pulled off the market in the United States 14 months later due to several reported cases of vaccine-associated intussusception. Two different vaccines are currently licensed for infants in the United States (RotaTeq and Rotarix), both having gone through rigorous clinical trials to prove their safety [93].

Meningococcus: meningococcal disease can refer to any disease caused by *Neisseria meningitidis* bacteria, an aerobic, gram-negative diplococcus that colonizes the human nasopharynx and is transmitted by respiratory tract droplets. Invasive disease may cause sepsis and meningitis and death. Sudden fever, headache, and stiff neck are typical symptoms along with nausea, vomiting, light sensitivity, rash, and confusion. Risk factors include crowding such as seen in military recruits or college students living in dormitories, tobacco smoke exposure, and alcohol-related behaviors. Persons who acquire the organism in the nasopharynx may develop a carrier state, but only a few develop invasive disease. The carrier state is common in college students. The overall case-fatality rate for invasive disease in the United States is 10–15%, even with appropriate antibiotics. Quadrivalent meningococcal vaccines protect against serogroups A, C, W, and Y and recommended to all children at ages 11–12 and 16 years and meningococcal serogroup B vaccine for those children at high risk and as a permissive recommendation for others [90].

Human papillomavirus (HPV): HPV is the most common sexually transmitted infection, and transmission occurs most frequently with sexual intercourse but can occur also with non-penetrative intimate contact. An estimated 14 million new infections occur per year, and an estimated 79 million persons are currently infected in the United States. HPV types 6 and 11 cause at least 90% of genital warts, and types 16 and 18 cause 70% of cervical cancers and 70% of genital cancers. Cancers of the penis, vagina, vulva, anus, rectum, and nasopharyngeal head and neck structures are caused by HPV. The first HPV vaccine was licensed in the United States in 2006. The nine-valent (9vHPV) vaccine (covering serotypes 6, 11, 16, 18, 31, 33, 45, 52, 58) is indicated for all adolescents ages 11–12 in a two-dose series, 6–12 months apart. For those who start the vaccination series between 15–26 years of age, a three-dose series is required for effective immune response [90].

Creation of the World Health Organization Global Recommendations for Vaccines

During the twentieth century, several international organizations devoted to health and welfare were created, but only a few survived post WWII. One group that persisted after the war, the Health Organization of the League of Nations (started in 1920), had been the weekly distributor of epidemiological information, using both

Geneva and a special bureau in Singapore as collecting posts. This health organization helped create an international public health system and expanded existing international epidemic control systems. Global disease management became more scientific, more technical, and less political under it than disease management was prior to WWII. The Health Organization of the League of Nations represented the beginning of social medicine, public health separation from politics, and global public health reform [94]. Eventually the United Nations (UN) proposed that even greater international organizational work and guidance was needed to combat the many diseases affecting people worldwide. The *World Health Organization* was proposed as a matter of international concern for "economic, social, cultural, educational, health and related matter" during the UN conference held in San Francisco, April 1945. One year later, an outline for the proposed constitution of the organization was proposed in 1946, but it wasn't until April 7, 1948, that all 26 signatures from all 26 member countries were obtained, officially documenting WHO's beginning [95].

The principle advisory group to the WHO for vaccines and immunization is the Strategic Advisory Group of Experts on Immunization (SAGE), established by the Director-General of the WHO in 1999. SAGE is charged with advising on overall global policies and strategies concerning all vaccine-preventable diseases. In 2005, the 58th World Health Assembly along with the United Nations Children's Emergency Fund (UNICEF) introduced the Global Immunization Vision and Strategy 2006–2015 (GIVS) as a framework for strengthening national immunization programs. SAGE was restructured to meet the needs of GIVS, reporting to the WHO Director-General, responsible for reviewing and approving all WHO policy recommendations, including the WHO position papers on vaccines. GIVS' goal was to reduce mortality due to vaccine-preventable diseases by two-thirds by 2015 compared to 2000 levels, equal to more than 40 million lives saved [16, 96]. There are four key objectives to achieve this goal:

1. To immunize more people against more diseases
2. To introduce a range of newly available vaccines and technologies
3. To integrate other critical health interventions with immunization
4. To manage vaccination programs within the context of global interdependence [96]

At the time of this publication, outcome data for GIVS is not yet available.

Beginnings of CDC

Centers for Disease Control and Prevention was established on July 1, 1946 in Atlanta, Georgia by Dr. Joseph W. Mountin of the US Public Health Services' Bureau of State Services. It was then called Communicable Disease Center (CDC). CDC had grown out of an organization called the Malaria Control in War Areas (MCWA), which had been established in 1942 to control malaria around military training bases in the United States. Initially CDC focused on MCWA's interests: fighting malaria, typhus, and other infectious diseases of concern post WWII. It had a three-fold primary mission: field investigation, training, and control of communicable diseases. Over the next 60 years, CDC's title changed several times (The National Communicable Disease Center, Center for Disease Control, Centers for Disease Control) to its name today, Centers for Disease Control and Prevention. Throughout its title changes, the initials "CDC" have remained the same [97]. Over time, under the leadership of chief epidemiologist Dr. Alexander Langmuir from 1949 to 1970, CDC's role in the United States grew dramatically, becoming a large federal agency. Today CDC helps to control epidemics within the United States. CDC tracks diseases and provides expert scientific advice on health issues to policy makers, serving as a reference laboratory to the states and informing the public about health issues through the *Morbidity and Mortality Weekly Report* (MMWR). Epidemiologists from CDC routinely assist state health departments in investigating and controlling outbreaks of infectious and noninfectious disease. On a larger scale, it has grown to provide leadership, often in partnership with the WHO in controlling emerging infectious disease worldwide [6].

Vaccine Recommendations in the United States

Today, all vaccine recommendations for American children and adults are made by CDC's Advisory Committee on Immunization Practices (ACIP) using evidence-based decision-making with input from many organizations and experts. Prior to the 1960s, this was not the case. In 1961, the main body making recommendations on vaccine use in the United States was the American Academy of Pediatrics' Committee on Infectious Diseases (COID) [98]. COID vaccine recommendations were first published in 1938 in a pamphlet with a red cover, giving rise to the publication's official nickname "Red Book." Red Book continues to be a major resource both for physicians and for government committees such as ACIP [99]. For children of the early 1960s, no formal nationwide immunization program existed. Vaccines were administered in private practices and local health departments and paid for out of pocket or provided by using state or local government funds with some support from federal Maternal and Child Health Block Grant funds. In 1962, the Vaccination Assistance Act (Section 317 of the Public Health Service Act) was passed to "achieve as quickly as possible the protection of the population, especially of all preschool children . . . through intensive immunization activity over a limited period of time. . ." The initial intention was to allow CDC to support mass, intensive vaccination campaigns. In addition, the Vaccination Assistance Act established a mechanism to provide ongoing financial support to state or local health departments and direct support "in lieu of cash." The direct support included provision of vaccines and of CDC public health advisors to assist in managing the programs. Section 317 has been reauthorized repeatedly since 1962 and remains one of the most important means of supporting health department immunization activities with federal funds [57]. At the initiation of the 317 funding program in 1963, there were few vaccines to consider. There were only three vaccines routinely recommended for children including diphtheria, tetanus, pertussis (DTP), oral polio (OPV), and smallpox. The measles vaccine was to be licensed later that year.

Vaccine recommendations until 1964 did not formally involve the federal government. The federal government involvement occurred through convening ad hoc expert advisory groups to address individual issues. One such issue was the adverse effect of paralysis related to poorly manufactured vaccines during the field trial of Jonas Salk's inactivated polio vaccine (IPV). Federal ad hoc groups were also formed to provide advice about the influenza pandemic of 1957, Albert Sabin's attenuated oral polio vaccine (OPV), and the measles vaccines prior to release. The frequency and complexity of issues requiring discussion and opinion statements from the federal government led CDC to propose an ongoing Advisory Committee on Immunization Practices. ACIP was established in 1964 and served as a technical advisory committee to the Public Health Service. It was initially comprised of eight members, including the CDC Director, who served as Chair [100, 101]. ACIP directed its recommendations to public health agencies.

Today, ACIP includes 15 voting members selected by the Secretary of the US Department of Health and Human Services and makes recommendations to CDC's director. Voting members are selected via an application and nomination process and serve voluntarily. Fourteen of the members have expertise in vaccinology, virology, immunology, pediatrics, internal medicine, family medicine, nursing, public health, infectious diseases, and/or preventive medicine. One member is a consumer representative to provide perspectives on the social and community aspects of vaccination. In addition, there are eight ex officio members who represent other federal agencies with immunization programs and 30 nonvoting representatives of liaison organizations. ACIP recommendations have major impact on immunization policies and practice in the United States as well as other countries. The committee meets three times a year in Atlanta at CDC, where it makes recommendations on how to use vaccines and related agents that are licensed by the US Food and Drug Administration (FDA) to control disease in the United States. These recommendations are then forwarded to CDC's director for approval, and once approved, they are published in CDC's MMWR. When data is available, specific rules of evidence, such as those followed by the US Preventive Services Task Force (USPSTF), are used to judge the quality of data and make decisions regarding the nature and strength of recommendations. ACIP recommendations on 17 vaccine-preventable diseases are published in the MMWR, the *Pink Book* (*Epidemiology and Prevention of Vaccine-Preventable Diseases*), the AAP *Red Book*, and in the US immunization schedules for children, adolescents, and adults. MMWR publication represents the final and official CDC recommendations for immunization of the US population [102].

Development of the Vaccines for Children Program

In 1993, a Childhood Immunization Initiative began with the goal of achieving, by 1996, 90% immunization coverage among preschool-aged children for vaccines recommended during the first 2 years of life. A critical part of the Childhood Immunization Initiative was to eliminate financial barriers to vaccination and ensure children could be vaccinated at their site of usual care (medical home). The vaccines for children (VFC) program was established through the Omnibus Reconciliation Act of 1993, as an entitlement program for vaccines recommended by ACIP. The program includes children who are Medicaid eligible, completely uninsured, or Native American Indian/Alaska Native. Those children, whose insurance does not cover vaccinations or who are underinsured, can receive vaccines at Federally Qualified Health Centers [103]. Coverage has grown to include approximately 45% of US children, including about 70% of African-American and Hispanic children. VFC authorizes ACIP to decide which vaccines will be covered [104].

The Childhood Immunization Initiative is also responsible for the development of the National Immunization Survey (NIS) in 1994, a program for documentation of vaccinations. Through random-digit dialing surveys, statistically valid immunization coverage rates for all 50 states and several urban areas were tracked. This helped improve progress toward meeting national immunization goals and identified problem areas requiring special interventions. The NIS documented in 1996 ≥ 90% coverage for the following vaccines routinely recommended for preschool-aged children: DTP (three or more doses), polio (three or more doses), MMR (one dose), and *Haemophilus influenzae* type b (Hib b) (three or more doses). The 70% coverage goal of three or more doses of hepatitis B vaccine was also met. NIS illustrated that racial and ethnic disparities in immunization rates, once as high as 20 percentage points for measles, had substantially narrowed [104]. To continue to ensure high coverage rates for immunizations for all ages, health plans today are required by law to cover recommended preventive services without charging a deductible, copayment, or coinsurance. This requirement is stipulated by the Affordable Care Act passed by Congress and signed into law by President Obama on March 23, 2010.

Up from a handful of vaccine recommendations for eight vaccine-preventable diseases in the 1980s, (Fig. 1.5) [105] today children in the United States receive vaccines to prevent 16 diseases (Table 1.1). Most diseases targeted by these vaccines have declined to historically low levels (Table 1.2) [106]. Familiar to most today, the current annual childhood schedule as endorsed by ACIP, AAP, and AAFP has been available since 1995. The annual updates since contain detailed information about the recommended vaccines, including specific age- and dosage-related information, catch-up schedules, and information about new vaccines as they are added to the schedule [107]. They can be found at https://www.cdc.gov/vaccines/schedules/.

TABLE 2. Recommended schedule for active immunization of normal infants and children*

Recommended age[1]	Vaccine(s)[§]	Comments
2 mos	DTP#1[1], OPV#1**	OPV and DTP can be given earlier in areas of high endemicity
4 mos	DTP#2, OPV#2	6-wk to 2-mo interval desired between OPV doses
6 mos	DTP#3	An additional dose of OPV at this time is optional in areas with a high risk of poliovirus exposure
15 mos[††]	MMR[‡‡], DTP#4, OPV#3	Completion of primary series of DTP and OPV
18 mos	HbCV[¶¶]	Conjugate preferred over polysaccharide vaccine***
4–6 yrs	DTP#5[†††], OPV#4	At or before school entry
14–16 yrs	Td[†††]	Repeat every 10 yrs throughout life

*See Table 3 for the recommended immunization schedules for infants and children up to their seventh birthday not immunized at the recommended times.
[1]These recommended ages should not be construed as absolute, e.g., 2 months can be 6–10 weeks. However, MMR should not be given to children <12 months of age. If exposure to measles disease is considered likely, then children 6 through 11 months old may be immunized with single-antigen measles vaccine. These children should be reimmunized with MMR when they are approximately 15 months of age.
[§]For all products used, consult the manufacturers' package enclosures for instructions regarding storage, handling, dosage, and administration. Immunobiologics prepared by different manufacturers can vary, and those of the same manufacturer can change from time to time. The package inserts are useful references for specific products, but they may not always be consistent with current ACIP and American Academy of Pediatrics immunization schedules.
[1]DTP=Diphtheria and Tetanus Toxoids and Pertussis Vaccine, Adsorbed. DTP may be used up to the seventh birthday. The first dose can be given at 6 weeks of age and the second and third doses given 4–8 weeks after the preceding dose.
**OPV=Poliovirus Vaccine Live Oral, Trivalent: contains poliovirus types 1, 2, and 3.
[††]Provided at least 6 months have elapsed since DTP#3 or, if fewer than 3 doses of DTP have been received, at least 6 weeks since the last previous dose of DTP or OPV. MMR vaccine should not be delayed to allow simultaneous administration with DTP and OPV. Administering MMR at 15 months and DTP#4 and OPV#3 at 18 months continues to be an acceptable alternative.
[‡‡]MMR=Measles, Mumps, and Rubella Virus Vaccine, Live. Counties that report ≥5 cases of measles among preschool children during each of the last 5 years should implement a routine 2-dose measles vaccination schedule for preschoolers. The first dose should be administered at 9 months or the first health-care contact thereafter. Infants vaccinated before their first birthday should receive a second dose at about 15 months of age. Single-antigen measles vaccine should be used for children aged <1 year and MMR for children vaccinated on or after their first birthday. If resources do not allow a routine 2-dose schedule, an acceptable alternative is to lower the routine age for MMR vaccination to 12 months.
[¶¶]HbCV=Vaccine composed of Haemophilus influenzae b polysaccharide antigen conjugated to a protein carrier. Children <5 years of age previously vaccinated with polysaccharide vaccine between the ages of 18 and 23 months should be revaccinated with a single dose of conjugate vaccine if at least 2 months have elapsed since the receipt of the polysaccharide vaccine.
***If HbCV is not available, an acceptable alternative is to give Haemophilus influenzae b polysaccharide vaccine (HbPV) at age ≥24 months. Children at high risk for Haemophilus influenzae type b disease where conjugate vaccine is not available may be vaccinated with HbPV at 18 months of age and revaccinated at 24 months.
[†††]Up to the seventh birthday.

1989 childhood immunization schedule

Fig. 1.5 1989 Recommendations (From: http://www.cdc.gov/vaccines/schedules/images/schedule1989s.jpg)

ACIP began publishing an annual adult schedule in 1984 [108] for those aged 19 years and older and is now developed with approval from the American College of Physicians (ACP), the AAFP, the American College of Obstetricians and Gynecologists (ACOG), and the American College of Nurse-Midwives (ACNM). There is one adult schedule organized by vaccine and age group and another schedule organized by medical and other indications. These schedules may be found at: http://www.cdc.gov/vaccines/schedules/hcp/adult.html.

Since their inception, immunization schedules have become more complicated (Fig. 1.6) and detailed, with separate catch-up schedules (Fig. 1.7) just as complex.

Table 1.1 Year of US licensure of selected childhood vaccines

Vaccine	Year of first US licensure
Tetanus toxoid	1943
Trivalent inactivated influenza	1945
Tetanus and diphtheria toxoids	1953 for children aged >7 years.; 1970 for children aged <7 years
Inactivated polio	1955
Oral polio	1963
Diphtheria-tetanus-pertussis	1970
Diphtheria-tetanus-acellular pertussis	1991
Measles-mumps-rubella	1963 (measles); 1967 (mumps); 1969 (rubella); 1971 (measles, mumps, rubella combined)
Hepatitis B	1981 (plasma derived); 1986 (recombinant)
Haemophilus influenzae type b conjugate	1987 for children aged ≥18 months; 1990 for infants
Hepatitis A	1995
Varicella	1995
Pneumococcal conjugate	2000 (7-valent); 2010 (13-valent)
Live attenuated influenza	2003
Tetanus-diphtheria-acellular pertussis	2005
Meningococcal conjugate	2006
Rotavirus	2006
Human papillomavirus	2006

Source: USIS (1967–1985); NHIS (1991–1993); CDC, NCHS, and NIS (1994–2009); CDC, NIP, and NCHS; no data during 1986–1990 due to cancelation of USIS because of budget reductions
Note: Children in the USIS and NHIS were 24–35 months of age. Children in the NIS were 19–35 months of age
https://www.cdc.gov/mmwr/preview/mmwrhtml/su6004a9.htm
Abbreviations: *MMR* measles-mumps-rubella, *DTP/DTaP* diphtheria and tetanus and acellular pertussis, *Hib Haemophilus influenzae* type b, *Heb B* hepatitis B, *PCV7* 7-valent pneumococcal conjugate vaccine, *USIS* US Immunization Survey, *NHIS* National Health Interview Survey, *NIS* National Immunization Survey, *NCHS* National Center for Health Statistics, *NIP* National Immunization Program, *NCIRD* National Center for Immunization and Respiratory Diseases
[a]DTP(3+) is not a Healthy People 2010 objective. DTaP(4) is used to assess Healthy People 2010 objectives

Schedules are color-coded for ease in interpretation. The comparison of the 1989 immunization recommendations highlighted in Fig. 1.5 in contrast to the 2017 recommendations illustrated in Fig. 1.6 epitomizes the incredible progress and increased complexity in vaccine science developing in just over 25 years. The necessary footnotes, determined with evidenced-based rigor, which give further guidance on the use of the recommended vaccines, now take up three full pages of small-type text (Fig. 1.8a, b, c, d) [105].

Table 1.2 Comparison of annual morbidity from vaccine-preventable diseases during the twentieth century and 2009

Disease	Twentieth century[a]	2010[c]	% Reduction
Diphtheria	21,053	0	100
Hepatitis A	117,333	8493[d]	93
Hepatitis B, acute	66,232	9419[d]	86
Haemophilus influenzae type b in children aged <5 years	20,000	240[e]	99
Measles	530,217	63	>99
Mumps	162,344	2612	98
Pertussis	200,752	27,538	86
Pneumococcus, invasive			
All ages	63,607	44,000[f]	30
<5 years	16,069	4700[f]	72
Poliomyelitis, paralytic	16,316	0	100
Rotavirus, hospitalizations	62,500[b]	28,125[d]	55
Rubella	47,745	5	>99
Congenital rubella syndrome	152	0	100
Smallpox	29,005	0	100
Tetanus	580	26	96
Varicella	4,085,120	408,572[d]	90

[a]Estimated annual average number of cases in the prevaccine era for each disease. Source: JAMA 2007;298:2155–63
[b]Source: MMWR 2009;58(No. RR-2)
[c]Source: MMWR 2011; 60(32):1088–1101
[d]2009 estimate
[e]23 type b and 223 unknown serotype (among children <5 years of age)
[f]Source: http://www.cdc.gov/abcs/reports-findings/survreports/spneu09.html
From: https://www.cdc.gov/mmwr/preview/mmwrhtml/su6004a9.htm

Summary

Morbidity and mortality conferred by infectious diseases have had devastating effects on the lives of people and populations, influencing social and political history throughout recorded time. Through modern medicine and technology, we can now prevent more infectious disease through immunizations than ever before. Vaccines save direct and indirect costs such as medical expenses to society and work days missed, with projected savings in the trillions of dollars in addition to over 700,000 lives saved in the United States for children born between 1995 and 2013 [14]. A historical review of infectious diseases in society, including the great pandemics and epidemics from 300 BCE through the early eighteenth century, helps highlight how infectious disease affects lives, civilizations, and culture. Smallpox

Figure 1. Recommended Immunization Schedule for Children and Adolescents Aged 18 Years or Younger—United States, 2017.

(FOR THOSE WHO FALL BEHIND OR START LATE, SEE T-HE CATCH-UP SCHEDULE [FIGURE 2]).

These recommendations must be read with the footnote: that follow. For those who fall behind or start late, provide catch-up vaccination at the earliest opportunity as indicated by the green bars in Figure 1.
To determine minimum intervals between doses, see the catch-up schedule (Figure 2). School entry and adolescent vaccine age groups are shaded in gray.

Vaccine	Birth	1 mo	2 mos	4 mos	6 mos	9 mos	12 mos	15 mos	18 mos	19-23 mos	2-3 yrs	4-6 yrs	7-10 yrs	11-12 yrs	13-15 yrs	16 yrs	17-18 yrs
Hepatitis B[1] (HepB)	1st dose	2nd dose			3rd dose												
Rotavirus[2] (RV) RV1 (2-dose series); RV5 (3-dose series)			1st dose	2nd dose	See footnote 2												
Diphtheria, tetanus, & acellular pertussis[3] (DTaP: <7 yrs)			1st dose	2nd dose	3rd dose		4th dose					5th dose					
Haemophilus influenzae type b[4] (Hib)			1st dose	2nd dose	See footnote 4		3rd or 4th dose, See footnote 4										
Pneumococcal conjugate[5] (PCV13)			1st dose	2nd dose	3rd dose		4th dose										
Inactivated poliovirus[6] (IPV: <18 yrs)			1st dose	2nd dose	3rd dose							4th dose					
Influenza[7] (IIV)							Annual vaccination (IIV) 1 or 2 doses							Annual vaccination (IIV) 1 dose only			
Measles, mumps, rubella[8] (MMR)							1st dose					2nd dose					
Varicella[9] (VAR)							1st dose					2nd dose					
Hepatitis A[10] (HepA)							2-dose series, See footnote 10										
Meningococcal[11] (Hib-MenCY ≥6 weeks; MenACWY-D ≥9 mos; MenACWY-CRM ≥2 mos)						See footnote 11								1st dose		2nd dose	
Tetanus, diphtheria, & acellular pertussis[12] (Tdap: ≥7 yrs)														Tdap			
Human papillomavirus[13] (HPV)													See footnote 13	See footnote 13			
Meningococcal B[11]															See footnote 11		
Pneumococcal polysaccharide[5] (PPSV23)														See footnote 5			

Legend:
- Range of recommended ages for all children
- Range of recommended ages for catch-up immunization
- Range of recommended ages for certain high-risk groups
- Range of recommended ages for non-high-risk groups that may receive vaccine, subject to individual clinical decision making
- No recommendation

NOTE: The above recommendations must be read along with the footnotes of this schedule.

Fig. 1.6 Childhood immunization schedule (from: https://www.cdc.gov/vaccines/schedules/downloads/child/0-18yrs-child-combined-schedule.pdf)

FIGURE 2. Catch-up immunization schedule for persons aged 4 months through 18 years who start late or who are more than 1 month behind—United States, 2017.

The figure below provides catch-up schedules and minimum intervals between doses for children whose vaccinations have been delayed. A vaccine series does not need to be restarted, regardless of the time that has elapsed between doses. Use the section appropriate for the child's age. Always use this table in conjunction with Figure 1 and the footnotes that follow.

Vaccine	Minimum Age for Dose 1	Minimum Interval Between Doses			
		Dose 1 to Dose 2	Dose 2 to Dose 3	Dose 3 to Dose 4	Dose 4 to Dose 5
Children age 4 months through 6 years					
Hepatitis B[1]	Birth	4 weeks	8 weeks *and at least 16 weeks after first dose.* Minimum age for the final dose is 24 weeks.		
Rotavirus[2]	6 weeks	4 weeks	4 weeks[2]		
Diphtheria, tetanus, and acellular pertussis[3]	6 weeks	4 weeks	4 weeks	6 months	6 months[3]
Haemophilus influenzae type b[4]	6 weeks	4 weeks if first dose was administered before the 1st birthday. 8 weeks (as final dose) if first dose was administered at age 12 through 14 months. No further doses needed if first dose was administered at age 15 months or older.	4 weeks[4] if current age is younger than 12 months **and** first dose was administered at younger than age 7 months, **and** at least 1 previous dose was PRP-T (ActHib, Pentacel, Hiberix) or unknown. 8 weeks *and age 12 through 59 months (as final dose)[4]* • if current age is younger than 12 months **and** first dose was administered at age 7 through 11 months; OR • if current age is 12 through 59 months **and** first dose was administered before the 1st birthday, **and** second dose administered at younger than 15 months; OR • if both doses were PRP-OMP (PedvaxHIB, Comvax) **and** were administered before the 1st birthday. No further doses needed if previous dose was administered at age 15 months or older.	8 weeks (as final dose) This dose only necessary for children age 12 through 59 months who received 3 doses before the 1st birthday.	
Pneumococcal[5]	6 weeks	4 weeks if first dose administered before the 1st birthday. 8 weeks (as final dose for healthy children) if first dose was administered at the 1st birthday or after. No further doses needed for healthy children if first dose was administered at age 24 months or older.	4 weeks if current age is younger than 12 months and previous dose given at <7 yrs old. 8 weeks (as final dose for healthy children) if previous dose given between 7–11 months (wait until at least 12 months old); OR if current age is 12 months or older and at least 1 dose was given before age 12 months. No further doses needed for healthy children if previous dose administered at age 24 months or older.	8 weeks (as final dose) This dose only necessary for children aged 12 through 59 months who received 3 doses before age 12 months or for children at high risk who received 3 doses at any age.	
Inactivated poliovirus[6]	6 weeks	4 weeks[6]	4 weeks[6]	6 months[6] (minimum age 4 years for final dose).	
Measles, mumps, rubella[8]	12 months	4 weeks			
Varicella[9]	12 months	3 months			
Hepatitis A[10]	12 months	6 months			
Meningococcal[11] (Hib-MenCY ≥6 weeks; MenACWY-D ≥9 mos; MenACWY-CRM ≥2 mos)	6 weeks	8 weeks[11]	See footnote 11	See footnote 11	
Children and adolescents age 7 through 18 years					
Meningococcal[11] (MenACWY-D ≥9 mos; MenACWY-CRM ≥2 mos)	Not Applicable (N/A)	8 weeks[11]	See footnote 11		
Tetanus, diphtheria; tetanus, diphtheria, and acellular pertussis[12]	7 years[12]	4 weeks	4 weeks if first dose of DTaP/DT was administered before the 1st birthday. 6 months (as final dose) if first dose of DTaP/DT or Tdap/Td was administered at or after the 1st birthday.	6 months if first dose of DTaP/DT was administered before the 1st birthday.	
Human papillomavirus[13]	9 years	Routine dosing intervals are recommended.[13]			
Hepatitis A[10]	N/A	6 months			
Hepatitis B[1]	N/A	4 weeks	8 weeks **and at least 16 weeks after first dose.**		
Inactivated poliovirus[6]	N/A	4 weeks	4 weeks[6]	6 months[6]	
Measles, mumps, rubella[8]	N/A	4 weeks			
Varicella[9]	N/A	3 months if younger than age 13 years. 4 weeks if age 13 years or older.			

NOTE: The above recommendations must be read along with the footnotes of this schedule.

Fig. 1.7 Catch-up schedule (from: https://www.cdc.gov/vaccines/schedules/downloads/child/0-18yrs-child-combined-schedule.pdf)

a   Footnotes — Recommended Immunization Schedule for Children and Adolescents Aged 18 Years or Younger, UNITED STATES, 2017

For further guidance on the use of the vaccines mentioned below, see: www.cdc.gov/vaccines/hcp/acip-recs/index.html.

For vaccine recommendations for persons 19 years of age and older, see the Adult Immunization Schedule.

Additional information

- For information on contraindications and precautions for the use of a vaccine and for additional information regarding that vaccine, vaccination providers should consult the ACIP General Recommendations on Immunization and the relevant ACIP statement, available online at www.cdc.gov/vaccines/hcp/acip-recs/index.html.
- For purposes of calculating intervals between doses, 4 weeks = 28 days. Intervals of 4 months or greater are determined by calendar months.
- Vaccine doses administered ≤4 days before the minimum interval are considered valid. Doses of any vaccine administered ≥5 days earlier than the min mum interval or minimum age should not be counted as valid doses and should be repeated as age-appropriate. The repeat dose should be spaced after the invalid dose by the recommended minimum interval. For further details, see Table 1, Recommended and minimum ages and intervals between vaccine doses, in MMWR, General Recommendations on Immunization and Reports / Vol. 60 / No. 2, available online at www.cdc.gov/mmwr/pdf/rr/rr6002.pdf.
- Information on travel vaccine requirements and recommendations is available at www.nc.cdc.gov/travel/.
- For vaccination of persons with primary and secondary immunodeficiencies, see Table 13, Vaccination of persons with primary and secondary immunodeficiencies, in General Recommendations on Immunization (ACIP), available at www.cdc.gov/mmwr/pdf/rr/rr6002.pdf; and Immunization in Special Clinical Circumstances, (American Academy of Pediatrics). In: Kimberlin DW, Brady MT, Jackson MA, Long SS, eds. Red Book: 2015 repo t of the Committee on Infectious Diseases. 30th ed. Elk Grove Village, IL: American Academy of Pediatrics; 2015:68-107.
- The National Vaccine Injury Compensation Program (VICP) is a no-fault alternative to the traditional legal system for resolving vaccine injury petitions. Created by the National Childhood Vaccine Injury Act of 1986, it provides compensation to people found to be injured by certain vaccines. All vaccines within the recommended childhood immunization schedule are covered by VICP except for pneumococcal polysaccharide vaccine (PPSV23). For more information; see www.hrsa.gov/vaccinecompensation/index.html.

1. Hepatitis B (HepB) vaccine. (Minimum age: birth)

Routine vaccination:

At birth:

- Administer monovalent HepB vaccine to all newborns within 24 hours of birth.
- For infants born to hepatitis B surface antigen (HBsAg)-positive mothers, administer HepB vaccine and 0.5 mL of hepatitis B immune globulin (HBIG) within 12 hours of birth. These infants should be tested for HBsAg and antibody to HBsAg (anti-HBs) at age 9 through 12 months (preferably at the next well-child visit) or 1 to 2 months after completion of the HepB series if the series was delayed.
- If mother's HBsAg status is unknown, within 12 hours of birth, administer HepB vaccine regardless of birth weight. For infants weighing less than 2,000 grams, administer HBIG in addition to HepB vaccine within 12 hours of birth. Determine mother's HBsAg status as soon as possible and, if mother is HBsAg-positive, also administer HBIG to infants weighing 2,000 grams or more as soon as possible, but no later than age 7 days.

Doses following the birth dose:

- The second dose should be administered at age 1 or 2 months. Monovalent HepB vaccine should be used for doses administered before age 6 weeks.
- Infants who did not receive a birth dose should receive 3 doses of a HepB-containing vaccine on a schedule of 0, 1 to 2 months, and 6 months, starting as soon as feasible (see figure 2).
- Administer the second dose 1 to 2 months after the first dose (minimum interval of 4 weeks); administer the third dose at least 8 weeks after the second dose AND at least 16 weeks after the **first** dose. The final (third or fourth) dose in the HepB vaccine series should be administered **no earlier than age 24 weeks.**

- Administration of a total of 4 doses of HepB vaccine is permitted when a combination vaccine containing HepB is administered after the birth dose.

Catch-up vaccination:

- Unvaccinated persons should complete a 3-dose series.
- A 2-dose series (doses separated by at least 4 months) of adult formulation Recombivax HB is licensed for use in children aged 11 through 15 years.
- For other catch-up guidance, see Figure 2.

2. Rotavirus (RV) vaccines. (Minimum age: 6 weeks for both RV1 [Rotarix] and RV5 [RotaTeq])

Routine vaccination:

Administer a series of RV vaccine to all infants as follows:

1. If Rotarix is used, administer a 2-dose series at ages 2 and 4 months.
2. If RotaTeq is used, administer a 3-dose series at ages 2, 4, and 6 months.
3. If any dose in the series was RotaTeq or vaccine product is unknown for any dose in the series, a total of 3 doses of RV vaccine should be administered.

Catch-up vaccination:

- The maximum age for the first dose in the series is 14 weeks, 6 days; vaccination should not be initiated for infants aged 15 weeks, 0 days, or older.
- The maximum age for the final dose in the series is 8 months, 0 days.
- For other catch-up guidance, see Figure 2.

3. Diphtheria and tetanus toxoids and acellular pertussis (DTaP) vaccine. (Minimum age: 6 weeks. Exception: DTaP-IPV [Kinrix, Quadracel]: 4 years)

Routine vaccination:

- Administer a 5-dose series of DTaP vaccine at ages 2, 4, 6, 15 through 18 months, and 4 through 6 years. The fourth dose may be administered as early as age 12 months.

provided at least 6 months have elapsed since the third dose.

- Inadvertent administration of fourth DTaP dose early: If the fourth dose of DTaP was administered at least 4 months after the third dose of DTaP and the child was 12 months of age or older, it does not need to be repeated.

Catch-up vaccination:

- The fifth dose of DTaP vaccine is not necessary if the fourth dose was administered at age 4 years or older.
- For other catch-up guidance, see Figure 2.

4. Haemophilus influenzae type b (Hib) conjugate vaccine. (Minimum age: 6 weeks for PRP-T [ActHIB, DTaP-IPV/Hib (Pentacel), Hiberix, and Hib-MenCY (MenHibrix)], PRP-OMP [PedvaxHIB])

Routine vaccination:

- Administer a 2- or 3-dose Hib vaccine primary series and a booster dose (dose 3 or 4, depending on vaccine used in primary series) at age 12 through 15 months to complete a full Hib vaccine series.
- The primary series with ActHIB, MenHibrix, Hiberix, or Pentacel consists of 3 doses and should be administered at ages 2, 4, and 6 months. The primary series with PedvaxHIB consists of 2 doses and should be administered at ages 2 and 4 months; a dose at age 6 months is not indicated.
- One booster dose (dose 3 or 4, depending on vaccine used in primary series) of any Hib vaccine should be administered at age 12 through 15 months.
- For recommendations on the use of MenHibrix in patients at increased risk for meningococcal disease, refer to the meningococcal vaccine footnotes and also to MMWR February 28, 2014 / 63(RR01):1-13, available at www.cdc.gov/mmwr/PDF/rr/rr6301.pdf.

Fig. 1.8 (a–d) Footnotes to childhood immunization schedule (Fig. 1.6) and catch-up schedule (Fig. 1.7) (from: https://www.cdc.gov/vaccines/schedules/downloads/child/0-18yrs-child-combined-schedule.pdf)

b For further guidance on the use of the vaccines mentioned below, see: www.cdc.gov/vaccines/hcp/acip-recs/index.html.

Catch-up vaccination:

- If dose 1 was administered at ages 12 through 14 months, administer a second (final) dose at least 8 weeks after dose 1, regardless of Hib vaccine used in the primary series.
- If both doses were PRP-OMP (PedvaxHIB or COMVAX) and were administered before the first birthday, the third (and final) dose should be administered at age 12 through 59 months and at least 8 weeks after the second dose.
- If the first dose was administered at age 7 through 11 months, administer the second dose at least 4 weeks later and a third (and final) dose at age 12 through 15 months or 8 weeks after second dose, whichever is later.
- If first dose is administered before the first birthday and second dose administered at younger than 15 months, a third (and final) dose should be administered 8 weeks later.
- For unvaccinated children aged 15–59 months, administer only 1 dose.
- For other catch-up guidance, see Figure 2. For catch-up guidance related to MenHibrix, see the meningococcal vaccine footnotes and also *MMWR* February 28, 2014 / 63(RR01):1–13, available at www.cdc.gov/mmwr/PDF/rr/rr6301.pdf.

Vaccination of persons with high-risk conditions:

Children aged 12 through 59 months who are at increased risk for Hib disease, including chemotherapy recipients and those with anatomic or functional asplenia (including sickle cell disease), human immunodeficiency virus (HIV) infection, immunoglobulin deficiency, or early component complement deficiency, who have received either no doses or only 1 dose of Hib vaccine before age 12 months, should receive 2 additional doses of Hib vaccine, 8 weeks apart; children who received 2 or more doses of Hib vaccine before age 12 months should receive 1 additional dose.

- For patients younger than age 5 years undergoing chemotherapy or radiation treatment who received a Hib vaccine dose(s) within 14 days of starting therapy or during therapy, repeat the dose(s) at least 3 months following therapy completion.
- Recipients of hematopoietic stem cell transplant (HSCT) should be revaccinated with a 3-dose regimen of Hib vaccine starting 6 to 12 months after successful transplant, regardless of vaccination history; doses should be administered at least 4 weeks apart.
- A single dose of any Hib-containing vaccine should be administered to unimmunized* children and adolescents 15 months of age and older undergoing an elective splenectomy; if possible, vaccine should be administered at least 14 days before procedure.
- Hib vaccine is not routinely recommended for patients 5 years or older. However, 1 dose of Hib vaccine should be administered to unimmunized* persons aged 5 years or older who have anatomic or functional asplenia

(including sickle cell disease) and unimmunized* persons 5 through 18 years of age with HIV infection.

*Patients who have not received a primary series and booster dose or at least 1 dose of Hib vaccine after 14 months of age are considered unimmunized.

5. **Pneumococcal vaccines. (Minimum age: 6 weeks for PCV13, 2 years for PPSV23)**

Routine vaccination with PCV13:

- Administer a 4-dose series of PCV13 at ages 2, 4, and 6 months and at age 12 through 15 months.

Catch-up vaccination with PCV13:

- Administer 1 dose of PCV13 to all healthy children aged 24 through 59 months who are not completely vaccinated for their age.
- For other catch-up guidance, see Figure 2.

Vaccination of persons with high-risk conditions with PCV13 and PPSV23:

- All recommended PCV13 doses should be administered prior to PPSV23 vaccination if possible.
- For children aged 2 through 5 years with any of the following conditions: chronic heart disease (particularly cyanotic congenital heart disease and cardiac failure); chronic lung disease (including asthma if treated with high-dose oral corticosteroid therapy); diabetes mellitus; cerebrospinal fluid leak; cochlear implant; sickle cell disease and other hemoglobinopathies; anatomic or functional asplenia; HIV infection; chronic renal failure; nephrotic syndrome; diseases associated with treatment with immunosuppressive drugs or radiation therapy, including malignant neoplasms, leukemias, lymphomas, and Hodgkin disease; solid organ transplantation; or congenital immunodeficiency:
  1. Administer 1 dose of PCV13 if any incomplete schedule of 3 doses of PCV13 was received previously.
  2. Administer 2 doses of PCV13 at least 8 weeks apart if unvaccinated or any incomplete schedule of fewer than 3 doses of PCV13 was received previously.
  3. The minimum interval between doses of PCV13 is 8 weeks.
  4. For children with no history of PPSV23 vaccination, administer PPSV23 at least 8 weeks after the most recent dose of PCV13.
- For children aged 6 through 18 years who have cerebrospinal fluid leak; cochlear implant; sickle cell disease and other hemoglobinopathies; anatomic or functional asplenia; congenital or acquired immunodeficiencies; HIV infection; chronic renal failure; nephrotic syndrome; diseases associated with treatment with immunosuppressive drugs or radiation therapy, including malignant neoplasms, leukemias, lymphomas, and Hodgkin disease; generalized malignancy; solid organ transplantation; or multiple myeloma:
  1. If neither PCV13 nor PPSV23 has been received previously, administer 1 dose of PCV13 now and 1 dose of PPSV23 at least 8 weeks later.

  2. If PPSV23 has been received previously but PPSV23 has not, administer 1 dose of PPSV23 at least 8 weeks after the most recent dose of PCV13.
  3. If PPSV23 has been received but PCV13 has not, administer 1 dose of PCV13 at least 8 weeks after the most recent dose of PPSV23.
- For children aged 6 through 18 years with chronic heart disease (particularly cyanotic congenital heart disease and cardiac failure), chronic lung disease (including asthma if treated with high-dose oral corticosteroid therapy), diabetes mellitus, alcoholism, or chronic liver disease, who have not received PPSV23, administer 1 dose of PPSV23. If PCV13 has been received previously, then PPSV23 should be administered at least 8 weeks after any prior PCV13 dose.
- A single revaccination with PPSV23 should be administered 5 years after the first dose to children with sickle cell disease or other hemoglobinopathies; anatomic or functional asplenia; congenital or acquired immunodeficiencies; HIV infection; chronic renal failure; nephrotic syndrome; diseases associated with treatment with immunosuppressive drugs or radiation therapy, including malignant neoplasms, leukemias, lymphomas, and Hodgkin disease; generalized malignancy; solid organ transplantation; or multiple myeloma.

6. **Inactivated poliovirus vaccine (IPV). (Minimum age: 6 weeks)**

Routine vaccination:

- Administer a 4-dose series of IPV at ages 2, 4, 6 through 18 months, and 4 through 6 years. The final dose in the series should be administered on or after the fourth birthday and at least 6 months after the previous dose.

Catch-up vaccination:

- In the first 6 months of life, minimum age and minimum intervals are only recommended if the person is at risk of imminent exposure to circulating poliovirus (i.e., travel to a polio-endemic region or during an outbreak).
- If 4 or more doses are administered before age 4 years, an additional dose should be administered at age 4 through 6 years and at least 6 months after the previous dose.
- A fourth dose is not necessary if the third dose was administered at age 4 years or older and at least 6 months after the previous dose.
- If both oral polio vaccine (OPV) and IPV were administered as part of a series, a total of 4 doses should be administered, regardless of the child's current age. If only OPV was administered, and all doses were given prior to age 4 years, 1 dose of IPV should be given at 4 years or older, at least 4 weeks after the last OPV dose.
- IPV is not routinely recommended for U.S. residents aged 18 years or older.
- For other catch-up guidance, see Figure 2.

C For further guidance on the use of the vaccines mentioned below, see: www.cdc.gov/vaccines/hcp/acip-recs/index.html.

7. Influenza vaccines. (Minimum age: 6 months for inactivated influenza vaccine [IIV], 18 years for recombinant influenza vaccine [RIV])

Routine vaccination:

- Administer influenza vaccine annually to all children beginning at age 6 months. For the 2016–17 season, use of live attenuated influenza vaccine (LAIV) is not recommended.

For children aged 6 months through 8 years:

- For the 2016–17 season, administer 2 doses (separated by at least 4 weeks) to children who are receiving influenza vaccine for the first time or who have not previously received ≥2 doses of trivalent or quadrivalent influenza vaccine before July 1, 2016. For additional guidance, follow dosing guidelines in the 2016–17 ACIP influenza vaccine recommendations (see MMWR August 26, 2016;65(5):1-54, available at www.cdc.gov/mmwr/volumes/65/rr/pdfs/rr6505.pdf).
- For the 2017–18 season, follow dosing guidelines in the 2017–18 ACIP influenza vaccine recommendations.

For persons aged 9 years and older:

- Administer 1 dose.

8. Measles, mumps, and rubella (MMR) vaccine. (Minimum age: 12 months for routine vaccination)

Routine vaccination:

- Administer a 2-dose series of MMR vaccine at ages 12 through 15 months and 4 through 6 years. The second dose may be administered before age 4 years, provided at least 4 weeks have elapsed since the first dose.
- Administer 1 dose of MMR vaccine to infants aged 6 through 11 months before departure from the United States for international travel. These children should be revaccinated with 2 doses of MMR vaccine, the first at age 12 through 15 months (12 months if the child remains in an area where disease risk is high), and the second dose at least 4 weeks later.
- Administer 2 doses of MMR vaccine to children aged 12 months and older before departure from the United States for international travel. The first dose should be administered on or after age 12 months and the second dose at least 4 weeks later.

Catch-up vaccination:

- Ensure that all school-aged children and adolescents have had 2 doses of MMR vaccine; the minimum interval between the 2 doses is 4 weeks.

9. Varicella (VAR) vaccine. (Minimum age: 12 months)

Routine vaccination:

- Administer a 2-dose series of VAR vaccine at ages 12 through 15 months and 4 through 6 years. The second dose may be administered before age 4 years, provided at least 3 months have elapsed since the first dose. If the second dose was administered at least 4 weeks after the first dose, it can be accepted as valid.

Catch-up vaccination:

- Ensure that all persons aged 7 through 18 years without evidence of immunity (see MMWR 2007;56[No. RR-4], available at www.cdc.gov/mmwr/pdf/rr/rr5604.pdf) have 2 doses of varicella vaccine. For children aged 7 through 12 years, the recommended minimum interval between doses is 3 months (if the second dose was administered at least 4 weeks after the first dose, it can be accepted as valid); for persons aged 13 years and older, the minimum interval between doses is 4 weeks.

10. Hepatitis A (HepA) vaccine. (Minimum age: 12 months)

Routine vaccination:

- Initiate the 2-dose HepA vaccine series at ages 12 through 23 months; separate the 2 doses by 6 to 18 months.
- Children who have received 1 dose of HepA vaccine before age 24 months should receive a second dose 6 to 18 months after the first dose.
- For any person aged 2 years and older who has not already received the HepA vaccine series, 2 doses of HepA vaccine separated by 6 to 18 months may be administered if immunity against hepatitis A virus infection is desired.

Catch-up vaccination:

- The minimum interval between the 2 doses is 6 months.

Special populations:

- Administer 2 doses of HepA vaccine at least 6 months apart to previously unvaccinated persons who live in areas where vaccination programs target older children, or who are at increased risk for infection. This includes persons travelling to or working in countries that have high or intermediate endemicity of infection; men having sex with men; users of injection and non-injection illicit drugs; persons who work with HAV-infected primates or with HAV in a research laboratory; persons with clotting-factor disorders; persons with chronic liver disease; and persons who anticipate close, personal contact (e.g. household or regular babysitting) with an international adoptee during the first 60 days after arrival in the United States from a country with high or intermediate endemicity. The first dose should be administered as soon as the adoption is planned, ideally, 2 or more weeks before the arrival of the adoptee.

11. Meningococcal vaccines. (Minimum age: 6 weeks for Hib-MenCY [MenHibrix], 2 months for MenACWY-CRM [Menveo], 9 months for MenACWY-D [Menactra], 10 years for MenB vaccines; MenB-4C [Bexsero] and MenB-FHbp [Trumenba])

Routine vaccination:

- Administer a single dose of Menactra or Menveo vaccine at age 11 through 12 years, with a booster dose at age 16 years.
- For children aged 2 months through 18 years with high-risk conditions, see "Meningococcal conjugate ACWY vaccination of persons with high-risk conditions and other persons at increased risk of disease" below.

Catch-up vaccination:

- Administer Menactra or Menveo vaccine at age 13 through 18 years if not previously vaccinated.
- If the first dose is administered at age 13 through 15 years, a booster dose should be administered at age 16 through 18 years, with a minimum interval of at least 8 weeks between doses.
- If the first dose is administered at age 16 years or older, a booster dose is not needed.
- For other catch-up guidance, see Figure 2.

Clinical discretion:

- Young adults aged 16 through 23 years (preferred age range is 16 through 18 years) who are not at increased risk for meningococcal disease may be vaccinated with a 2-dose series of either Bexsero (0, ≥1 month) or Trumenba (0, 6 months) vaccine to provide short-term protection against most strains of serogroup B meningococcal disease. The two MenB vaccines are not interchangeable; the same vaccine product must be used for all doses.
- If the second dose of Trumenba is given at an interval of <6 months, a third dose should be given at least 6 months after the first dose; the minimum interval between the second and third doses is 4 weeks.

Meningococcal conjugate ACWY vaccination of persons with high-risk conditions and other persons at increased risk:

Children with anatomic or functional asplenia (including sickle cell disease), children with HIV infection, or children with persistent complement component deficiency (includes persons with inherited or chronic deficiencies in C3, C5-9, properdin, factor D, factor H, or taking eculizumab [Soliris]):

- Menveo

  o Children who initiate vaccination at 8 weeks. Administer doses at ages 2, 4, 6, and 12 months.

  o Unvaccinated children who initiate vaccination at 7 through 23 months. Administer 2 primary doses, with the second dose at least 12 weeks after the first dose AND after the first birthday.

  o Children 24 months and older who have not received a complete series. Administer 2 primary doses at least 8 weeks apart.

- MenHibrix

  o Children who initiate vaccination at 6 weeks. Administer doses at ages 2, 4, 6, and 12 through 15 months.

  o If the first dose of MenHibrix is given at or after age 12 months, a total of 2 doses should be given at least 8 weeks apart to ensure protection against serogroups C and Y meningococcal disease.

Fig. 1.8 (continued)

d For further guidance on the use of the vaccines mentioned below, see: www.cdc.gov/vaccines/hcp/acip-recs/index.html.

- **Menactra**
  - o **Children with anatomic or functional asplenia or HIV infection**
    - — *Children 24 months and older who have not received a complete series.* Administer 2 primary doses at least 8 weeks apart. If Menactra is administered to a child with asplenia (including sickle cell disease) or HIV infection, do not administer Menactra until age 2 years and at least 4 weeks after the completion of all PCV13 doses.
  - o **Children with persistent complement component deficiency**
    - — *Children 9 through 23 months.* Administer 2 primary doses at least 12 weeks apart.
    - — *Children 24 months and older who have not received a complete series.* Administer 2 primary doses at least 8 weeks apart.
  - o **All high-risk children**
    - — If Menactra is to be administered to a child at high risk for meningococcal disease, it is recommended that Menactra be given either before or at the same time as DTaP.

Meningococcal B vaccination of persons with high-risk conditions and other persons at increased risk of disease:
Children with anatomic or functional asplenia (including sickle cell disease) or children with persistent complement component deficiency (includes persons with inherited or chronic deficiencies in C3, C5-9, properdin, factor D, factor H, or taking eculizumab [Soliris]):
- o *Persons 10 years or older who have not received a complete series.* Administer a 2-dose series of Bexsero, with doses at least 1 month apart, or a 3-dose series of Trumenba, with the second dose at least 1–2 months after the first and the third dose at least 6 months after the first. The two MenB vaccines are not interchangeable; the same vaccine product must be used for all doses.

For children who travel to or reside in countries in which meningococcal disease is hyperendemic or epidemic, including countries in the African meningitis belt or the Hajj:
- Administer an age-appropriate formulation and series of Menactra or Menveo for protection against serogroups A and W meningococcal disease. Prior receipt of MenHibrix is not sufficient for children traveling to the meningitis belt or the Hajj because it does not contain serogroups A or W.

For children at risk during an outbreak attributable to a vaccine serogroup:
- For serogroup A, C, W, or Y: Administer or complete an age- and formulation-appropriate series of MenHibrix, Menactra, or Menveo.

- For serogroup B: Administer a 2-dose series of Bexsero, with doses at least 1 month apart, or a 3-dose series of Trumenba, with the second dose at least 1–2 months after the first and the third dose at least 6 months after the first. The two MenB vaccines are not interchangeable; the same vaccine product must be used for all doses.

For MenACWY booster doses among persons with high-risk conditions, refer to *MMWR* 2013;62(RR02):1-22, at www.cdc.gov/mmwr/preview/mmwrhtml/rr6202a1.htm, *MMWR* June 20, 2014 / 63(24):527-530, at www.cdc.gov/mmwr/pdf/wk/mm6324.pdf, and *MMWR* November 4, 2016 /65(43):1189-1194, at www.cdc.gov/mmwr/volumes/65/wr/pdfs/mm6543a3.pdf.

For other catch-up recommendations for these persons and complete information on use of meningococcal vaccines, including guidance related to vaccination of persons at increased risk of infection, see meningococcal *MMWR* publications, available at: www.cdc.gov/vaccines/hcp/acip-recs/vacc-specific/mening.html.

12. **Tetanus and diphtheria toxoids and acellular pertussis (Tdap) vaccine. (Minimum age: 10 years for both Boostrix and Adacel)**
Routine vaccination:
- Administer 1 dose of Tdap vaccine to all adolescents aged 11 through 12 years.
- Tdap may be administered regardless of the interval since the last tetanus and diphtheria toxoid-containing vaccine.
- Administer 1 dose of Tdap vaccine to pregnant adolescents during each pregnancy (preferably during the early part of gestational weeks 27 through 36), regardless of time since prior Td or Tdap vaccination.

Catch-up vaccination:
- Persons aged 7 years and older who are not fully immunized with DTaP vaccine should receive Tdap vaccine as 1 dose (preferably the first) in the catch-up series; if additional doses are needed, use Td vaccine. For children 7 through 10 years who receive a dose of Tdap as part of the catch-up series, an adolescent Tdap vaccine dose at age 11 through 12 years may be administered.
- Persons aged 11 through 18 years who have not received Tdap vaccine should receive a dose, followed by tetanus and diphtheria toxoids (Td) booster doses every 10 years thereafter.
- **Inadvertent doses of DTaP vaccine:**
  - If administered inadvertently to a child aged 7 through 10 years, the dose may count as part of the catch-up series. This dose may count as the adolescent Tdap dose, or the child may receive a Tdap booster dose at age 11 through 12 years.
  - If administered inadvertently to an adolescent aged 11 through 18 years, the dose should be counted as the adolescent Tdap booster.
  - For other catch-up guidance, see Figure 2.

13. **Human papillomavirus (HPV) vaccines. (Minimum age: 9 years for 4vHPV [Gardasil] and 9vHPV [Gardasil 9])**
Routine and catch-up vaccination:
- Administer a 2-dose series of HPV vaccine on a schedule of 0, 6-12 months to all adolescents aged 11 or 12 years. The vaccination series can start at age 9 years.
- Administer HPV vaccine to all adolescents through age 18 years who were not previously adequately vaccinated. The number of recommended doses is based on age at administration of the first dose.
- For persons initiating vaccination before age 15, the recommended immunization schedule is 2 doses of HPV vaccine at 0, 6-12 months.
- For persons initiating vaccination at age 15 years or older, the recommended immunization schedule is 3 doses of HPV vaccine at 0, 1–2, 6 months.
- A vaccine dose administered at a shorter interval should be readministered at the recommended interval.
  - ▪ In a 2-dose schedule of HPV vaccine, the minimum interval is 5 months between the first and second dose. If the second dose is administered at a shorter interval, a third dose should be administered a minimum of 12 weeks after the second dose and a minimum of 5 months after the first dose.
  - ▪ In a 3-dose schedule of HPV vaccine, the minimum intervals are 4 weeks between the first and second dose, 12 weeks between the second and third dose, and 5 months between the first and third dose. If a vaccine dose is administered at a shorter interval, it should be readministered after another minimum interval has been met since the most recent dose.

Special populations:
- For children with history of sexual abuse or assault, administer HPV vaccine beginning at age 9 years.
- Immunocompromised persons*, including those with human immunodeficiency virus (HIV) infection, should receive a 3-dose series at 0, 1–2, and 6 months, regardless of age at vaccine initiation.
- Note: HPV vaccination is not recommended during pregnancy, although there is no evidence that the vaccine poses harm. If a woman is found to be pregnant after initiating the vaccination series, no intervention is needed; the remaining vaccine doses should be delayed until after the pregnancy. Pregnancy testing is not needed before HPV vaccination.

*See *MMWR* December 16, 2016;65(49):1405-1408, available at www.cdc.gov/mmwr/volumes/65/wr/pdfs/mm6549a5.pdf.

CS270457-C

Fig. 1.8 (continued)

was an undeniable influence on the Americas from its beginning as Europeans colonized the New World. Inoculation by variolation was instrumental in the eventual eradication of smallpox and served as the first form of vaccination. Vaccines, first attributed to Edward Jenner, with his trials and experiments using what we now call "evidence-based medicine" were developed by way of the scientific method. Vaccine development through the nineteenth and twentieth centuries has resulted in the eradication of smallpox, is close to eradicating polio, and is responsible for the elimination of many diseases locally and regionally. In the United States, there has been a 99% decrease in incidence of the nine diseases for which vaccines have been recommended for decades accompanied by a similar decline in mortality and disease sequelae [9]. These diseases include smallpox, diphtheria, tetanus, pertussis, paralytic poliomyelitis, measles, mumps, rubella (including congenital rubella syndrome), and *Haemophilus influenzae* type b. Today, there are 26 different diseases listed by the WHO for which there exist vaccines to prevent them. These vaccines are available worldwide with many more VPD vaccines (24 to date) in development, many with likely approval within the next few years to the next decade.

References

1. Recommendations of the Immunization Practices Advisory Committee (ACIP) General Recommendations on Immunization [Internet]. Available from: http://www.cdc.gov/mmwr/preview/mmwrhtml/00001372.htm
2. Catalog Record: Public health in New York state. Report of... | Hathi Trust Digital Library [Internet]. Available from: https://catalog.hathitrust.org/Record/001581709
3. Francis T. Approach to control of poliomyelitis by immunological methods. Bull N Y Acad Med [Internet]. 1955;31(4):259–74. [cited 2016 Sep 3]. Available from: http://www.ncbi.nlm.nih.gov/pubmed/14364073
4. Lambert SM, Markel H. Making history: Thomas Francis, Jr, MD, and the 1954 Salk Poliomyelitis Vaccine Field Trial. Arch Pediatr Adolesc Med [Internet]. 2000;154(5):512–7. [cited 2016 Sep 3]. Available from: http://www.ncbi.nlm.nih.gov/pubmed/10807305
5. André FE. Vaccinology: past achievements, present roadblocks and future promises. Vaccine [Internet]. 2003;21(7–8):593–5. [cited 2016 Sep 4]. Available from: http://www.ncbi.nlm.nih.gov/pubmed/12531323
6. Nelson KE, Williams CF. Early history of infectious disease. Available at: http://www.jblearning.com/samples/0763728799/28799_CH01_001_022.pdf
7. Epidemic Diseases and their Effects on History, Christian W. McMillen, Last Modified: 24 July 2013, doi: 10.1093/OBO/9780199743292-0155. Epidemic Diseases and their Effects on History – International Relations – Oxford Bibliographies [Internet]. Available from: http://www.oxfordbibliographies.com/view/document/obo-9780199743292/obo-9780199743292-0155.xml
8. Armstrong GL, Conn LA, Pinner RW. Trends in infectious disease mortality in the United States during the 20th century. JAMA [Internet]. 1999;281(1):61. [cited 2016 Sep 5]. Available from: http://jama.jamanetwork.com/article.aspx?doi=10.1001/jama.281.1.61
9. Achievements in Public Health, 1900–1999 Impact of Vaccines Universally Recommended for Children – United States, 1990–1998 [Internet]. Available from: http://www.cdc.gov/mmwr/preview/mmwrhtml/00056803.htm
10. Achievements in Public Health, 1900–1999: Control of Infectious Diseases [Internet]. Available from: http://www.cdc.gov/mmwr/preview/mmwrhtml/mm4829a1.htm

11. Centers for Disease Control and Prevention (CDC). Ten great public health achievements – United States, 2001–2010. MMWR Morb Mortal Wkly Rep [Internet]. 2011;60(19):619–23. [cited 2016 Sep 1]. Available from: http://www.ncbi.nlm.nih.gov/pubmed/21597455

12. MMWR / August 28, 2015 / Vol. 64 / No. 33.

13. Dayan GH, Ortega-Sánchez IR, LeBaron CW, Quinlisk MP. The cost of containing one case of measles: the economic impact on the public health infrastructure – Iowa, 2004. Pediatrics. 2005;116(1):e1–4.

14. Whitney CG, Zhou F, Singleton J, Schuchat A. Benefits from Immunization during the vaccines for children program era – United States, 1994–2013. Weekly [Internet]. 2014;63(16);352–5. Available from: http://www.cdc.gov/mmwr/preview/mmwrhtml/mm6316a4.htm

15. Smith PJ, Chu SY, Barker LE. Children who have received no vaccines: who are they and where do they live? Pediatrics [Internet]. 2004; 114(1):187–95. [cited 2016 Sep 17]. Available from: http://www.ncbi.nlm.nih.gov/pubmed/15231927

16. Philippe D, Jean-Marie O-B, Marta G-D, Thomas C, Bilous J, Eggers R, et al. Global immunization: status, progress, challenges and future. BMC Int Health Hum Rights [Internet]. 2009; 9(Suppl 1):S2. [cited 2016 Aug 27]. Available from: http://bmcinthealthhumrights.biomedcentral.com/articles/10.1186/1472-698X-9-S1-S2

17. Measles | History of Measles | CDC [Internet]. Available from: http://www.cdc.gov/measles/about/history.html

18. Reported. Vol. 29.

19. Sencer DJ, Dull HB, Langmuir AD. Epidemiologic basis for eradication of measles in 1967. Public Health Rep [Internet]. 1967;82(3):253–6. [cited 2016 Sep 8]. Available from: http://www.ncbi.nlm.nih.gov/pubmed/4960501

20. Notifiable Diseases/Deaths in Selected Cities Weekly Information [Internet]. Available from: http://www.cdc.gov/mmwr/preview/mmwrhtml/00056175.htm

21. Challenges in global immunization and the Global Immunization Vision and Strategy 2006–2015. Wkly Epidemiol Rec [Internet]. 2006;81(19):190–5. [cited 2016 Aug 27]. Available from: http://www.ncbi.nlm.nih.gov/pubmed/16696156

22. Simons E, Ferrari M, Fricks J, Wannemuehler K, Anand A, Burton A, et al. Assessment of the 2010 global measles mortality reduction goal: results from a model of surveillance data. Lancet (London, England) [Internet]. 2012; 379(9832):2173–8. [cited 2016 Sep 3]. Available from: http://www.ncbi.nlm.nih.gov/pubmed/22534001

23. Progress Toward Regional Measles Elimination – Worldwide, 2000–2014 [Internet]. Available from: http://www.cdc.gov/mmwr/preview/mmwrhtml/mm6444a4.htm

24. McNeill WH. Plagues and peoples. New York: Anchor Books; 1989.

25. Sabbatani S, Fiorino S. [The Antonine Plague and the decline of the Roman Empire]. Infez Med [Internet]. 2009;17(4):261–75. [cited 2016 Aug 8]. Available from: http://www.ncbi.nlm.nih.gov/pubmed/20046111

26. Geib GW. Justinian's Flea: Plague, Empire, and the Birth of Europe, by William Rosen, Viking, 2007. 2013. [cited 2016 Aug 27]. Available from: http://digitalcommons.butler.edu/las_bookreviews/131

27. Lindemann M. The black death 1346–1353: the complete history (review). Renaiss Q. 2006;59(2):599–601.

28. Khan IA. Plague: the dreadful visitation occupying the human mind for centuries. Trans R Soc Trop Med Hyg. 2004;98(5):270–7.

29. Scott S, Duncan CJ. Return of the black death: the world's greatest serial killer. Chichester: Wiley; 2004. 310 p

30. Price R. State church charity and smallpox: an epidemic crisis in the City of Mexico 1797–98. J R Soc Med [Internet]. 1982;75(5):356–67. [cited 2016 Sep 4]. Available from: http://www.ncbi.nlm.nih.gov/pubmed/7042974

31. Henderson DA, Moss B. Smallpox and vaccinia. In: Plotkin SA, Orenstein WA, editors. Vaccines. 3rd ed. Philadelphia: Saunders; 1999. Chapter 6. Available from: https://www.ncbi.nlm.nih.gov/books/NBK7294/

32. BBC – History – British History in depth: Smallpox: eradicating the scourge [Internet]. Available from: http://www.bbc.co.uk/history/british/empire_seapower/smallpox_01.shtml

33. King LS. Princes and peasants: smallpox in history. JAMA J Am Med Assoc [Internet]. 1984;252(1):106. [cited 2016 Aug 28]. Available from: http://jama.jamanetwork.com/article. aspx?doi=10.1001/jama.1984.03350010066034

34. Hopkins DR. Smallpox: ten years gone. Am J Public Health [Internet]. 1988;78(12):1589–95. [cited 2016 Sep 5]. Available from: http://www.ncbi.nlm.nih.gov/pubmed/2461102

35. Blower S, Bernoulli D. An attempt at a new analysis of the mortality caused by smallpox and of the advantages of inoculation to prevent it. Rev Med Virol [Internet]. 1766;14(5):275–88. [cited 2016 Aug 7]. Available from: http://www.ncbi.nlm.nih.gov/pubmed/15334536

36. Buck C. Smallpox inoculation – should we credit Chinese medicine? Complement Ther Med [Internet]. 2003;11(3):201–2. [cited 2016 Aug 17]. Available from: http://www.ncbi.nlm.nih. gov/pubmed/14659400

37. Historic Dates and Events Related to Vaccines and Immunization [Internet]. Available from: http://www.immunize.org/timeline/

38. Plotkin SA. Vaccines: past, present and future. Nat Med Suppl. 2005;11(4):S5–11.

39. Odier L. Inoculation against smallpox in England. Bull N Y Acad Med [Internet]. 1975; 51(7):889–90. [cited 2016 Sep 5]. Available from: http://www.ncbi.nlm.nih.gov/pubmed/ 19312934

40. Rusnock AF. Vital accounts quantifying health and population in eighteenth-century. Cambridge: Cambridge University Press; 2002.

41. Edward Jenner – Jenner Institute [Internet]. Available from: http://www.jenner.ac.uk/ edward-jenner

42. White PJ, Shackelford PG. Edward Jenner, MD, and the scourge that was. Am J Dis Child [Internet]. 1983;137(9):864–9. [cited 2016 Aug 27]. Available from: http://www.ncbi.nlm. nih.gov/pubmed/6351592

43. Pead PJ. Benjamin Jesty: new light in the dawn of vaccination. Lancet (London, England) [Internet]. 2003;362(9401):2104–9. [cited 2016 Aug 27]. Available from: http://www.ncbi. nlm.nih.gov/pubmed/14697816

44. Hammarsten JF, Tattersall W, Hammarsten JE. Who discovered smallpox vaccination? Edward Jenner or Benjamin Jesty? Trans Am Clin Climatol Assoc. 1979;90:44–55.

45. The first recorded Smallpox vaccination [Internet]. Available from: http://www.thedorset-page.com/history/smallpox/smallpox.htm

46. Rusnock AA. Historical context and the roots of Jenner's discovery [Internet]. Vol. 12, Human vaccines and immunotherapeutics. Taylor & Francis; 2016. p. 2025–8. [cited 2016 Aug 18]. Available from: https://www.tandfonline.com/doi/full/10.1080/21645515.2016.1158369

47. George Washington Papers at the Library of Congress, 1741–1799. Series 4. General Correspondence. 1697–1799 [Internet]. Available from: http://memory.loc.gov/cgi-bin/amp age?collId=mgw4&fileName=gwpage034.db&recNum=315

48. BLAKE JB. Smallpox inoculation in Colonial Boston. J Hist Med Allied Sci [Internet]. 1953;8(3):284–300. [cited 2016 Aug 27]. Available from: http://www.ncbi.nlm.nih.gov/ pubmed/13069694

49. Grabenstein JD, Pittman PR, Greenwood JT, Engler RJ. Immunization to protect the US Armed forces: heritage, current practice, and prospects. Epidemiol Rev. 2006;28:3–26. Epub 2006 Jun 8.

50. Artenstein AW, Opal JM, Opal SM, Tramont EC, Usa M, Peter G, et al. History of U.S. military contributions to the study of vaccines against infectious diseases. Mil Med. 2005;170(4):3–11.

51. Byerly CR. Of smallpox and empire. [Review of: Fenn, EA. Pox Americana: the great smallpox epidemic of 1775–82. New York: Hill and Wang, 2001]. Rev Am Hist [Internet]. 2002;30(2):204–11. [cited 2016 Aug 8]. Available from: http://www.ncbi.nlm.nih.gov/ pubmed/12166479

52. USAMRIID [Internet]. Available from: http://www.usamriid.army.mil/

53. CDC Smallpox Vaccine Overview [Internet]. Available from: https://emergency.cdc.gov/agent/smallpox/vaccination/facts.asp

54. Smallpox Vaccination Program Questions and Answers.

55. Parkman F. The conspiracy of Pontiac: and the Indian war after the conquest of Canada: Parkman, Francis, 1823–1893: Free Download and Streaming: Internet Archive [Internet]. Available from: https://archive.org/details/conspiracyofpont01park

56. CDC Smallpox | Abstract: Smallpox as a Biological Weapon: Medical and Public Health Management [Internet]. Available from: https://emergency.cdc.gov/agent/smallpox/smallpox-biological-weapon-abstract.asp

57. Vaccine-Preventable Diseases, Immunizations, and MMWR – 1961–2011 [Internet]. Available from: http://www.cdc.gov/mmwr/preview/mmwrhtml/su6004a9.htm

58. Research C for BE and. Questions about Vaccines – Smallpox.

59. Smith KA. Louis pasteur, the father of immunology? Front Immunol [Internet]. 2012;3:68. [cited 2016 Aug 29]. Available from: http://www.ncbi.nlm.nih.gov/pubmed/22566949

60. Bazin H. Pasteur and the birth of vaccines made in the laboratory. In: History of vaccine development [Internet]. New York: Springer New York; 2011. p. 33–45. [cited 2016 Aug 27]. Available from: http://link.springer.com/10.1007/978-1-4419-1339-5_6

61. Sternbach G. The history of anthrax. J Emerg Med. 2003;24(4):463–7.

62. Historical Perspectives a Centennial Celebration: Pasteur and the Modern Era of Immunization [Internet]. Available from: http://www.cdc.gov/mmwr/preview/mmwrhtml/00000572.htm

63. Baxter D. Active and passive immunity, vaccine types, excipients and licensing. Occup Med (Lond) [Internet]. 2007;57(8):552–6. [cited 2016 Aug 29]. Available from: http://www.ncbi.nlm.nih.gov/pubmed/18045976

64. Services USD of H and H. Vaccines.gov.

65. WHO | DNA vaccines. WHO. 2011;

66. WHO | Zika virus vaccine product development. WHO. 2016;

67. Pinkbook | Tetanus | Epidemiology of Vaccine Preventable Diseases | CDC [Internet]. Available from: http://www.cdc.gov/vaccines/pubs/pinkbook/tetanus.html

68. Frierson JG. The yellow fever vaccine: a history. Yale J Biol Med [Internet]. 2010;83(2):77–85. [cited 2016 Sep 13]. Available from: http://www.ncbi.nlm.nih.gov/pubmed/20589188.

69. Boire AN, Riedel VAA, Parrish NM, Riedel S. Tuberculosis: from an untreatable disease in antiquity to an untreatable disease in modern times? J Anc Dis Prev Remedies [Internet]. 2013;1(2). [cited 2016 Aug 28]. Available from: http://www.esciencecentral.org/journals/tuberculosis-from-an-untreatable-disease-in-antiquity-to-an-untreatable-disease-in-modern-times-2329-8731.1000106.php?aid=14234

70. Gheorghiu M, Lagranderie M, Balazuc A-M. Tuberculosis and BCG. In: Vaccines: a biography [Internet]. New York: Springer New York; 2010. p. 125–40. [cited 2016 Sep 3]. Available from: http://link.springer.com/10.1007/978-1-4419-1108-7_8

71. WHO | Tuberculosis vaccine development. WHO. 2015;

72. Luca S, Mihaescu T. History of BCG vaccine. Mædica [Internet]. 2013;8(1):53–8. [cited 2016 Sep 25]. Available from: http://www.ncbi.nlm.nih.gov/pubmed/24023600

73. Scheindlin S. The flu in retrospect: etiology and immunization. Mol Interv [Internet]. 2009; 9(6):284–90. [cited 2016 Sep 14]. Available from: http://www.ncbi.nlm.nih.gov/pubmed/20048132

74. Flu.gov. Pandemic Flu History.

75. Shrestha SS, Swerdlow DL, Borse RH, Prabhu VS, Finelli L, Atkins CY, et al. Estimating the burden of 2009 pandemic influenza A (H1N1) in the United States (April 2009–April 2010). Clin Infect Dis [Internet]. 2011;52 Suppl 1:S75–82. [cited 2016 Oct 9]. Available from: http://www.ncbi.nlm.nih.gov/pubmed/21342903

76. Baicus A. History of polio vaccination. World J Virol [Internet]. 2012;1(4):108–14. [cited 2016 Aug 28]. Available from: http://www.ncbi.nlm.nih.gov/pubmed/24175215

77. Polio | U.S. Polio Elimination | CDC [Internet]. Available from: http://www.cdc.gov/polio/us/index.html

78. Epidemiologic Notes and Reports Follow-Up on Poliomyelitis – United States, Canada, Netherlands [Internet]. Available from: http://www.cdc.gov/mmwr/preview/mmwrhtml/00050435.htm

79. Vaccines: VPD-VAC/Polio/Disease FAQs [Internet]. Available from: http://www.cdc.gov/vaccines/vpd-vac/polio/dis-faqs.htm

80. Gallagher KM, Plotkin SA, Katz SL, Orenstein WA. Measles, mumps, and rubella. In: Vaccines: a biography [Internet]. New York: Springer New York; 2010. p. 223–47. [cited 2016 Aug 28]. Available from: http://link.springer.com/10.1007/978-1-4419-1108-7_13

81. Mumps – History of Vaccines [Internet]. Available from: http://www.historyofvaccines.org/content/articles/mumps

82. Plotkin SA. The history of rubella and rubella vaccination leading to elimination. Clin Infect Dis. 2006;43(Supplement 3):S164–8.

83. What is the history of measles vaccine in America–National Vaccine Information Center [Internet]. Available from: http://www.nvic.org/vaccines-and-diseases/measles/history-measles-vaccine.aspx

84. Flaherty DK. The vaccine-autism connection: a public health crisis caused by unethical medical practices and fraudulent science. Ann Pharmacother [Internet]. 2011; 45(10):1302–4. [cited 2016 Aug 28]. Available from: http://www.ncbi.nlm.nih.gov/pubmed/21917556

85. Wakefield AJ, Murch SH, Anthony A, Linnell J, Casson DM, Malik M, et al. Ileal-lymphoid-nodular hyperplasia, non-specific colitis, and pervasive developmental disorder in children. Lancet (London, England) [Internet]. 1998;351(9103):637–41. [cited 2016 Sep 3]. Available from: http://www.ncbi.nlm.nih.gov/pubmed/9500320

86. Demicheli V, Rivetti A, Debalini MG, Di Pietrantonj C. Vaccines for measles, mumps and rubella in children. Cochrane Database Syst Rev [Internet]. 2012;(2):CD004407. [cited 2016 Aug 28]. Available from: http://www.ncbi.nlm.nih.gov/pubmed/22336803

87. Mr Justice Mitting: Procedural history. 2012.

88. Dyer C. Texas court dismisses defamation case brought by Andrew Wakefield against The BMJ. BMJ [Internet]. 2014;349:g5998. [cited 2016 Aug 28]. Available from: http://www.ncbi.nlm.nih.gov/pubmed/25288504

89. Poland GA. MMR vaccine and autism: vaccine nihilism and postmodern science. Mayo Clin Proc [Internet]. 2011; 86(9):869–71. [cited 2016 Aug 28]. Available from: http://www.ncbi.nlm.nih.gov/pubmed/21878599

90. Shots Immunizations [Internet]. [cited 2017 Jan 2]. Available from: http://shotsonline.immunizationed.org/html/vaccine.html#&ui-state=dialog

91. Issued. Pneumococcal 7-valent Conjugate Vaccine (Diphtheria CRM 197 Protein) Prevnar ® FOR PEDIATRIC USE ONLY.

92. Research C for BE and. Approved Products – Prevnar 13.

93. Ask the Experts about Rotavirus Vaccines – CDC experts answer Q&As [Internet]. Available from: http://www.immunize.org/askexperts/experts_rota.asp

94. Sealey PA. The League of Nations Health Organisation and the Evolution of Transnational Public Health. DISSERTATION. Presented in Partial Fulfillment of the Requirements for the Degree Doctor of Philosophy in the in the Graduate School of The Ohio State University. 2011.

95. Charles J. Origins, history, and achievements of the World Health Organization. Br Med J [Internet]. 1968;2(5600):293–6. [cited 2016 Sep 5]. Available from: http://www.ncbi.nlm.nih.gov/pubmed/4869199

96. Global Immunization Vision and Strategy – Gavi, the Vaccine Alliance [Internet]. Available from: http://www.gavi.org/about/ghd/givs/

97. Our History – Our Story I About I CDC [Internet]. Available from: http://www.cdc.gov/about/history/ourstory.htm

98. Pickering LK, Peter G, Shulman ST. The Red Book through the ages. Pediatrics [Internet]. 2013;132(5):898–906. [cited 2016 Sep 18]. Available from: http://www.ncbi.nlm.nih.gov/pubmed/24127477

99. Walton LR, Orenstein WA, Pickering LK. The history of the United States Advisory Committee on Immunization Practices (ACIP). Vaccine [Internet]. 2015;33(3):405–14. [cited 2016 Sep 18]. Available from: http://www.ncbi.nlm.nih.gov/pubmed/25446820

100. ACIP | Home | Advisory Committee on Immunization Practices | CDC [Internet]. Available from: http://www.cdc.gov/vaccines/acip/index.html
101. Smith JC, Snider DE, Pickering LK, Advisory Committee on Immunization Practices. Immunization policy development in the United States: the role of the Advisory Committee on Immunization Practices. Ann Intern Med [Internet]. 2009;150(1):45–9. [cited 2016 Sep 3]. Available from: http://www.ncbi.nlm.nih.gov/pubmed/19124820
102. ACIP Vaccine Recommendations, Schedules and GRADE | CDC [Internet]. Available from: https://www.cdc.gov/vaccines/acip/recs/index.html
103. Santoli JM, Rodewald LE, Maes EF, Battaglia MP, Coronado VG. Vaccines for Children program, United States, 1997. Pediatrics [Internet]. 1999;104(2):e15. [cited 2016 Sep 3]. Available from: http://www.ncbi.nlm.nih.gov/pubmed/10429133
104. Status Report on the Childhood Immunization Initiative: National, State, and Urban Area Vaccination Coverage Levels Among Children Aged 19–35 Months – United States, 1996 [Internet]. Available from: https://www.cdc.gov/mmwr/preview/mmwrhtml/00048503.htm
105. Past Immunization Schedules | CDC [Internet]. Available from: http://www.cdc.gov/vaccines/schedules/past.html
106. Vaccine-Preventable Diseases, Immunizations, and MMWR – 1961–2011 [Internet]. Available from: https://www.cdc.gov/mmwr/preview/mmwrhtml/su6004a9.htm
107. The Development of the Immunization Schedule – History of Vaccines [Internet]. Available from: http://www.historyofvaccines.org/content/articles/development-immunization-schedule
108. Update on Adult Immunization Recommendations of the Immunization Practices Advisory Committee (ACIP) [Internet]. Available from: http://www.cdc.gov/mmwr/preview/mmwrhtml/00025228.htm

Chapter 2
Vaccine Science and Immunology

Jennifer L. Hamilton

The history of vaccination and inoculation can be traced to the observation that infection with some diseases conferred lifelong immunity to the survivors. Deliberate infection with what was hoped to be a mild form of smallpox was an early attempt at preventing more serious disease; this was later replaced with inoculation with a related virus, cowpox (*vaccinia*), which caused a much milder illness while also providing immunity to smallpox. Many of the first vaccines introduced—such as those against rabies and pertussis—were based on killed or weakened viruses and bacteria. More recently introduced vaccines provide immunity using only a portion of the proteins or polysaccharide (complex sugar) shells associated with these infectious agents. These newer vaccines are able to generate a more targeted immune response. Because they include only a few features of the infectious organism for the immune system to learn, the subunit vaccines are able to generate immunity while having a lower risk of vaccination-associated reactions, such as fever and malaise. The development of these more recent vaccines is based on understanding how the immune system is able to recognize and respond to infection.

Immunology Review

The immune system is highly complex, with many different branches and functions. One of the more fundamental distinctions is between the innate immune system and the adaptive immune system. The innate system consists of those defenses that function for wide categories of threats, rather than for specific targets: this includes

J.L. Hamilton, MD, PhD (✉)
Department of Family, Community, and Preventive Health, Drexel University College of Medicine, Philadelphia, PA, USA
e-mail: jennifer.hamilton@drexelmed.edu

© Springer International Publishing AG 2017
P.G. Rockwell (ed.), *Vaccine Science and Immunization Guideline*,
DOI 10.1007/978-3-319-60471-8_2

physical barriers (skin, mucus); white blood cells with receptors that respond to bacterial cell walls; and natural killer cells that identify and destroy cells that are so deranged they no longer display the "self" signal of the major histocompatibility complex. These defenses are present even before a given threat is encountered; they require no prior contact with an infectious organism. The adaptive immune system, in contrast, develops the ability to react to specific targets, creating a defense based on characteristics of the bacteria, virus, fungus, or parasite being encountered.

What follows is not meant to be a comprehensive review of immunology; that would be well beyond the scope of this book. Instead, this will serve as an introduction (or a review) of the adaptive response to bacterial and viral infection. For this discussion, we can think of three different tasks of the adaptive immune system: how it identifies a threat, how it deals with the current infection, and how it eventually maintains surveillance against a recurrence of the same infection. This overview of those aspects of the immune system will then lead to discussion of how vaccination engages those key pathways to produce a lasting immune memory.

The adaptive immune system features multiple types of cells to encounter and identify threats, to produce antibodies to mark dangers, to destroy foreign organisms, and (perhaps most important for vaccines) to prime a renewed response for the next time those same threats are seen. Many of these cells are named based on the tissues in which they were first identified. *T cells* mature in the thymus after being generated in the liver. *B cells* were first studied in birds, which have an immune organ called the "bursa of Fabricius." In mammals, these cells generally mature in the bone marrow and the fetal liver. Different subgroups of T cells and B cells have different functions, but both lineages feature cells that recognize threats.

This recognition requires that certain chemical signatures of the threat bind to receptors on the surface of immune cells. The full structure identified as a threat is called an antigen; ideally, antibodies produced by the immune system will react to foreign antigens. Examples of antigens include part of the sugary polysaccharide coating of *Streptococcus pneumonia* bacteria or the changing protein structure of a given year's influenza virus. An *epitope* is that portion of the antigen bound by antibodies. There are also receptors (called B cell receptors [BCRs] or T cell receptors [TCRs] depending on the cells on which they're found) that bind to antigens. For example, a B cell with receptors that bind a particular epitope may go on to produce antibodies to the same structure.

The specific defining shape of BCRs and TCRs is set before the cell ever encounters its corresponding target. The immune proteins, or immunoglobulins (Igs), on the surface of these cells take their shapes through a reshuffling of the individual cell's genes that code for different parts of these Igs. This recombination allows for the immune system to generate receptors against millions of different epitopes, without needing specific genes for each one.

To give an idea of the complexity that can be generated from repeated instances of simple structures, consider the basic shapes that can be generated from four squares arranged to form polygons. These shapes may be familiar from the video game Tetris (see Fig. 2.1). Building a sequence of the 7 different shapes shown, 7 shapes long, can give over 823,000 combinations if simply placed end to end; more combinations would result if the chain branched along the way.

Fig. 2.1 Developing complex structures from simple shapes. The top row shows seven different continuous arrangements of four squares; lower rows illustrate some of the myriad varying shapes that can be constructed using seven of the shapes to form a larger pattern

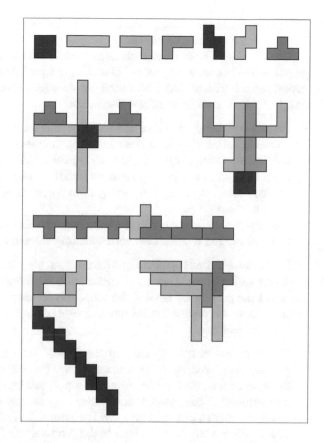

Some of the resulting combinations will match normal, healthy parts of the body. Ideally, cells with these receptors will be destroyed before fully maturing and entering the circulation. (If any escape this process, autoimmune disease could result.) Some of the combinations will match common infectious threats encountered in the environment. Some will remain on surveillance for their entire life span, never finding the specific epitope that would lead them to trigger a full immune response.

Rather than circulating randomly though the bloodstream, B cells cluster in the spleen, lymph nodes, and mucosal-associated lymphoid tissue in the intestines. Patterns of blood flow in these regions increase the chances that a novel antigen will pass through; thus, a given B cell is more likely to encounter its matching antigen in these secondary lymphoid tissues than elsewhere. Other specialized immune cells, also found in the secondary lymphoid tissues, work in concert with the B cells to help ensure that threatening antigens are recognized while enforcing safeguards to limit autoimmunity. Further types of cells from the innate immune system, dendritic cells and macrophages, maintain surveillance in the peripheral tissues. Dendritic cells take up extracellular fluid from the periphery before traveling to the lymphoid tissues where T cells are found. Once there, these cells can display the antigens they encountered in the periphery to the T cells. Macrophages, in contrast, do not travel;

they may activate circulating T cells. (Macrophages also engulf and destroy threats that have been tagged with antibodies.)

Once a B cell links to enough copies of its matching antigen, it activates in response and begins a process of "clonal expansion." The cell rapidly divides and makes more copies of itself, with each copy initially sharing the same BCR as the ancestor cell. These copies later differentiate:

- *Plasma B cells* rapidly make antibodies, which go on to mark or tag their corresponding antigens, making it easier for other immune system cells to recognize and destroy them. These cells have life spans of a few days.
- *Long-lived plasma B cells* generate antibodies more slowly, but live for months or years after migrating from the germinal centers of the secondary lymphoid tissue to the bone marrow.
- *Memory B cells* do not generate antibodies, but can divide to create a new population of plasma B cells if the corresponding antigen is re-encountered.

T cells have a similar process by which a matching antigen is encountered, leading to activation of a cell and reproduction of a line with the same TRC. Again, the details of the process are beyond the scope of this chapter. Still, some key features of the process, as compared to the development of plasma cells and memory B cells, need to be mentioned:

- T cells do not activate by recognizing "naked" antigens. They respond only to proteins displayed by other immune cells, dendritic cells, and macrophages. Because of this, they cannot respond to polysaccharides or lipids; but because they respond to processed proteins, they may be better able to identify epitopes which are hidden or buried on a viral structure.
- The T cell process does not lead to the production of antibodies. Instead, *cytotoxic T lymphocytes* (CTLs) result; these cells can destroy virus-infected cells which display the matching antigen.
- Central memory T cells (TCM) stay within the lymph nodes; effector memory T cells (TEM) are located peripherally, near where contact with the antigen occurred (and could be expected to occur again).

See Table 2.1 for a summary of B cell and T cell features.

Types of Vaccines

Understanding how the immune system develops the ability to target specific antigens helps us understand the development of vaccines and reveals strengths and limitations of different kinds. The first modern vaccine, in which cowpox infection was used to protect against smallpox, is now known to be a type of *live virus* vaccine. The cowpox/smallpox pair, with an intact, wild-type virus that causes mild disease that can serve as an immunization for a more deadly disease, is highly unusual. A much more common variation is to use a *weakened live virus*, which has been cultured over time to select for strains that don't cause disease in healthy

Table 2.1 Summary of key events in B cell, T cell lineages of adaptive immune system

	Identification of threat	Current infection	Surveillance/memory
B cell lineage	Cluster in secondary lymphoid tissue Encounter blood-borne antigens Links with several copies of antigen OR fewer copies plus T helper cell Responds to polysaccharides and proteins	Plasma B cells generate antibodies; live for days Long-lived plasma B cells generate antibodies; live for months/years	Memory B cell population regenerates plasma B cells when needed
T cell lineage	Cluster in secondary lymphoid tissue Needs processed protein carried by antigen-presenting cell	Cytotoxic T lymphocytes attack infected cells	Central memory T (TCM) cells in lymph nodes Effector memory T (TEM) cells in periphery

people. Examples of this type of vaccine include those for rubella, varicella (chicken pox), the oral polio vaccine, and some influenza vaccines. The use of an intact, replicating virus helps ensure a strong immunologic response from both the humoral (antibody based, derived from B cells) and cell-mediated parts of the adaptive immune system. Because of concerns regarding the use of a potentially infectious agent, weakened live virus vaccines generally come into use when attempts to develop a vaccine by other means have failed. *Killed virus vaccines*, sometimes called *inactivated virus vaccines*, are those in which the viral agent cannot replicate in the body; formaldehyde or similar chemicals are often used to kill the viruses. Examples of killed-virus vaccines include the injected polio vaccine and some versions of the influenza vaccine.

Similarly, some vaccines are based on entire bacteria. The bacillus Calmette–Guérin (BCG) vaccine used in many countries to protect against tuberculosis is derived from an attenuated strain of *Mycobacterium bovis*. The pertussis (whooping cough) vaccine used in the USA through the 1990s is an example of a *killed whole-cell vaccine*: it was made from whole bacterial cells, which were then killed. The wide variety of antigenic targets associated with an entire bacterium helps the immune system to develop multiple different types of antibodies that would all respond to infection when needed.

Some vaccines prime the immune system not to respond to infectious agents but to the harmful toxins they produce. The vaccines against diphtheria and tetanus are based on inactivated toxins, called *toxoids*. A toxoid-based vaccine against botulism has been developed, but is no longer licensed in the USA [1].

More recently developed vaccines target only certain features of the infectious agent in question. The bacterium *Streptococcus pneumoniae*, a cause of pneumonia, septicemia, and meningitis, has a polysaccharide coating outside the bacteria itself. This capsule limits the effectiveness of any vaccine directed against characteristics of the bacteria's cell wall. Two types of vaccine are currently in use: one derived from purified capsules only (*polysaccharide* vaccine, US brand name Pneumovax) and one in which polysaccharides from different strains of *S. pneumoniae* are linked to, or conjugated with, an altered nontoxic form of diphtheria toxoid protein (*conjugate* vaccine, US brand name Prevnar). Recall from the discussion of the immune system that polysaccharides do not provoke a response from T cells, which includes the development of effector memory T cells. TEM cells, unlike cells that generate antibodies, are located in peripheral tissues. Thus, it should not be surprising that although both the pneumococcal conjugate and polysaccharide vaccines protect against invasive disease (bacteremia, meningitis, etc.), it appears that for represented strains of *S. pneumoniae*, the conjugate vaccine provides better protection from mucosal disease such as nonbacteremic pneumonia [2].

Some vaccine components are now produced by recombinant genetic technology, rather than through bacterial or viral culture. The initial vaccine against hepatitis B, brand name Heptavax, was derived from hepatitis B surface antigen (HBsAg) drawn from HBV-infected blood donors [3]. Concerns about the safe use of a blood product only increased when it was later recognized that one group of HBV carriers, gay men, were also at risk for the infection now identified as HIV [4]. In 1986, a new version of the vaccine, based on HBsAg grown recombinantly in yeast, was approved by the FDA [5]. Recombinantly derived antigens are not associated with a full genome and cannot cause infection. Similar techniques are now used to manufacture vaccine for human papilloma virus as well.

Techniques under development may offer the ability to replace existing vaccines with better ones (more immunogenic, perhaps, or with fewer side effects); the hope of using vaccine technology to coax the immune system to respond to noninfectious threats such as cancers also persists. Advances in manipulating DNA and RNA enabled the creation of recombinant yeast to produce viral proteins as mentioned above. More recently, these techniques have been used to create a chimeric virus: the attenuated strain of yellow fever virus used in the yellow fever vaccine was modified to produce proteins from the Japanese encephalitis virus [6]. The resulting live attenuated virus is used as the basis of the IMOJEV Japanese encephalitis vaccine, which is licensed in Australia and several Asian nations [7].

Another technique under development involves the use of so-called naked DNA. In this approach, a DNA segment that codes for a protein associated with a threat is introduced to the body, where it is taken up by antigen-presenting cells. The cells then create the protein coded for by the DNA and present that protein to T cells [8]. Messenger RNA (mRNA) may be similarly used [9]. It is hoped that nucleic acid vaccines may someday be effective not only for infectious agents but also for cancers, autoimmune diseases, and severe allergies [8].

A list of vaccines commonly used in the USA and their method of manufacture is given in Table 2.2.

As can be noted, there may be more than one type of vaccine for a given pathogen. In these cases, the selection of which vaccine to use may depend upon the prevalence of the disease, the availability of different vaccine types, and the health and immune status of the person receiving the vaccine.

Table 2.2 Sources for common US-licensed vaccines

Disease	Vaccine(s)	Vaccine source(s)
Diphtheria	DT DTaP DTaP-IPV DTaP-HepB-IPV DTaP-IPV/Hib Td Tdap	Toxoid
Haemophilus influenzae type B	DTaP-IPV/Hib Hib Hib-HepB Hib-MenCY	Conjugated polysaccharides
Hepatitis A	HepA HepA-HepB	Inactivated virus
Hepatitis B	DTaP-HepB-IPV HepA-HepB HepB Hib-HepB	Recombinant proteins
Human papilloma virus (HPV)	2vHPV 4vHPV 9vHPV	Recombinant proteins
Influenza	IIV	Inactivated virus
Influenza	RIV3	Recombinant proteins
Influenza	LAIV	Live attenuated virus
Japanese encephalitis	JE	Inactivated virus
Measles	MMR MMRV	Live attenuated virus
Meningococcus serogroup B	MenB-4C (brand Bexsero)	Recombinant proteins with filtered killed bacterial components
Meningococcus serogroup B	MenB-FHbp (brand Trumenba)	Recombinant proteins
Meningococcus serogroups A, C, W, Y	MenACWY	Conjugated polysaccharides
Meningococcus serogroups C, Y	Hib-MenCY	Conjugated polysaccharides
Meningococcus serogroups A, C, W, Y	MPSV4	Polysaccharides
Mumps	MMR MMRV	Live attenuated virus
Pneumococcus, 13 serotypes	PCV13	Conjugated polysaccharides
Pneumococcus, 23 serotypes	PPSV23	Polysaccharides
Polio	DTaP-IPV DTaP-HepB-IPV DTaP-IPV/Hib IPV	Inactivated virus
Rotavirus	RV1 (monovalent) RV5 (pentavalent)	Live attenuated virus

(continued)

Table 2.2 (continued)

Disease	Vaccine(s)	Vaccine source(s)
Rubella	MMR MMRV	Live attenuated virus
Tetanus	DT DTaP Tdap DTaP-IPV DTaP-HepB-IPV DTaP-IPV-Hib	Toxoid
Tuberculosis	BCG	Live attenuated bacteria
Typhoid	ViCPS	Polysaccharides
Typhoid	Ty21a	Live attenuated bacteria
Varicella	VAR MMRV	Live attenuated virus
Yellow fever	YF	Live attenuated virus
Zoster (varicella)	HZV	Live attenuated virus

- The weakened virus oral polio vaccine (OPV) is more effective at producing an immune response than the killed-virus injected vaccine (IPV) [10]. IPV soon fell out of use in the USA once OPV was introduced in the early 1960s. However, in approximately 1/1,000,000 doses, the weakened OPV virus can spontaneously change back to a form that can cause paralysis. To minimize this risk, the USA switched to using only the killed-virus vaccine in 2003 [11]. In areas where wild polio is still endemic, however, the oral vaccine is preferred. IPV and OPV both protect the vaccine recipient against paralysis, but only OPV provides mucosal immunity [12]. Preventing replication of the virus in the intestine prevents fecal–oral transmission of the disease. IPV will prevent paralysis in an immunized individual; OPV prevents paralysis *and* stops transmission of the wild virus to others.
- Two vaccines against *S. pneumoniae* are recommended for use in the USA: a polysaccharide vaccine that covers 23 different strains of the bacterium (PPSV23, brand name Pneumovax) and a conjugate vaccine that protects against 13 strains (PCV13, brand name Prevnar). Both vaccines are recommended for use in adults over age 65. However, because toddlers are generally unable to mount a full immune response to polysaccharides, PPSV23 is not recommended even for children at high risk of infection until the age of at least 2 years [13].
- Influenza vaccine was initially developed as an inactivated virus vaccine; in 2003, an inhaled live attenuated virus vaccine (LAIV) was introduced (brand name FluMist) [14]. Early studies indicated that LAIV was more effective at preventing influenza in children than inactivated influenza virus vaccines (IIV) were, and for the 2014–2015 influenza season, the CDC recommended that children ages 2–8 years old receive LAIV if available [15]. However, in more recent flu seasons, LAIV has been significantly less protective than IIV. In June 2016, after reviewing data suggesting that LAIV provided minimal if any protection in

the 2015–2016 season, the CDC's Advisory Committee on Immunization Practices (ACIP) recommended against the use of LAIV [16] pending further investigation.

- Influenza virus for live attenuated vaccines and for inactivated virus vaccines is cultured in chicken eggs. Proteins from the eggs may persist into the vaccines, potentially causing anaphylaxis in those allergic to eggs. An influenza vaccine based on recombinant hemagglutinin subunits (RIV, US brand name FluBlok) avoids the use of eggs at any stage of manufacture and contains no egg proteins. Another inactivated virus vaccine is cultured in mammalian cells (ccIIV, US brand name Flucelvax) rather than in hen's eggs; it may contain traces of egg protein from the initial "seed" virus used in manufacture.

Inactivated influenza virus vaccines are also available in "regular strength" and "high-dose" versions; the high-dose version, with four times the hemagglutinin content of the standard vaccine, was designed for use in elderly patients and is approved for use in patients aged 65 and older.

Immunizing Special Populations

Why do older patients need special vaccines? Geriatric patients face different risks than children or younger adults. The differences may be due to the natural history of the infection itself (e.g., consider how varicella causes chicken pox in children and shingles in the elderly) or to changes in the immune system that come with aging. Several factors that contribute to immunosenescence have been identified. The number of naive T cells produced falls, and the population of T effector cells relatively increases; T cell receptor diversity decreases. The number of natural killer cells (part of the innate immune system) remains stable or may even increase, but the effectiveness of each cell declines [17, 18]. Overall, the immune system shifts from specific responses targeting particular antigens to nonspecific, less effective methods of defense such as inflammation. Thus, older patients are more vulnerable to infection and would conceivably benefit from vaccination more than the population at large; but the same changes that increase their risk also make vaccination less effective.

Several strategies have been suggested to reduce the risk from infectious disease in geriatric patients. One is to make the vaccines themselves more immunogenic, to compensate for the reduced ability of the immune system to respond to novel threats. The use of high-dose flu vaccines is one example of this [19]; a similar technique is the use of PCV13 followed by PPSV23 a year later to protect against pneumococcal disease. The use of intradermal, rather than intramuscular, vaccines is being researched [20]. Another route is to ensure that patients develop immunity to disease that affects seniors before immunosenescence develops: healthcare professionals can review patient needs for immunization regularly, reducing the chances that opportunities to vaccinate are overlooked. While this approach will not help for novel infections such as seasonal flu, it can help with zoster, pneumococcal disease, and other disease.

One more approach is to reduce the chances that the elderly will encounter infections by immunizing those around them. Although there are no legal requirements for employees of nursing homes, assisted living centers, or hospitals to have documented vaccinations, many such facilities recommend or require influenza vaccine for their employees. Preventive health measures intended for other age groups have been demonstrated to benefit seniors as well: reduction in pneumococcal disease associated with the serotypes found in pneumococcal conjugate vaccine was demonstrated in those ages 65 and over shortly after the vaccine was recommended for use in children (and before it was recommended for adults) [21].

In many ways, immunosenescence can be similar to more general mild immune suppression. Patients may have weakened immune systems for many reasons, resulting from trauma (asplenia), disease (HIV, leukemias), inherited immunodeficiencies (Wiskott–Aldrich syndrome), or medical intervention/treatment (cancer chemotherapy, antirejection medications posttransplant). The exact pathways by which the immune system is weakened alter the specific recommendations for patient care, but the general principles remain the same: the anticipated benefit from vaccination should exceed the risks of not vaccinating.

If immune suppression can be predicted before it begins—for example, in the case of a young child with sickle cell disease who may be anticipated to lose splenic function or a patient with worsening renal disease who may someday receive a kidney transplant—vaccinations may often be given while the immune system is still intact. (Recommendations regarding BCG vaccine, the attenuated whole-cell vaccine against tuberculosis, are an exception to this general rule: if a patient is expected to become immunosuppressed, BCG vaccine should not be used [22].) Vaccination for meningococcal and pneumococcal disease is recommended for many patients with immune disorders and may be suggested at a lower age than would be appropriate otherwise.

In many cases, the concern is that vaccination will be merely ineffective in patients with weakened immune systems. However, some vaccines may be hazardous. Vaccines based on live viruses or bacteria should not be used in those with immune deficiencies: these include the varicella vaccine, the rotavirus vaccine, the attenuated live influenza vaccine, and others. Antiviral medication or other appropriate therapy may be used if infection develops. Vaccination of household contacts, although not appropriate in all circumstances, may be a valuable adjunct in these circumstances.

Another special population to consider when discussing vaccination is the very young. Although we often associate immunizations with childhood, special challenges exist early in life that shape the recommended timing and spacing of vaccines.

Newborns have a component of their immune system not found at other ages: large amounts of antibodies derived from their mothers. These may have crossed the placenta in utero or be contained in breast milk. These antibodies help protect neonates and infants from infection—indeed, current vaccine guidelines recommend vaccinating pregnant women against pertussis to foster this temporary immunity in their children. However, these antibodies will also respond to antigens deliberately introduced, reducing the effectiveness of vaccines given early in life. In addition, the newborn's immune system is less able to develop memory and make its own antibodies than it would be later in infancy.

These factors contribute to a balance that influences the age at which vaccines are recommended. What is the risk of developing the disease if no vaccination is given, and how severe would that disease be? Can an immune response be generated? How long would that response last?

As an example, consider pertussis. Over 28,000 cases were reported in the USA in 2013 [23]; the disease is more severe in younger children. Vaccination of the mother during pregnancy is recommended to help prevent the illness in newborns, with a series of immunizations for the child beginning at age 2 months to promote long-term immunity. Before 2 months, the vaccine is ineffective.

Vaccinations for several diseases of childhood (rotavirus, diphtheria, pneumococcal infection, and others) are recommended starting at age 2 months, when risk of serious outcome from infection is high and maternal contribution to immunity, if any, begins to wane. Even so, these vaccines must be administered multiple times at staged intervals in order to produce immunity.

Before the introduction of the measles vaccine, its incidence occurred at ages 3–6 at different US cities; however, the highest mortality rate was found in younger children [24]. This would suggest the need for an early vaccination. Initial studies, however, noted that maternal antibodies against measles persisted beyond the age of 6 months; later clinical experience demonstrated that those antibodies persisted beyond age 11 months in a substantial proportion of infants [25, 26]. The current US vaccination schedule recommends vaccination starting at age 12 months [13]. (If travel to a measles-endemic area is planned, or during an outbreak, a dose may be given as early as 6 months; however, this does not replace the 12-month dose.) [13].

Given the difficulties of developing immunity from early vaccination, why is the hepatitis B vaccine recommended for the first day of life? Here, the concern is that the mother will not pass immunity to the child, but may pass the disease itself. It is not expected that the vaccination at birth will provide long term immunity; instead, it's given as part of sequence that continues with more vaccinations during infancy. Because children born to hepatitis B-infected mothers have a high risk of becoming infected themselves, and because these infections can result in early death from cirrhosis or liver cancer [27], the need for early protection surpasses concern for impermanent immunity.

Immunization Scheduling

This discussion may also clarify why most vaccine-preventable illnesses require more than one dose of vaccine. Many vaccines are administered in two distinct stages: one or more doses in early childhood to establish immunity, followed by so-called booster doses later in life.

The initial spacing of vaccines in early childhood is limited by immaturity of the immune system. Generally speaking, those vaccines started earlier require more doses to establish an immune response. Vaccination with pneumococcal conjugate vaccine in infancy is recommended to begin at age 2 months and requires four doses; the same vaccine given in adulthood to those with no prior pneumococcal immunization is recommended for a single dose only. Children aged 6 months to 8 years receiving their first seasonal influenza vaccine are recommended for two doses 4 weeks apart.

Once immunity is established, boosters may be needed. They may promote long-lasting immunity; a second vaccination may lead to immunity for those who, for some reason, did not develop immunity from the first dose; or a renewed vaccination may be needed to respond to changes in the pathogen being protected against.

Immunity from both the tetanus [28] and diphtheria vaccine fades over time, and repeated booster doses every 10 years are recommended in the USA. The need for continued revaccination against diphtheria can be inferred from the epidemic that struck countries of the former USSR in the 1990s: although the disease was largely controlled in the 1980s with only 0.34 cases per 100,000 reported in 1989 [29], the Soviet Union did not generally recommend adult booster vaccines. After the breakup of the USSR, vaccination of children faltered; cases of the disease increased dramatically. From 1990 through 1998, over 157,000 cases of diphtheria were reported among nations of the former USSR with over 5000 deaths [29]; more than half the cases were reported among adults.

In contrast to the case with the tetanus and diphtheria vaccines, vaccination against measles after the age of 12 months is thought to provide long-standing immunity—for those who receive any benefit. When the use of a second dose at ages 4–6 years was introduced in 1998, it was not done to counteract waning immunity; instead, it was a response to the observation that around 5% of children do not develop immunity with only a single vaccination [30]. (Discussion of herd immunity, later in this chapter, will highlight the difficulty with a measles vaccine that is at best 95% effective.)

Annual vaccination for influenza is needed for a third reason—in this case, revaccination is recommended yearly as different strains of the influenza virus become more or less common. If a universal influenza vaccine is ever developed, it will likely not require annual dosing.

An additional concern with timing and spacing of vaccines concerns the way in which one may interfere with another. Live virus vaccines for MMR and varicella may be administered on the same day without any reduction in effect; but if given on different days within 28 days of each other, the second vaccine will have reduced effect [31]. Variations in timing and spacing of other types of vaccines, when studied, have generally been found to have no impact on vaccine efficacy, but a few exceptions are worth noting:

- When both pneumococcal conjugate vaccine (PCV7 or PCV13) and pneumococcal polysaccharide vaccine (PPSV23) are appropriate for a patient, administer the conjugate vaccine first. Giving PCV13 before PPSV23 has been found to enhance immune response to the serotypes shared between the two vaccines. In contrast, giving PPSV23 first blunted the later response to PCV13 [32].

- One of the meningococcal conjugate vaccines, MenACWY-D (Menactra), was found to blunt the response to pneumococcal conjugate vaccine when the two are administered simultaneously. No interaction between MenACWY-CRM (Menveo) and PCV7/PCV13 has been noted [33].

The effect of co-administration of different vaccines is not researched for all possible combinations. Generally, combinations are investigated if the vaccines involved are intended for use in the same special population (as meningococcal and pneumococcal vaccines might be used in asplenic patients) or age group. Because there can be unexpected interactions between vaccines, and not all timing intervals have been evaluated, there may be unforeseen shortcomings in using alternate immunization schedules.

Adjuvants and Additives

Given the need to protect against infections in infancy, when the immune system may not respond as effectively to threats as later in life, the immunogenicity of a vaccine is a key factor in its development. How well will a given antigen provoke an immune response? And will this provide long-term protection against disease, or will booster vaccines be needed?

Recall that, for many infections, more than one type of vaccine has been developed—even if only a single variety is in current use. The whole-cell vaccine against pertussis was replaced with an acellular version; influenza vaccines include attenuated virus, inactivated virus, and recombinant subunit varieties. An ideal vaccine would provide the long-lasting immune response characteristic of a live virus or whole cell and the minimal adverse reactions more common of subunit vaccines. Is there some way to increase the ability of the immune system to "notice" a given immunization or to prolong its effects—other than changing the type of vaccine being used?

One way to increase the immunogenicity of a vaccine is introduce additional material, unrelated to the particular infection being targeted, specifically to provoke a stronger immune response. These substances are called adjuvants (from Latin, to help). The group of adjuvants in most common use, aluminum salts, dates back to research done in the 1920s with toxoid-type vaccines [34]. Why risk working with potentially infectious bacteria if developing an immune response to respond to an altered toxin would be enough? The first adjuvant of this type, potassium aluminum sulfate (also called potassium alum), was thought at the time to have its effect by forming a depot, delaying the rate of absorption of the injected vaccine into the body [34]. This would extend the time the antigen was available to promote an immune response. Since then, alum and related aluminum salts have also been found to increase uptake of antigens by antigen-presenting cells (recall that T cells respond not to "naked" antigens but only to proteins displayed by immune cells such as dendritic cells) [35]. These salts also increase production of complement, part of the innate immune system [35]. Aluminum-based adjuvants currently in use in the USA include aluminum hydroxide, aluminum potassium sulfate, aluminum hydroxyphosphate sulfate, and aluminum phosphate.

The use of aluminum-based adjuvants is sometimes called into question, since aluminum is known to be toxic at certain levels. These adjuvants have been used for generations, beginning with the diphtheria and tetanus toxoid vaccines; they are also used in several other vaccines introduced more recently (see Table 2.3). During this time, they have been associated with rare localized reactions such as erythema, subcutaneous nodules, and granulomatous inflammation [35]. As the number of vaccines using aluminum adjuvants has increased, popular concern for possible aluminum-associated neurotoxicity has grown as well. Individual vaccines are limited to at most 1.25 mg aluminum/dose, but of those vaccines which contain aluminum, most do not reach this limit. Reviewing the aluminum content of each vaccine and the ACIP-recommended childhood vaccination schedule, it is possible to determine that the maximum single day's vaccination-related aluminum in the first year of life would be 1.2 mg (at 2 months and again at 4 months); the maximum total aluminum from vaccines in the first year would be 4.225 mg [36].

As a comparison, many varieties of infant formula have an average aluminum content of 0.225 mg/L [35]. For those who are concerned that the aluminum received on a single day is higher than that from dietary sources, recall that one of the functions of aluminum adjuvants is to form a depot. The aluminum from the vaccine stays localized and enters the broader body compartments only over time. This means that any single day's vaccines contribute to the overall aluminum level or aluminum body burden slowly—in a manner more like dietary aluminum [36].

Two adjuvants unrelated to aluminum are also used in the USA: monophosphoryl lipid A (MPLA) and MF59. MPLA was introduced in the Cervarix bivalent HPV vaccine in 2009. A derivative of lipopolysaccharide from bacterial cell walls may exert its effect by bolstering the function of antigen-presenting cells [37]. In Cervarix it is used in conjunction with alum, which increases its effectiveness as an adjuvant by preventing it from dissociating from the vaccine antigen [38].

MF59, an oil-in-water adjuvant based on squalene, was approved for use in the USA as part of the Fluad inactivated influenza virus vaccine in 2016. (Fluad has been used elsewhere since 1997 [39].) The chemical squalene occurs in all animals; an unsaturated hydrocarbon is a precursor to the synthesis of cholesterol, vitamin D, and steroid hormones. In tests, MF59 was shown to improve the immunogenicity of inactivated influenza vaccine compared to the use of non-adjuvanted vaccine. Further, the use of the adjuvant may also help protect against not only the exact three strains of influenza used in the vaccine but also against variants created by genetic drift [40]. Fluad demonstrates the use of adjuvants to address weakened immune systems: it is approved in the USA only for use in those aged 65 or older.

Some vaccine products contain preservatives. This is not a function of the vaccine design, the immune status of the patient, or the disease being addressed.

Table 2.3 Additives found in some US vaccines

Vaccine	Source: product insert dated	Adjuvants						Preservatives			Antibiotics					Potential allergens		
		Aluminum hydroxide	Aluminum potassium sulfate	Aluminum hydroxyphosphate sulfate	Aluminum phosphate	MF59	MPLA	Phenol	2-phenoxyethanol	Thim.	Neo	Poly	Kana	Genta	Strepto	Egg	Gelatin	Latex
DT (Sanofi)	Jun-13				x					Trace								
DTaP (Daptacel)	Oct-13				x				x									
DTaP (Infanrix)	Apr-16	x																Tip caps
DTaP-IPV (Kinrix)	Apr-16	x									x	x						Tip caps
DTaP-HepB-IPV (Pediarix)	Apr-16	x			x						x	x						Tip caps
DTaP-IPV/Hib (Pentacel)	Oct-13				x				x		x	x						
Hib (ActHIB)	Dec-15																	Diluent stopper vial
Hib (Hiberix)	Feb-16																	
Hib (PedvaxHIB)	Dec-10			x				x										Vial stopper
Hib/Hep B (Comvax)	Dec-10		x	x				x										vial stopper
Hib/Mening. CY (MenHibrix)	2012																	
Hep A (Havrix)	May-16	x																Tip caps
Hep A (Vaqta)	Feb-14			x														Vial stopper, plunger stopper, tip cap
Hep B (Engerix-B)	May-16	x																Tip caps

(continued)

Table 2.3 (continued)

Vaccine	Source: product insert dated	Adjuvants						Preservatives			Antibiotics					Potential allergens		
		Aluminum hydroxide	Aluminum potassium sulfate	Aluminum hydroxyphosphate sulfate	Aluminum phosphate	MF59	MPLA	Phenol	2-phenoxyethanol	Thim.	Neo	Poly	Kana	Genta	Strepto	Egg	Gelatin	Latex
Hep B (Recombivex)	Nov-14		x	x														Vial stopper, plunger stopper, tip cap
Hep A/Hep B (Twinrix)	May-16	x			x						x							Tip caps
HPV (Cervarix)	Apr-16	x					x											Tip caps
HPV (Gardasil 9)	Dec-15			x														
Influenza (Afluria)	Dec-13									Multi only	x	x				x		
Influenza (Agriflu)	Oct-13										x		x			x		
Influenza (Fluad)	Mar-16					x					x		x			x		
Influenza (Fluarix)	Jul-05													x		x		
Influenza (Flublok)	Mar-14																	
Influenza (Flucelvax)	Apr-16															******		Syringe cap
Influenza (Fluvirin)	Mar-16									Multi: yes prefilled, trace	x	x				x		Syringe cap
Influenza (Flulaval)	May-16									x						x	x	
Influenza (Fluzone)	May-15									Multi only						x	x	

Vaccine	Date														Notes
Influenza LAIV (FluMist)	Jul-16								x		x	x			
MenACWY (Menactra)	Aug-14														
MenACWY (Menveo)	Aug-13														
MenACWY (Menomune)	Apr-13				Multi only										Vial stoppers
MenB (Bexsero)	2015	x													Tip caps
MenB (Trumenba)	Apr-16														
MMR (MMR-II)	Oct-15					x					x	x			
MMRV (ProQuad)	Oct-15					x					x	x			
Pneumococcal (Prevnar 13)	Jan-14	x													
Pneumococcal (Pneumovax)	May-15			x											
Polio (IPV—Ipol)	Aug-15		x			x	x	x							
Rotavirus (RotaTeq)	Nov-14														
Rotavirus (Rotarix)	Apr-16														Tip caps
Td (Decavac)	Mar-11	x													Tip caps
Td (Tenivac)	Apr-13	x													Tip caps
Td (Mass Biologics)	Feb-11	x			Trace										
Tdap (Adacel)	Mar-14	x		x											Tip caps
Tdap (Boostrix)	Apr-16	x													Tip caps

(continued)

Table 2.3 (continued)

Vaccine	Source: product insert dated	Adjuvants						Preservatives			Antibiotics					Potential allergens		
		Aluminum hydroxide	Aluminum potassium sulfate	Aluminum hydroxyphosphate sulfate	Aluminum phosphate	MF59	MPLA	Phenol	2-phenoxyethanol	Thim.	Neo	Poly	Kana	Genta	Strepto	Egg	Gelatin	Latex
Typhoid (Typhim Vi)	Mar-14							x										
Typhoid (Vivotif)	Sep-13																x	
Varicella (Varivax)	Jul-14										x						x	
Zoster (Zostavax)	Feb-16										x						x	

MPLA monophospholipid A, *thim* thiomersal, *neo* neomycin and neomycin sulfate, *poly* polymyxin B, *kana* kanamycin, *strepto* streptomycin
Note that the Flucelvax influenza vaccine contains under 5×10^{-8} μg egg protein

Instead, it's about packaging: single-dose units can be produced without needing preservatives, but if the barrier on the vial containing the vaccine will be repeatedly pierced by needles drawing out contents, a preservative is needed. Agents including phenol and phenoxyethanol are used (see Table 2.3), but the most familiar one is likely thiomersal. This mercury-containing compound came to public attention in the USA in 1990s, when the FDA was directed to assess how much mercury was contained in vaccines and other products. At the time, three vaccines recommended during infancy contained thiomersal. The combined mercury content of these three did not exceed Food and Drug Administration (FDA) recommendations, but did exceed guidelines from the Environmental Protection Agency (EPA) [35]. The EPA guidelines of the time were based on the experience of pregnant women who were inadvertently exposed to methylmercury during their pregnancies. Thiomersal, in contrast, is metabolized to *ethyl*mercury, which is excreted from the body roughly seven times faster [35]. Thus, the EPA guidelines overstated the risk associated with thiomersal.

Unlike adjuvants, which are needed for vaccine efficacy, thiomersal could be readily removed from vaccine products by manufacturing them in unit doses. This raised prices—a concern in some parts of the world—but it was thought that in the USA, those who were concerned about mercury could be reassured when they learned it was possible to give entire childhood vaccination series without thiomersal-containing products. Instead, removing the agent may have contributed to the belief that thiomersal plays a role in the development of autism [35].

Antibiotics are used in some vaccines to protect against bacterial contamination [35]. These are generally found in vaccines against illnesses caused by viruses. Viral strains used to produce live or inactivated virus vaccines must be grown in cells; this introduces the possibility that the cells may be infected with bacteria. Several different antibiotics may be used (see Table 2.3). Most commonly used are aminoglycosides (i.e., antibiotics in the "-mycin" family, such as neomycin, streptomycin, gentamicin). Of these, only neomycin can be found in detectable quantities in the final vaccine. There have been case reports of uneventful administration of neomycin-containing vaccines to patients who have had prior allergic reactions to the antibiotic [41]. Still, a prior *anaphylactic* reaction to any vaccine component is a contraindication to its use.

For those concerned about possible allergic reactions, egg proteins and gelatin may be additional concerns. Influenza viral cultures used in many flu vaccines are grown on chicken eggs. The final vaccine product may contain small amounts of egg protein. Deaths from anaphylaxis following influenza vaccination have been reported in egg-allergic patients [42]. For this reason, it is general practice to ask about egg allergies before flu vaccination. Anaphylaxis following immunization is rare, occurring at approximately one case per million doses of any vaccine [43]. Anaphylaxis associated with influenza vaccine in egg-allergic patients is rarer still: a 2009 review found no cases in the literature for the prior two decades [43], and literature review for this chapter found no cases since then. This low case rate may be because of reduction in the amount of egg protein found in the vaccines; awareness of the risk may also be a factor.

Case reports suggest that at least some patients with prior anaphylactic reactions to egg, and positive skin patch testing, can nonetheless safely receive influenza vaccine grown on eggs [44]. If patient can tolerate a small amount of cooked egg, any of the current flu vaccines can be safely used. Current ACIP guidelines suggest that all approved influenza vaccines, regardless of origin, now contain small enough amounts of egg protein for safe use in egg-allergic patients "in a medical setting... supervised by a health care provider who is able to recognize and manage severe allergic conditions"[45]. Still, clinicians may prefer to use vaccines cultured in mammalian cells or grown recombinantly for patients who don't tolerate egg at all.

The viruses used for measles and mumps vaccines are grown in chicken fibroblast cultures. Because of this origin, there may be trace amounts of egg protein present in the MMR and MMRV vaccines, but these are on the order of nano- or picograms [46]. Studies have found that children with even severe egg allergies may safely receive these vaccines [41, 46, 47].

Gelatin is used in some vaccines as stabilizer against heat and cold [35]. It is found most often in live virus vaccines. An oral typhoid vaccine, Vivotif, is given in gelatin capsule. As is the case with egg proteins, gelatin can provoke serious allergic reactions [48]. Indeed, some of the allergic reactions once attributed to the egg component of the MMR vaccine were later attributed to gelatin instead [41].

Herd Immunity

Thus far, we've looked at immunity at the level of the individual: the functioning of the immune system, the changes in the immune system with aging and with medical conditions, and how vaccines are developed with ingredients to produce a long-lasting, beneficial immune response.

Immunity can also be considered at the population level, rather than at the level of an individual. Before the vaccine era, it was common for many infectious diseases to come through a given area every few years. A contagious disease would spread through a population; those who were vulnerable to the disease would become infected and eventually develop immunity (if they survived). The community of now-disease-resistant people would not see another outbreak of the same illness for some number of years. For a while, if someone within the community becomes infected with the disease (perhaps by travel to an area with an active outbreak and then returning home), there would not be enough of an at-risk population to start spreading the infection widely. Over time, more nonimmune people would be added to the community, usually through births. When the population had a high enough proportion of nonimmune population, the chances that any given infected person can spread the disease to another nonimmune person increase—and another epidemic can begin. These repeating outbreaks had long been noted in "childhood" diseases such as measles and varicella [49]. The number of cases between outbreaks can approach zero in small regions with limited population, such as a city; national statistics, which may incorporate several peak/minimum cycles across a wide geographic range, may show valleys without ever approaching zero (see Figs. 2.2 and 2.3).

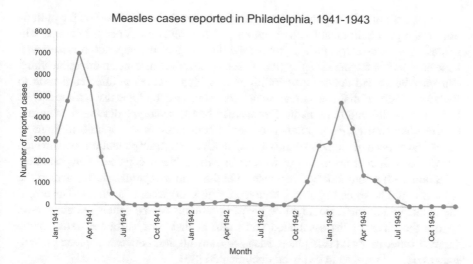

Fig. 2.2 Measles incidence in Philadelphia, 1941–1943. Note recurrent spikes in incidence (Table based on data from Ref. [49])

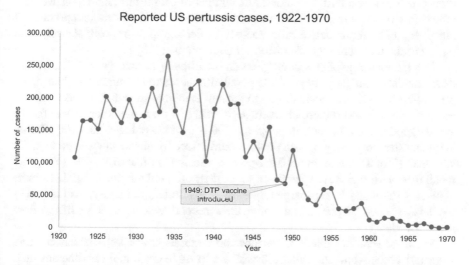

Fig. 2.3 US pertussis cases, 1922–1970. Note periodic spikes which persist even after the introduction of DTP vaccine (Data from the Centers for Disease Control and Prevention (CDC), http://www.cdc.gov/pertussis/surv-reporting/cases-by-year.html, cited August 6, 2016)

When a disease is novel to most of a population, rather than just those who have been added to the group in the last few years, the morbidity and mortality can be catastrophic. Estimates of deaths from the 1918 to 1918 "Spanish flu" influenza pandemic vary from 24.7 million upward; data from European countries with established public health reporting suggest an excess mortality of 1.1% during the pandemic [50]. Other regions had higher influenza-associated mortality: estimates of population [51] and deaths [52] lead to an estimated mortality of over 4% in India.

The spread of a disease through a population, then, is based in part on the proportion of the population that has no immunity to the infection. A novel infection will spread rapidly; an infection will not spread if enough of the population is immune. Disease-specific factors also play a role. At one extreme, imagine an infection which can only be spread under rare conditions or which causes the infected person to withdraw from social contact or which is otherwise biologically, culturally, or behaviorally difficult to transmit. Rabies may be the prototype disease for this end of the spectrum: although human-to-human transmission is possible [53], more cases have been documented involving inadvertent transplantation of infected organs [54] than from exposure to human saliva. Next, consider a hypothetical infection with a long interval between infection and symptoms, during which the disease could be spread by casual contact, fomites, or airborne methods. The example at this end of the scale might be measles: patients can be contagious for 4 days before the onset of the associated rash; during that time, airborne transmission (among other modes) takes place. Measles transmission between airplane passengers seated 17 rows apart has been documented [55].

Cumulative data suggest that a single person with measles can infect as many as 18 others, if the people he or she contacts are not immune. Rubella is less contagious; each case results in 6–7 more. The number of people one person, on average, infects in an environment where no one is immune is called the "basic reproductive ratio," R_0. (The reproductive ratio appears in demography, as well; R_0 may also represent the number of female births per adult woman [56].)

With a knowledge of how contagious an infection is, as measured by R_0, we can then calculate what percentage of the population needs to be immune—either from prior infection or from vaccination—to prevent epidemic spread. A disease will not spread if an infected person, on average, infects less than one other person (or, to avoid hypothetical fragments of people, if 100 people infect fewer than 100 others). With measles, for example, each person could infect 18 others; so we need to make sure that 17 of 18 are immune. That gives a vaccination rate of 94.4%. (You may recall from earlier in the chapter that a single dose of MMR vaccine at age 12 months generates immunity in approximately 95%. Because that immunity level is barely the level needed to prevent an outbreak, a second vaccine later in life is now recommended.)

As can be seen in Table 2.4, measles and pertussis have comparatively high R_0 values. If vaccination rates fall, outbreaks are likely to occur in these illnesses first. The French measles epidemic of 2008–2011 provides an example of what may happen when the vaccination rate falls and the percentage of the population that is susceptible to infection increases.

In France, a two-tiered system of vaccination was used: some vaccines, such as those for polio or diphtheria, were required; others, including MMR, were recommended but not required [58, 59]. This has parallels to the USA, where some states require public school students to be vaccinated unless granted a medical exemption and others allow exemptions for religious or philosophical reasons as well.

A two-dose MMR schedule has been used in France since 1996 [60]. The incidence of measles in France dropped overall during 2000–2007, from approximately

Table 2.4 Estimated basic reproduction number R_0 for different diseases, with corresponding percent immune needed for herd immunity

Disease	Estimated basic reproduction number R_0	Crude community immunity threshold (%)
Diphtheria	6–7	83–85
Influenza (varies with strain)	1.4–4	30–75
Measles	12–18	92–94
Mumps	4–7	75–86
Pertussis	5–17	92–94
Rubella	6–7	83–85

From Ref. [57]

10,000 cases in 2000 to only 47 reported in 2007 [60]. Overlaid with this, however, was a relatively low vaccination rate: national vaccination rates for the first dose of MMR, to be given by the age of 2, did not reach 90% at any time between 2005 and 2008 [61].

Figure 2.4 shows vaccination rates in France in 2005–2008, with the most recent data available before the beginning of the epidemic. As can be seen, most of the countries did not reach the 94% immunization rate needed to prevent transmission if the disease appeared.

In the spring of 2008, outbreaks were identified among students at certain private religious schools at which few children received vaccines. Although Ministry of Health representatives met with parents, many continued to decline to vaccine their children [60, 61]. The outbreak soon spread geographically. In 2008, the highest incidence rates were found in Vendee on the Atlantic Coast (which had under 85% coverage), neighboring Deux-Sevres (under 90%), and the more central department Allier (under 90%). Over time, the disease moved toward the southeast, with an incidence rate of over 30 cases per 100,000 in some departments before the epidemic was brought under control. At the peak of the epidemic in March 2011, over 3600 cases were reported in a single month [61] (see Fig. 2.5).

Even 2 years after the start of the epidemic, vaccination rates remained low. A study of 17-year-olds in Poitou-Charentes, a larger region containing Deux-Sevres, conducted between June 2010 and May 2011, found that only 83% had received two doses of MMR [59] (Fig. 2.5).

Overall, more than 21,600 cases of measles were reported between October 2008 and September 2011. This included 4980 hospitalized patients. Of those who were diagnosed with measles, 28% of infants under 1 year of age required hospitalization; over 30% of affected adults were hospitalized. Complications of measles were significant, with more than 1000 cases of pneumonia and 26 cases of encephalitis. Ten deaths were reported [61].

At the time of this epidemic in France, other outbreaks were occurring elsewhere in Europe. Over 30,000 cases of measles were reported to EUVAC, a European surveillance network, in 2010 [62]. Editorials at the time contrasted the ongoing European cases with the successful efforts against measles in the Americas, where

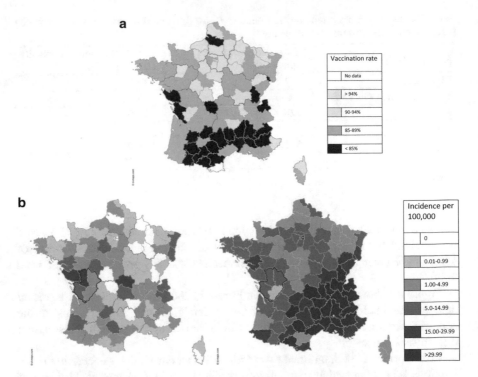

Fig. 2.4 (**a**) Immunization rates in France, 2005–2008 (Redrawn from [61], with map outline from http://www.d-maps.com/m/europa/france/france/france48.svg). (**b**) Measles incidence in France, October 2008–September 2009 (*left*) and October 2010–September 2011 (*right*). Outlined region is Poitou-Charentes, where vaccination rates among 17-year-olds were surveyed during outbreak (see text) (Redrawn from [61], with map outline from http://www.d-maps.com/m/europa/france/france/france48.svg)

the disease was virtually eliminated by 2002 [62]. Recent incidents, however, have demonstrated that herd immunity (also called community immunity) may falter in regions of the USA as well. In 2014, an outbreak of 383 cases of measles was associated with a largely unvaccinated Amish community in Ohio; the Disneyland-related measles outbreak in 2015 sickened 125, including 110 California residents. Childhood immunization rates vary greatly across California. On average, only 2.5% of kindergarten students had received personal belief exemptions in the 2014–2015 school year—but in 4 of its 58 counties reported exemption rates of at least 10% (source: California Health Department data, downloaded from [63]).

The emphasis on complete eradication of a disease such as measles should not obscure the community benefits that can come to a vulnerable population through even limited immunization. Consider an infection that has an R_0 of 3. One person

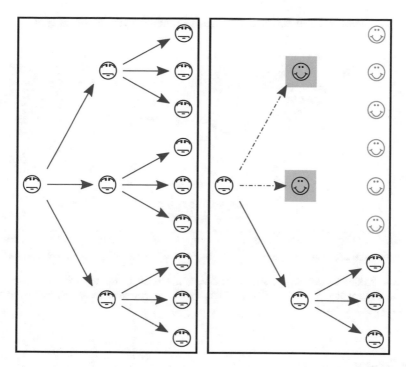

Fig. 2.5 *Left side* of diagram shows spread of disease with $R_0 = 3$ through nonimmune population. *Right side* shows limited spread when some of the population (*shaded*) is vaccinated. *Smiling* figures are those who did not become ill

can be expected to infect three vulnerable people; those three can be expected to infect nine (see Fig. 2.5). Now imagine that two of the three who would otherwise be infected by the index patient are immune. Not only are they protected, but those who they would go on to infect also do not get the disease.

This limited or partial form of herd immunity has been observed. One striking example of the protection of one group by immunization of others within a larger community is the reduction of invasive pneumococcal disease in those aged 65 and above that has taken place as children under the age of 2 have received PCV7 or PCV13 ("Prevnar") immunizations (Fig. 2.6). In the USA, PCV7 vaccination with a series of immunizations beginning at age 2 months was recommended starting in 2000; PCV13 was introduced in 2010. Although pneumococcal conjugate vaccine was not recommended for those 65+ until 2014, invasive pneumococcal disease caused by the serotypes represented in PCV13 in the elderly has decreased dramatically since 2000. This drop-off has not been seen in the non-PCV13 serotypes, further suggesting that the reduced incidence is due to the vaccination of children rather than to other factors.

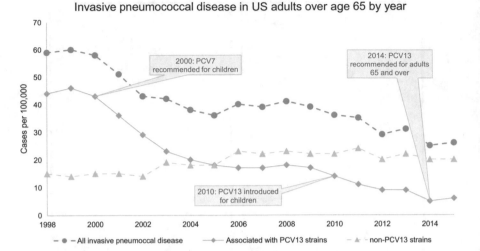

Fig. 2.6 Decline in invasive pneumococcal disease in US adults over age 65 (From Centers for Disease Control and Prevention (CDC), at http://www.cdc.gov/pneumococcal/surveillance.html. Cited August 15, 2016)

Summary

The reduction of disease shown in Fig. 2.6 brings together many of the concepts of this chapter. Two different types of pneumococcal vaccine were introduced. The first was based on unconjugated polysaccharides; the second conjugated the polysaccharides with a protein. Addressing the limitations of the vaccine based on unconjugated polysaccharides required an understanding of the immune system: polysaccharide antigens do not prompt the development of effector memory T cells. Without the involvement of TEM cells, the immune response generated by vaccination is based on secondary lymphoid tissues. The unconjugated polysaccharide vaccine protects against invasive disease—bacteremia and meningitis—but is less effective against infections that have not reached the bloodstream. The addition of a protein component to the vaccine antigen allows the antigen to be processed by antigen-presenting cells. The involvement of APCs then triggers the development of T cells, including TEM cells found in the periphery. The resulting conjugate vaccine provides enhanced protection against pneumococcal infection of mucosal tissues—pneumonia and otitis media—while also protecting against systemic infection.

Recommendations for the use of these vaccines are based on an understanding of the maturation of the immune system in children and later immunosenescence in the geriatric population. The polysaccharide vaccine is not recommended for children under 2 years of age, even those at high risk of infection, because the ability to respond appropriately to polysaccharide antigens does not develop earlier. Later in life, vaccination against pneumococcus is recommended for those at increased risk of disease: smokers, for example, or patients without a spleen. In recognition of the reduced ability of the immune system to ward off infection with increasing age, the two different types of pneumococcal vaccine are recommended for those 65 years old or older. Pneumococcal conjugate vaccine also contains an adjuvant to increase its ability to promote immunity.

Lastly, the declining incidence of pneumococcal disease shown in Fig. 2.6 highlights the key reason for vaccines: their use reduces rates of disease. Vaccination protects immunized individuals from infection and helps protect vulnerable unvaccinated people as well. Continued use of vaccines fosters ongoing protection of the individual and of broader populations as well.

References

1. Webb RP, Smith LA. What next for botulism vaccine development? Expert Rev Vaccines. 2013;12(5):481+.
2. Plosker GL. 13-valent pneumococcal conjugate vaccine: a review of its use in adults. Drugs. 2015;75(13):1535–46.
3. Szmuness W, Stevens CE, Zang EA, Harley EJ, Kellner A. A controlled clinical trial of the efficacy of the hepatitis B vaccine (heptavax B): a final report. Hepatology. 1981;1(5):377–85.
4. Francis DP, Feorino PM, McDougal S, et al. The safety of the hepatitis b vaccine: inactivation of the AIDS virus during routine vaccine manufacture. JAMA. 1986;256(7):869–72.
5. Center for Disease Control (CDC). Recommendations of the immunization practices advisory committee update on hepatitis B prevention. MMWR Morb Mortal Wkly Rep. 1987;36(23):353–66.
6. Appaiahgari MB, Vrati S. IMOJEV ®: a yellow fever virus-based novel Japanese encephalitis vaccine. Expert Rev Vaccines. 2010;9(12):1371–84.
7. World Health Organization (WHO). Global Advisory Committee on Vaccine Safety, 11–12 December 2013. Wkly Epidemiol Rec. 2014;89(7):53–60.
8. Liu MA. DNA vaccines: a review. J Intern Med. 2003;253(4):402–10.
9. Geall AJ, Mandl CW, Ulmer JB. RNA: the new revolution in nucleic acid vaccines. Semin Immunol. 2013;25(2):152–9.
10. ACIP: poliomyelitis prevention: enhanced-potency IPV [Internet]. [cited 2016 Aug 14]. Available from: http://wonder.cdc.gov/wonder/prevguid/m0025216/m0025216.asp
11. Recommended childhood and adolescent immunization schedule/United States, 2003. MMWR Morb Mortal Wkly Rep. 2003;52(4):Q1.
12. Estívariz CF, Pallansch MA, Anand A, Wassilak SG, Sutter RW, Wenger JD, et al. Poliovirus vaccination options for achieving eradication and securing the endgame. Curr Opin Virol. 2013;3(3):309–15.
13. Advisory Committee on Immunization Practices (ACIP), ACIP Child/Adolescent Immunization Work Group. Advisory Committee on immunization practices recommended immunization schedules for persons aged 0 through 18 years – United States, 2016. MMWR Morb Mortal Wkly Rep. 2016;65(4):86–7.
14. Harper SA, Fukuda K, Cox NJ, Bridges CB. Using live, attenuated influenza vaccine for prevention and control of influenza: supplemental recommendations of the Advisory Committee on Immunization Practices (ACIP). Morb Mortal Wkly Rep. 2003:1–8.

15. Grohskopf LA, Olsen SJ, Sokolow LZ, Bresee JS, Cox NJ, Broder KR, et al. Prevention and control of seasonal influenza with vaccines: recommendations of the Advisory Committee on Immunization Practices (ACIP) – United States, 2014–15 influenza season. MMWR Morb Mortal Wkly Rep. 2014;63(32):691–7.
16. CDC Press Releases [Internet]. CDC. 2016. [cited 2016 Aug 14]. Available from: http://www.cdc.gov/media/releases/2016/s0622-laiv-flu.html
17. Del Giudice G, Weinberger B, Grubeck-loebenstein B. Vaccines for the elderly. Gerontology. 2015;61(3):203–10.
18. Pera A, Campos C, López N, Hassouneh F, Alonso C, Tarazona R, et al. Immunosenescence: implications for response to infection and vaccination in older people. Maturitas. 2015; 82(1):50–5.
19. DiazGranados CA, Robertson CA, Talbot HK, Landolfi V, Dunning AJ, Greenberg DP. Prevention of serious events in adults 65 years of age or older: a comparison between high-dose and standard-dose inactivated influenza vaccines. Vaccine. 2015;33(38):4988–93.
20. Pileggi C, Mascaro V, Bianco A, Nobile CGA, Pavia M. Immunogenicity and safety of intradermal influenza vaccine in the elderly: a meta-analysis of randomized controlled trials. Drugs Aging. 2015;32(10):857–69.
21. Moore MR, Link-Gelles R, Schaffner W, Lynfield R, Lexau C, Bennett NM, et al. Effect of use of 13-valent pneumococcal conjugate vaccine in children on invasive pneumococcal disease in children and adults in the USA: analysis of multisite, population-based surveillance. Lancet Infect Dis. 2015;15(3):301–9.
22. World Health Organization (WHO). Global Advisory Committee on Vaccine Safety, 3–4 December 2009/Comité consultatif mondial de la Sécurité vaccinale, 3–4 décembre 2009. Wkly Epidemiol Rec. 2010;85(5):29–33.
23. Centers for Disease Control and Prevention (CDC). Final 2013 reports of nationally notifiable infectious diseases. MMWR Morb Mortal Wkly Rep. 2014;63(32):702.
24. Langmuir AD. Medical importance of measles. Arch Pediatr Adolesc Med. 1962;103(3):224.
25. Albrecht P, Ennis FA, Saltzman EJ, Krugman S. Persistence of maternal antibody in infants beyond 12 months: mechanism of measles vaccine failure. J Pediatr. 1977;91(5):715–8.
26. Krugman RD, Rosenberg R, McIntosh K, Herrmann K, Witte JJ, Ennis FA, et al. Further attenuated live measles vaccines: the need for revised recommendations. J Pediatr. 1977;91(5):766–7.
27. Centers for Disease Control and Prevention (CDC). Newborn hepatitis B vaccination coverage among children born January 2003–June 2005 – United States. Morb Mortal Wkly Rep. 2008;57(30):825–8.
28. Simonsen O, Badsberg JH, Kjeldsen K, Moller-Madsen B, Heron I. The fall-off in serum concentration of tetanus antitoxin after primary and booster vaccination. Acta Pathol Microbiol Immunol Scand, Sect C Immunol. 1986;94(2):77–82.
29. Dittmann S, Wharton M, Vitek C, Ciotti M, Galazka A, Guichard S, et al. Successful control of epidemic diphtheria in the states of the former Union of Soviet Socialist Republics: lessons learned. J Infect Dis. 2000;181(Suppl 1):S10–22.
30. Watson JC, Hadler SC, Dykewicz CA, Reef S, Phillips L. Measles, mumps, and rubella – vaccine use and strategies for elimination of measles, rubella, and congenital rubella syndrome and control of mumps: recommendations of the Advisory Committee on Immunization Practices (ACIP). Morb Mortal Wkly Rep Recomm Rep. 1998;47(RR-8):i–57.
31. Centers for Disease Control and Prevention (CDC). Simultaneous administration of varicella vaccine and other recommended childhood vaccines – United States, 1995–1999. MMWR Morb Mortal Wkly Rep. 2001;50(47):1058–61.
32. Greenberg RN, Gurtman A, Frenck RW, Strout C, Jansen KU, Trammel J, et al. Sequential administration of 13-valent pneumococcal conjugate vaccine and 23-valent pneumococcal polysaccharide vaccine in pneumococcal vaccine-naive adults 60–64 years of age. Vaccine. 2014;32(20):2364–74.
33. Sanofi Pasteur. Menactra Product Insert [Internet]. 2014. [cited 2016 Aug 28]. Available from: http://www.fda.gov/downloads/BiologicsBloodVaccines/Vaccines/ApprovedProducts/UCM131170.pdf

34. Glenny AT, Pope CG, Waddington H, Wallace U. The antigenic value of toxoid precipitated by potassium alum. J Pathol Bacteriol. 1926;26:38–9.
35. Offit PA, Jew RK. Addressing parents' concerns: do vaccines contain harmful preservatives, adjuvants, additives, or residuals? Pediatrics. 2003;112(6):1394–402.
36. Mitkus RJ, King DB, Hess MA, Forshee RA, Walderhaug MO. Updated aluminum pharmacokinetics following infant exposures through diet and vaccination. Vaccine. 2011;29(51):9538–43.
37. De Becker G. The adjuvant monophosphoryl lipid a increases the function of antigen-presenting cells. Int Immunol. 2000;12(6):807–15.
38. Brito LA, Malyala P, O'Hagan DT. Vaccine adjuvant formulations: a pharmaceutical perspective. Semin Immunol. 2013;25(2):130–45.
39. Press Announcements – FDA approves first seasonal influenza vaccine containing an adjuvant [Internet]. [cited 2016 Aug 19]. Available from: http://www.fda.gov/NewsEvents/Newsroom/PressAnnouncements/ucm474295.htm
40. Broker M, Beyer C. Adjuvantien für Humanvakzinen. Pharm Unserer Zeit. 2008;37(1):42–51.
41. Latshman R, Finn A. MMR vaccine and allergy. Arch Dis Child. 2000;82(2):93–5.
42. Bierman CW, Shapiro GG, Pierson WE, Taylor JW, Foy HM, Fox JP. Safety of influenza vaccination in allergic children. J Infect Dis. 1977;136:S652–5.
43. Erlewyn-Lajeunesse M, Brathwaite N, Lucas JSA, Warner JO. Recommendations for the administration of influenza vaccine in children allergic to egg. BMJ. 2009;339:b3680.
44. Webb L, Petersen M, Boden S, LaBelle V, Bird JA, Howell D, et al. Single-dose influenza vaccination of patients with egg allergy in a multicenter study. J Allergy Clin Immunol. 2011;128(1):218–9.
45. ACIP. Summary recommendations: prevention and control of influenza with vaccines: Recommendations of the Advisory Committee on Immunization Practices – (ACIP) – United States, 2013–14 [Internet]. [cited 2016 Sep 25]. Available from: http://www.cdc.gov/flu/professionals/acip/2013-summary-recommendations.htm#egg-allergy
46. Cox JE, Cheng TL. Egg-based vaccines. Pediatr Rev. 2006;27(3):118–9.
47. Aickin R, Hill D, Kemp A. Measles immunisation in children with allergy to egg. BMJ. 1994;309(6949):223–5.
48. Sakaguchi M, Nakayama T, Fujita H, Toda M, Inouye S. Minimum Estimated incidence in Japan of anaphylaxis to live virus vaccines including gelatin. Vaccine. 2000;19(4–5):431–6.
49. Bartlett M. The critical community size for measles in the United States. J R Stat Soc. 1960;123(1):37–44.
50. Ansart S, Pelat C, Boelle P-Y, Carrat F, Flahault A, Valleron A-J. Mortality burden of the 1918–1919 influenza pandemic in Europe. Influenza Other Respir Viruses. 2009;3(3):99–106.
51. Census of India: Census Reports 1921 [Internet]. [cited 2016 Aug 20]. Available from: http://www.censusindia.gov.in/Census_And_You/old report/census_1921.aspx
52. Chandra S, Kuljanin G, Wray J. Mortality from the influenza pandemic of 1918–1919: the case of India. Demography. 2012;49(3):857–65.
53. Fekadu M, Endeshaw T, Alemu W, Bogale Y, Teshager T, Olson JG. Possible human-to-human transmission of rabies in Ethiopia. Ethiop Med J. 1996;34(2):123–7.
54. Maier T, Schwarting A, Mauer D, Ross RS, Martens A, Kliem V, et al. Management and outcomes after multiple corneal and solid organ transplantations from a donor infected with rabies virus. Clin Infect Dis. 2010;50(8):1112–9.
55. Edelson PJ. Patterns of measles transmission among airplane travelers. Travel Med Infect Dis. 2012;10(5–6):230–5.
56. Heesterbeek JAP. A brief history of R_0 and a recipe for its calculation. Acta Biotheor. 2002;50(3):189–204.
57. Fine PE. Herd immunity: history, theory, practice. Epidemiol Rev. 1993;15(2):265–302.
58. Haverkate M, D'Ancona F, Giambi C, Johansen K, Lopalco PL, Cozza V, et al. Mandatory and recommended vaccination in the EU, Iceland and Norway: results of the VENICE 2010 survey on the ways of implementing national vaccination programmes. Euro Surveill BullEuropean Commun Dis Bull. 2012;17(22):pii: 20183.

59. Roblot F, Robin S, Chubilleau C, Giraud J, Bouffard B, Ingrand P. Vaccination coverage in French 17-year-old young adults: an assessment of mandatory and recommended vaccination statuses. Epidemiol Infect. 2016;144(3):612–7.
60. Parent du Chatelet I, Antona D, Waku-Kouomou D, Freymuth F, Maine C, Lévy-Bruhl D. La rougeole en France en 2008: bilan de la déclaration obligatoire. Bull Épidémiologique Hebd. 2009, 2009:39, 415–40, 419.
61. Antona D, Lévy-Bruhl D, Baudon C, Freymuth F, Lamy M, Maine C, et al. Measles elimination efforts and 2008–2011 outbreak. France Emerg Infect Dis. 2013;19(3):357–64.
62. Cottrell S, Roberts RJ. Measles outbreak in Europe. BMJ 2011;342(Jun15 1):d3724–d3724.
63. Immunization Levels [Internet]. [cited 2016 Aug 21]. Available from: https://www.cdph.ca.gov/programs/immunize/Pages/ImmunizationLevels.aspx

Chapter 3
Immunization Recommendations and Guidelines: From Development to CDC Recommendations

Margot Latrese Savoy

Overview

When family physicians think about vaccines, typically they imagine the colorful vaccine schedule tables that are updated by the Advisory Committee on Immunization Practices and published annually in February across the medical specialty journals like *American Family Physician*, *Pediatrics*, and the *Annals of Internal Medicine*. The journey from the bench to the guideline is a long and often unsuccessful process typically requiring an estimated half of a billion dollars and over a decade of research and development [1, 2]. An overview of the process is shown in Fig. 3.1.

Currently there are many vaccines licensed for use by the US Food and Drug Administration (FDA) for use in humans in the United States manufactured by several pharmaceutical companies from around the world. The US vaccine manufacturers and their products are listed in Table 3.1 [3].

This chapter will review the process of vaccine development from the early stages of research and development through regulatory review and ultimately recommendation and widespread use in the United States.

Research and Development

Vaccine research and development is a time-consuming and expensive process encompassing a wide range of scientists, locations, and funding sources. Researchers often focus on pathogens with significant disease and economic burden that have either suboptimal or no vaccine available; however, a significant

M.L. Savoy, MD, MPH, FAAFP, FABC, CPE, CMQ (✉)
Christiana Care Health System, Department of Family & Community Medicine,
Wilmington, DE, USA
e-mail: MSavoy@christianacare.org

© Springer International Publishing AG 2017
P.G. Rockwell (ed.), *Vaccine Science and Immunization Guideline*,
DOI 10.1007/978-3-319-60471-8_3

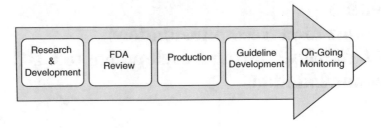

Fig. 3.1 Overall process of immunization development and use

Table 3.1 US vaccine manufacturers (as of June 2016) [3]

Company	Product(s)
Emergent Biosolutions	Anthrax vaccine adsorbed (BioThrax)
GSK Vaccines	DTaP (Infanrix); DTaP + IPV (Kinrix); DTaP + Hepatitis B + IPV (Pediarix); Hepatitis A (Havrix); Hepatitis B (Engerix-B); Hepatitis A + Hepatitis B (Twinrix); Hib (Hiberix); Hib + Meningococcal Groups C and Y (Menhibrix); HPV (Cervarix); Influenza (Fluarix and FluLaval); Meningococcal-MCV4 (Menveo); Meningococcal serogroup B vaccine (Bexsero); Rabies (RabAvert); Rotavirus (Rotarix); Tdap (Boostrix)
MedImmune, Inc. (parent company AstraZeneca)	Influenza (FluMist)
Merck & Co., Inc.	Hib (PedvaxHIB); Hib + Hepatitis B (Comvax); Hepatitis A (VAQTA); Hepatitis B (Recombivax-HB); HPV (Gardasil and Gardasil 9); Measles, Mumps, and Rubella (M-M-R II); MMR+Varicella (ProQuad); Pneumococcal-PPV23 (Pneumovax 23); Rotavirus (RotaTeq); Varicella (Varivax); Zoster (Zostavax)
PaxVax	Typhoid, live oral Ty21a (Vivotif)
Pfizer	Meningococcal serogroup B vaccine (Trumenba); Pneumococcal-PCV13 (Prevnar 13)
Protein Sciences Corporation	Influenza (Flublok)
Sanofi Pasteur	DTaP (Daptacel); DTaP + Hib + IPV (Pentacel); DTaP + IPV (Quadracel); DT (pediatric); Hib (ActHIB); Influenza (Fluzone); Meningococcal-MPSV4 (Menomune A/C/Y/W-135); Meningococcal-MCV4 (Menactra); Poliovirus, inactivated (IPOL); Rabies (Imovax); Smallpox (ACAM2000); Td (DECAVAC); Td (TENIVAC); Tdap (Adacel); Typhoid Vi, inactivated, injectable (TYPHIM Vi); Yellow Fever (YF-Vax)
Seqirus	Influenza (Afluria, Flucelvax, Fluvirin)
Valneva (Intercell USA)	Japanese encephalitis vaccine (IXIARO)

amount of work is also invested in identifying novel ways to deliver, refine, or improve the effectiveness of existing vaccines as well. Vaccine development research occurs in university, industry, government, and not-for-profit organization laboratories. Depending on the type of pathogen or the approach being employed, a wide range of research expertise may be required to create the final product including, but not limited to, cellular or molecular biology, chemistry, biochemistry, virology, microbiology, and immunology.

Prioritization for Research and Development

Deciding which diseases and conditions are suitable for vaccine development is a complicated process that involves a number of considerations. Because vaccine development is time and resource intensive, establishing and understanding priorities for development and encouraging collaboration between stakeholders are essential in addressing the challenges of developing new and improved vaccines [4].

On a global scale, the World Health Organization's Initiative for Vaccine Research (IVR) facilitates vaccine research and development (R&D) against pathogens with significant disease and economic burden, with a particular focus on low- and middle-income countries [5]. In general, when prioritizing vaccines at global scale, the World Health Organization (WHO) focuses on prioritizing vaccines that will address diseases that impact low- and middle-income countries [6]. So, for example, while malaria and dengue vaccines would likely be a low priority in a country like the United States, the WHO works to ensure that the research activity remains a priority since the countries most affected would likely be unable to develop such a vaccine on their own. In addition, the WHO remains involved in the regulatory standards that govern the appropriate and ethical conduct of research in developing countries who may be particularly vulnerable for clinical trial of investigational products [6].

In the United States most vaccine research and development occurs as a result of a collaboration of partners in the academic, government, manufacturing, and public health arenas. By leveraging public-private partnerships that include researchers, government, manufacturers, purchasers, and policy makers who work together to create a shared plan for directing resources into developing targeted high-priority vaccines, new vaccines have been moved through the development pipeline more efficiently and granted licensure for broad use [7]. The National Vaccine Advisory Committee recommends research priorities and other measures the Director of the National Vaccine Program should take to enhance the safety and efficacy of vaccines. The US National Vaccine Plan was established in 2010 and among its five overarching goals includes developing new and improved vaccines and increasing global prevention of death and disability through safe and effective vaccination [4].

Because of the growing number of factors that could impact the decision to pursue a particular vaccine, the National Academy of Sciences (specifically the National Academy of Engineering and the Institute of Medicine) has developed, tested, and launched "SMART Vaccines: Strategic Multi-Attribute Ranking Tool for Vaccines" [8]. This decision-support software aids in prioritizing new potential vaccine targets using demographic, economic, health, scientific, business, programmatic, social, policy, and related factors [8]. Version 1.1 is available for download at no cost from www.nap.edu/smartvaccines.

Exploratory Stage

The initial phase of vaccine development is typically called the exploratory stage. Occurring "at the bench" over 2–4 years, scientists work to identify potential antigens that could be used to prevent or treat a particular disease. While many ideas may be generated at this stage, only a select number of antigens will progress from this stage to continue the process of being developed as candidate vaccines.

Preclinical Stage

Antigens with high potential to be developed continue on for an additional 1–2 years of preclinical research. At this stage the animal models can be used to assess the safety of the antigen and further narrow down best options for continued candidate vaccine development.

Case in Point: Zika virus

Although not a widely known virus in the United States before 2015, *Zika virus* (ZIKV) has been known to be circulating in areas of Africa and Southeast Asia for decades. By some accounts ZIKV was initially discovered in Uganda in 1947, while other accounts report it was first isolated from a Nigerian child with fever and headache in 1952; later, an experimental inoculation of a human subject reproduced a mild self-limited febrile illness [9, 10]. Though estimated seroprevalence was noted to be as high as 48–56% in Nigeria, it was uncharacteristic for ZIKV to cause major outbreaks. The first ZIKV outbreak came in 2007 in the Yap Island in Micronesia and was followed by a larger outbreak in French Polynesia. ZIKV became a major concern in the United States after the Pan American Health Organization issued an alert over transmission in Brazil. This alert has now spread to several countries in South and Central America, the Caribbean islands (including Puerto Rico and the US Virgin Islands), and to the mainland of the continental United States [11].

Zika virus is a member of the *Flavivirus* family related to dengue, yellow fever, and West Nile fever. It is primarily transmitted to humans through the bite of infected *Aedes aegypti* mosquitoes, but can also be transmitted from an infected pregnant woman to her baby during pregnancy or around the time of birth, via sexual transmission by males, and through blood transfusion. Only 20% of infected people become ill; symptoms resemble a mild viral syndrome and include fever, rash, joint pain, and conjunctivitis, lasting several days to weeks. The alarming concern is that infection with *Zika virus* during pregnancy is linked to microcephaly and other severe fetal brain defects.

The National Institute of Allergy and Infectious Disease (NIAID) is collaborating with the government, academia, pharmaceutical, and biotechnology partners to accelerate our understanding of *Zika virus* including disease transmission, prevention, diagnosis, and treatment strategies [12]. Because researchers have been studying flaviviruses for some time now, NIAID and the National Institutes of Health (NIH) are hoping that they have a good foundation for developing new ideas. In 2016 they issued calls to the research community announcing an interest in expanding funding research on *Zika virus*, including:

- Developing sensitive, specific, and rapid clinical diagnostic tests for *Zika virus*
- Creating treatments for *Zika virus* and broad-spectrum antiviral drugs that would be effective against multiple flaviviruses
- Developing and testing vaccines to protect against *Zika virus* infection and advancing new vaccination strategies
- Conducting basic research to understand *Zika virus* infection, replication, pathogenesis, and transmission, as well as the biology of the mosquito vectors
- Developing animal models that mimic *Zika virus* infection in people, so that researchers can investigate the progression of disease
- Pursuing studies on the evolution and emergence of *Zika virus*, including the identification of factors that affect host range and virulence
- Performing surveillance studies of the distribution and natural history of *Zika virus*
- Evaluating the relative immune responses to Zika and other flaviviruses that may occur in the same geographical regions (especially dengue virus and yellow fever virus)
- Investigating how *Zika virus* infection affects reproduction, pregnancy, and the developing fetus

There are a number of ZIKV candidate vaccines currently under development; however, of the 23 ZIKV candidates reported at the February 2016 Advisory Committee on Immunization Practices (ACIP) meeting, only one vaccine had moved from the discovery/in vitro phase to preclinical phase.

According to the NIAID [13] they are in the process of developing multiple vaccine candidates:

- A DNA-based vaccine that uses a strategy similar to an investigational flavivirus vaccine for West Nile virus infection. That vaccine, which was developed by scientists at the NIAID Vaccine Research Center, was found to be safe and induced an immune response when tested in a phase 1 clinical trial.
- A live-attenuated (live but weakened virus, so that it cannot cause disease) investigational Zika virus vaccine building on a similar vaccine approach for the closely related dengue virus. The dengue vaccine candidate was shown to be safe and immunogenic in early-phase trials and is currently being evaluated in a large phase III study in Brazil.
- An investigational Zika virus vaccine that uses a genetically engineered version of vesicular stomatitis virus (VSV) - an animal virus that primarily affects cattle. VSV was successfully used in an investigational Ebola vaccine tested by NIAID. This vaccine approach is at an early stage with plans underway to evaluate the Zika virus vaccine candidate in tissue culture and animal models.

- A whole-particle inactivated Zika virus vaccine based on a similar vaccine approach used by the Walter Reed Army Institute of Research (WRAIR) to develop vaccines against the related Japanese encephalitis and dengue viruses.

In August 2016, NIAID announced that the first stage I clinical trials have begun to evaluate the NIAID *Zika virus* investigational DNA vaccine's safety and ability to generate an immune system response in at least 80 healthy volunteer participants aged 18–35 years in three study sites in the United States [14]. Even with this accelerated work, a safe, effective, licensed ZIKV vaccine is not expected to be available to the public for several more years.

Clinical Development Stage

A candidate vaccine that successfully makes it through the preclinical stage becomes an investigational vaccine in the clinical development stage. Because this is the first time the vaccine is administered to humans, it is at this stage that the FDA becomes involved. Typically, this is the longest and most detailed time of research and development, spanning on average of 6–8 years. The majority of investigational vaccines will *not* successfully make it through this process.

Overview of the Federal Drug Administration

Like the Centers for Disease Control and Prevention (CDC) and Centers for Medicare and Medicaid Services, the FDA is an agency within the US Department of Health and Human Services (HHS). The FDA has a wide scope of influence, and in vaccine development, its role is to protect the public health by ensuring that human and veterinary drugs and vaccines and other biological products and medical devices intended for human use are safe and effective. FDA's responsibilities extend to the 50 United States, the District of Columbia, Puerto Rico, Guam, the Virgin Islands, American Samoa, and other US territories and possessions. A full organization chart of the FDA is available on its website (http://www.fda.gov/downloads/AboutFDA/CentersOffices/OrganizationCharts/UCM432556.pdf). A simplified version is shown in Fig. 3.2. The Center for Biologics Evaluation and Research (CBER) oversees the regulation of vaccines and biologics.

CBER's mission is "to protect and enhance the public health through the regulation of biological and related products including blood, vaccines, allergenics, tissues, and cellular and gene therapies" [15]. Unlike medications and drugs that are chemically synthesized, biologic agents and vaccines are derived from living sources (such as humans, animals, and microorganisms). These new products are often on the leading edge of biomedical research and technology.

Fig. 3.2 Simplified organizational chart of the federal drug administration

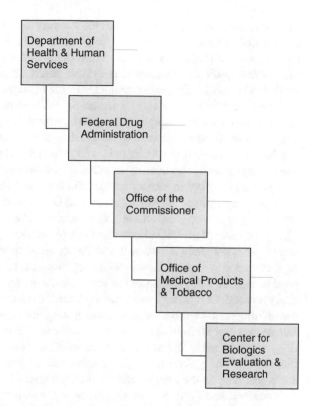

CBER carefully evaluates scientific and clinical data submitted by manufacturers to determine whether the product meets the standards for approval. They also monitor the clinical trial process to ensure that researchers are adhering to the FDA's regulations for the conduct of clinical trials established in the 1970s to ensure consistent use of the principles of good clinical practices (GCPs), including adequate human subject protection (HSP). After thoroughly assessing the data, CBER renders a decision by balancing the risk-benefit for the intended population and the product's intended use. FDA's Bioresearch Monitoring Program (BIMO) ensures the protection of research subjects and the integrity of data submitted to the agency in support of a marketing application by conducting on-site inspections of both clinical and nonclinical studies [15].

Clinical Trial Process

Before administering an investigational vaccine or biological product to a human subject, clinical researchers must submit an official request for authorization called an Investigational New Drug (IND) Application to CBER [16]. The IND describes the vaccine, its method of manufacture, and quality control tests for release. It also includes information about the vaccine's safety and immunogenicity (ability to elicit a protective immune response) in animal testing, as well as the proposed clinical protocol for studies in humans. At any stage of the clinical or animal studies, if data raise significant concerns about either safety or effectiveness, the FDA may request additional information or studies or may halt ongoing clinical studies.

There are two IND categories (research and commercial) and three IND types including investigator, emergency use, and treatment. If a physician intends to directly administer or dispense the investigational drug and is the one who both initiates and conducts the study, it is considered an investigator IND. This scenario is common when a physician has an interest in studying an unapproved drug or attempting to use an approved drug but in a new population or for a new indication.

A physician might submit a research IND to propose studying an unapproved drug or an approved product for a new indication or in a new patient population. Emergency use of an IND allows the FDA to authorize the use of an experimental drug in an emergency situation that does not allow time for submission of an IND in accordance with law. Under certain circumstances, an emergency IND can be used to include a population of patients who do not meet the criteria of an existing study protocol or if an approved study protocol does already not exist. If an experimental drug shows promise in clinical testing for a serious or immediately life-threatening condition, a treatment IND facilitates the availability of promising new drugs to desperately ill patients as early in the drug development process as possible, even before general marketing begins, while ongoing trials continue to obtain additional data on the drug's safety and effectiveness.

The Food and Drug Administration Safety and Innovation Act (FDASIA) was signed into law on July 9, 2012 [16]. It expanded the FDA's authority to expedite the review process and promote innovation that speeds patient access to safe and effective products. It allows investigators to apply for a breakthrough therapy (BT) designation from CBER which expedites the development and review process for serious or life-threatening conditions. Qualification for BT designation requires preliminary clinical evidence that demonstrates the drug may have substantial improvement on at least one clinically significant endpoint over currently available therapy.

Case in Point: Meningococcal B Vaccine [17, 18]

Neisseria meningitidis is a leading cause of bacterial meningitis. The bacteria are transmitted from person to person through respiratory or throat secretions (e.g., by coughing, kissing, or sharing eating utensils). Even with appropriate antibiotics and intensive care, between 10 and 15% of people who develop meningococcal disease die from the infection. Another 10–20% suffer permanent complications, such as brain damage or limb loss. According to the CDC 160 of the approximately 500 total cases of meningococcal disease reported in the United States in 2012 were caused by serogroup B. In 2013, eight cases of serogroup B meningococcal disease at Princeton University and four cases at University of California, Santa Barbara were reported. In the wake of these outbreaks, two vaccines which were already approved in 2013 for use in the European Union, Canada, and Australia were granted breakthrough therapy designations to expedite drug development and review by the FDA. In October 2014, the FDA licensed the first serogroup B meningococcal (MenB) vaccine (MenB-FHbp [Trumenba, Wyeth Pharmaceuticals, Inc.]) as a three-dose series. In January 2015, the FDA licensed a second MenB vaccine (MenB-4C [Bexsero, Novartis Vaccines]) as a two-dose series. Both vaccines were approved for use in persons aged 10–25 years [18].

Having the designation of BT provided the manufacturers more intensive FDA guidance on an efficient MenB development program; it facilitated the scientific evaluation during the IND application stage, offered an organizational commitment involving senior managers, and a "rolling" submission of the Biologics License Application (BLA). Acquiring the status of BT allows sponsors to submit sections of the BLA to FDA for review as they are completed, as opposed to waiting to submit the complete BLA at one time.

The Expanded Access to Investigational New Drug protocol made it possible for a CDC-sponsored clinical trial to be conducted in more than 15,000 individuals at Princeton University and the University of California, Santa Barbara (UCSB) during meningitis B outbreaks on these college campuses. In addition to helping to abort the outbreaks and save lives, the expedited process provided data that supported the accelerated FDA approval of both vaccines for the public market in the United States [19]. On February 26, 2015, the ACIP recommended the use of MenB vaccines among certain groups of persons aged ≥ 10 years who are at increased risk for serogroup B meningococcal disease [17]. In June, 2015, the ACIP further recommended that adolescents and young adults aged 16–23 years may be vaccinated with a serogroup B meningococcal (MenB) vaccine to provide short-term protection against most strains of serogroup B meningococcal disease [18].

Phases of Clinical Testing

In phase I of the clinical testing, 10–100 volunteer human subjects are given the investigational vaccine, and then they are monitored closely for safety. Often phase I trials occur over 6 months to a year in hospital settings. Researchers at this stage are typically looking to confirm that the vaccine is generally safe, to identify side effects, and to confirm if the vaccine causes the expected immune response in a human subject.

In phase II of clinical testing, an additional 100–3000 volunteer human subjects are given the investigational candidate vaccine and undergo a careful evaluation of their immune response. Typically volunteers are healthy; however, if the vaccine is to be used in a population with a particular medical condition, attention will be paid to recruiting participants who resemble the intended population to receive the vaccine. Matching participants for characteristics such as age and physical health are common at this stage. Phase II clinical researchers are looking to verify how well the vaccine works, to monitor for any new safety signals or side effects that emerge as a larger population is exposed to the vaccine, and to identify optimal dosing and administration of the vaccine.

In phase III of clinical testing, a 1–4-year large-scale test of the investigational vaccine's efficacy and tolerance is conducted in hospitals, clinics, or physician offices on an additional 3000–40,000 volunteer human subjects. Like in phase II, most volunteers will be healthy, but volunteers with diseases or medical conditions can be included. Phase III clinical researchers continue confirming the effectiveness of the vaccine, monitoring for any new safety signals or side effects, and for the first time, they begin comparing the vaccine to existing vaccines or other commonly used treatments.

Vaccines that successfully complete phase III clinical trials will be presented to the FDA for licensing review; however, many vaccines will continue to undergo research in what is called phase IV of clinical testing. Phase IV studies are often referred to as post-licensure studies and are valuable for refining indications and confirming the effectiveness of the vaccine as a larger population begins to receive the vaccine in real-world conditions. More about phase IV clinical trials can be found in the post-licensure section.

FDA Regulatory Review: Biologics License Application

If an investigational vaccine successfully completes the three clinical trial phases, it can move forward for regulatory review. During the regulatory approval phase, all of the available preclinical and clinical data are submitted to the FDA as a Biologics License Application (BLA) [20]. The BLA is reviewed by a multidisciplinary FDA review team which includes but is not limited to medical officers, microbiologists, chemists, and biostatisticians. The review team carefully examines the efficacy and safety data, completes a risk/benefit assessment, and makes the decision to recommend or oppose the approval of a vaccine. Concurrent to the safety/efficacy review, an initial facility inspection is performed, and the vaccine manufacturing production process is examined closely.

Vaccines and Related Biological Products Advisory Committee

The next step of the process includes a presentation of final report from the FDA review and the vaccine's sponsor presentation to the Vaccines and Related Biological Products Advisory Committee (VRBAC) [21]. VBRAC is a 15-person committee external to the FDA comprised of appointed experts knowledgeable in the fields of immunology, molecular biology, rDNA, virology, bacteriology, epidemiology or biostatistics, vaccine policy, vaccine safety science, federal immunization activities, vaccine development including translational and clinical evaluation programs, allergy, preventive medicine, infectious diseases, pediatrics, microbiology, and biochemistry [21]. The role of the VBRAC is to review the data being offered on the safety, effectiveness, and appropriate use of vaccines/biological products seeking FDA licensure or a new indication. They offer an important unbiased final review of all the applicable data and have the opportunity to consider the quality and relevance of the FDA's research. All of this work serves to ensure the final recommendation provided to the Commissioner of Food and Drugs is appropriate and based on the sufficient scientific support [21].

Vaccine Labeling

Because the vaccine label provides the most widely accessible collection of information about the indications, potential risks and benefits, adverse effects, and supporting information for a particular vaccine, the FDA takes the labeling process very seriously [22]. Many clinicians use the vaccine's product labeling to communicate with patients and parents and to make decisions about providing the vaccine safely to their patients. The process of vaccine labeling occurs in two major steps: preapproval review of labeling and post-approval surveillance.

Preapproval Review [23]

Vaccine manufacturers submit proposed vaccine labeling to FDA as part of the initial BLA process, or in the event of a later change, as a part of a BLA supplement (BLS) and transmittal form. During the preapproval review, the FDA determines whether the information presented in the labeling is scientifically accurate, conforms to current regulatory requirements, and includes any previously requested revisions.

The labeling review is not limited to the physical label on the vaccine vial but also includes a review of the outer packaging and the package insert for adequacy and accuracy. If the preliminary review uncovers concerns such as a lack of adequate warnings, use instructions, and/or precautionary information, the manufacturer is notified and offered the opportunity to submit a revision. Once all identified concerns have been sufficiently revised to include current information regarding the nature and extent of the dangers posed by such vaccines, the FDA formally approves the final draft labeling.

Post-Approval Surveillance

A vaccine's product label is not a static document. Even after approval and licensure, the FDA conducts surveillance and reviews whether there are changes to existing or new warnings, use instructions, and precautionary information [22]. In addition to the standing label requirements, the FDA uses epidemiological information contained in *Morbidity and Mortality Weekly Reports* (MMWR), published by the CDC, reports in the medical literature, and summaries from the Vaccine Adverse Event Reporting System (VAERS) to identify new information on a vaccine's safety and efficacy post-licensure. FDA reviews the new data, determines whether package inserts and other labeling should be revised to include this new information, and then notifies manufacturers if their package inserts do not reflect currently available information regarding the warnings, use instructions, and precautionary information.

Case in Point: 9-Valent Human Papillomavirus Vaccine [24, 25]

There are over 150 different types of human papillomaviruses of which around 40 of them are known to infect the genital areas of men and women. Human papilloma virus (HPV) infection is highly prevalent with some studies showing that 27% of women aged 14–59 tested positive for one or more strains of HPV and over 80% of women will have been infected with genital HPV by the time they reach age 50. Two particular strains of the virus are responsible for nearly 70% of cervical cancers which accounts for approximately 500,000 new cases and 270,000 deaths worldwide each year. There are about a dozen other high-risk HPV strains that collectively account for the other 30% of cervical cancers [24, 25]. The first vaccine licensed by the FDA for HPV was Gardasil (HPV4) in 2006, a Merck vaccine, providing protection for four strains of HPV including 6, 11, 16, and 18. Cervarix (HPV2) from GlaxoSmithKline, which protects against two high-risk types of HPV [16, 18], was licensed in 2009. A 9-valent vaccine (HPV9, Gardasil 9) was approved in 2014. Today, only the HPV9 vaccine is available for use in the US.

At the time of the initial FDA approval for HPV9, available data showed that in both females and males, >99% seroconverted to all nine HPV vaccine types, and geometric mean titers of antibody (GMT) in males were non-inferior to those in females and males aged 9–15 years. Because study results were only available for these certain age ranges, HPV9 was initially licensed for use in females aged 9–26 years and males aged 9–15 years. Fortunately, as ongoing research studies concluded that immunogenicity in males aged 16 through 26 years was comparable with females of the same age group, the data was reviewed by the FDA and the ACIP, and on December 14, 2015, the FDA extended the age indication by including males aged 16–26 years [24, 25].

Vaccine Production

Concurrent with the licensing process, the FDA reviews and oversees the production and manufacturing process that will be used to produce the vaccine. Practically, having a licensed vaccine that a manufacturer is unable to produce safely and reliably would not be beneficial to society. Traditionally vaccines are produced using eggs or mammalian cells; however, advances in biotechnology are exploring novel production mechanisms using plant, insect cells, and bacteria cultures [26]. As we continue to develop more complicated vaccine combinations, new adjuvants for stability, and augmented processes to increase speed and volume of production, it will remain critical to assess that we are producing vaccines with the safe (or better) safety profiles and potency that we have come to expect from our traditional approaches. It can take up to 22 months to produce a single batch of vaccine, so faulty practices that contaminate or cause a vaccine lot to be wasted not only cost significant loss of money and resources, but also can create critical shortages to vaccine supply. This is one of the driving reasons that nearly 70% of vaccine production time is dedicated to quality control and confirmation measures [26].

Manufacturing

To ensure safety, the FDA oversees vaccine production and manufacturing processes after licensure. As long as a manufacturer holds a license for a product, they are subject to regular monitoring of the product and of production activities including periodic facility inspections. At times the FDA may request data from the manufacturer's required ongoing monitoring results around the potency, safety, and purity for each vaccine lot and the manufacturer may be expected to randomly submit samples of each vaccine lot to the FDA for testing. If a manufacturer is able to demonstrate continued assurance of safety, purity, and potency, the FDA may determine that routine submission of lot release protocols and samples is no longer necessary [23].

The Centers for Disease Control and Prevention Advisory Committee on Immunization Practice

The ACIP is a group of 15 individuals appointed by the Secretary of HHS to develop recommendations on the use of vaccines in the United States.

Authority and Oversight of the ACIP

The authority and scope of the ACIP is established under Section 222 of the Public Health Service Act (42 U.S.C. §2l7a) [27]. The Secretary of HHS delegates the CDC Director to "assist states and their political subdivisions in the prevention and control of communicable diseases; to advise the states on matters relating to the preservation and improvement of the public's health; and to make grants to states and, in consultation with the state health authorities, to agencies and political subdivisions of states to assist in meeting the costs of communicable disease control programs" [27]. To make these decisions, the CDC Director relies in part on guidance and advice from the ACIP regarding use of vaccines and related agents for effective control of vaccine-preventable diseases in the civilian population of the United States. While our military population of the United States often follows similar guidance, the actual authority for determining immunization requirements for military personnel resides with the Department of Defense and follows a parallel approval process.

ACIP recommendations are presented to the CDC Director for review and if adopted are published as official CDC/HHS recommendations in the *Morbidity and Mortality Weekly Report* (MMWR). HHS Secretary and Assistant Secretary for Health are briefed on immunization recommendations by the CDC Director.

Scope of ACIP Recommendations and Guidance

ACIP guidance and recommendations are expected to provide advice on the control of diseases for which a vaccine is licensed in the United States. In addition, there are times when circumstances may warrant the committee develop and provide guidance for use of unlicensed vaccines [27]. In addition to vaccine recommendations, the committee may also provide recommendations for administration of immune globulin preparations and/or antimicrobial therapy during times of vaccine-preventable disease exposure or outbreaks.

Vaccine-Specific Recommendations

Guidance for each vaccine typically includes brief overviews of the scientific data supporting the included recommendations, consideration of disease epidemiology and burden of disease, vaccine efficacy and effectiveness, vaccine safety, economic analyses, and implementation issues with specific advice about:

- Population groups and/or circumstances in which a vaccine or related agent is recommended
- Guidance on route, dose, and frequency of administration of the vaccine, associated immune globulin, or antimicrobial agent

- Recommendations on contraindications and precautions for use of the vaccine and related agents' information on recognized adverse events

The ACIP reviews and updates guidance as new information on disease epidemiology, vaccine effectiveness or safety, economic considerations, or other data become available, and the committee may revise or withdraw their recommendation(s) regarding a particular vaccine if warranted.

Case in Point: Live Attenuated Influenza Vaccine

CDC has recommended an annual influenza vaccination for everyone ages 6 months and older since February 24, 2010. Each year the ACIP provides an updated seasonal influenza recommendation published in the MMWR based on the circulating influenza strains anticipated for the upcoming season and available products available in the United States [28]. On June 22, 2016, many in the immunization community were surprised to witness the removal of an increasingly popular option, the live attenuated influenza nasal spray vaccine (FluMist®, MedImmune/AstraZeneca) from the recommended list of vaccines for use during the 2016–2017 season as ongoing efficacy studies had found the vaccine less effective against circulating influenza viruses than other available influenza vaccines [29]. While some viewed the reversal of the nasal spray vaccine recommendation as a visible failure of the ACIP's decision-making process, those most familiar with the committee recognized it as the process working exactly as it was intended to do.

A New Way to Deliver Vaccine

Although relatively new to the market, the live attenuated intranasal influenza vaccine had been a work in progress for nearly 60 years. In 1960, in response to an influenza A virus subtype H2N2 pandemic, the NIH and the US Army invested resources at the University of Michigan to study novel influenza vaccination strategies that included development of a live attenuated vaccine option. The goal was to stimulate a broader immune response than the available injectable influenza vaccine (which contained proteins from inactivated viruses) by allowing the body to respond to a weakened live version of the influenza virus. The endeavor proved successful in 1967 when Dr. Hunein Maassab of the University of Michigan developed a live, cold-adapted flu virus for use in a vaccine. The cold adaption process developed involved selectively growing live vaccine viruses over multiple generations in increasing cooler temperatures; this process ultimately prevented the virus from spreading beyond the relatively cool atmosphere in the human upper respiratory tract. This novel vaccine, administered via a spray mist to the nose, quickly became a popular option among children and needle-avoidant adults.

An Unexpected Lack of Effectiveness

Initial data appeared to support the expected boosted immunity when using the live inactivated formulation over the inactivated injected formulation in younger children [30]. After reviewing the initial data, during the 2014–2015 influenza season, the CDC and ACIP released a preferential recommendation for nasal spray vaccine for young children. The 2014–2015 influenza season was a difficult one in the US, fraught with poor vaccine effectiveness across all seasonal influenza vaccines, including inactivated vaccines and FluMist Quadrivalent. The vaccines' lower than expected effectiveness that season has been attributed primarily to the spread of a "drifted" strain of influenza A (H3N2) that did not match well with the H3N2 strain used in the vaccines [31]. While typically overall effectiveness for all influenza vaccines for any season is around 50–60%, in that season, it was estimated at only 23% [31].

ACIP reviewed all available data including effectiveness data, and they downgraded their advice during the subsequent 2015–2016 season, to return to recommending influenza vaccination without any preference for one vaccine type or formulation over another [32]. The ACIP influenza workgroup continued to review the data, and when preliminary data showed poor or relatively lower effectiveness of LAIV from 2013 through 2016 in the children ages 2 through 17 years, ACIP voted to suspend use of the vaccine for the 2016–2017 season. FDA continues to find that the benefits of FluMist Quadrivalent outweighed any potential risks and has determined that no specific regulatory action is warranted [33]. As the FDA continues to work closely with MedImmune to determine the cause of the lower than expected effectiveness of FluMist Quadrivalent observed in recent years, the influenza workgroup will continue to review and provide revised policy recommendations for review by the ACIP [34]. A brief timeline of intranasal influenza vaccine use in the United States can be found in Table 3.2.

General Recommendations

In addition to vaccine-specific guidance, the ACIP provides recommendations addressing the general use of vaccines and immune globulin preparations as a class of biologic agents. General recommendations typically address principles that govern administration technique; dose and dosing intervals; recognized contraindications and precautions; reporting adverse events; correct storage, handling, and recording of vaccines and immune globulin preparations; and special situations or populations that may warrant modification of the routine recommendations. Examples of currently published ACIP general recommendations include General Recommendations on Immunization and Immunization of Health-Care Personnel.

Table 3.2. Brief timeline of intranasal influenza vaccine use in the United States

2016–2017	ACIP votes to no longer recommend for use of intranasal influenza vaccine in any population for the 2016–2017 influenza season after review showing poor or relatively lower effectiveness of LAIV from 2013 through 2016
May 2016	Preliminary data on the effectiveness of LAIV among children 2–17 years during 2015–2016 season became available from the US Influenza Vaccine Effectiveness Network, and the observational studies showed lower than expected effectiveness
2015–2016	CDC and ACIP modify the preferential recommendation to no preference after vaccine effectiveness studies suggest the anticipated benefit was not being observed in post-licensure studies
2014–2015	CDC and ACIP briefly had a preferential recommendation for nasal spray vaccine for young children based on initial studies
February 2012	FDA approves FluMist Quadrivalent, a formulation containing two *Influenza A* subtype viruses and two type B viruses for use in persons 2–49 years of age
2007–2008	CAIV-T is approved for use during the flu season
August 2006	The FDA approves CAIV-T, an unfrozen refrigerated version for the same age group (ages 5–49) following completion of phase 3 clinical trials
Winter 2003–2004	FluMist is available for use for the first time to health adults and children ages 5 through 49 years
June 2003	The FDA approves FluMist for healthy adults and children ages 5 through 49 years
December 2002	The FDA's Vaccines and Related Biological Products Advisory Committee again evaluates the safety and efficacy of FluMist. The committee recommends that the FDA approve FluMist for healthy children and adults ages 5–49 years. MedImmune continues to work with the FDA to answer the committee's questions about the safety and efficacy of FluMist for children under 5 and adults 50 and older.
January 2002	MedImmune, Inc. acquires FluMist when it purchases Aviron
July 2001	The FDA's Vaccines and Related Biological Products Advisory Committee evaluates the safety and efficacy of FluMist. The majority of the committee members agree that while there are adequate data to show the vaccine works in healthy people ages 1–64 years, the analysis of the safety data is incomplete. Aviron continues to work with the FDA to provide additional clinical and manufacturing data to support the licensing of FluMist
October 2000	Aviron submits an application for FluMist to the Food and Drug Administration (FDA), seeking approval for FluMist as an annual vaccine for healthy individuals 1–64 years old
1999	Aviron enters an agreement with Wyeth Lederle Vaccines of Philadelphia for marketing FluMist in the United States and worldwide
1998–2003	The NIAID sponsors a large, multiyear trial with FluMist to test a popular theory: If a critical number of children, about 70%, are vaccinated against influenza, the spread of the virus within a community can be stopped, resulting in a kind of "community immunity." In Temple, Texas, researchers vaccinate more than 14,000 children with FluMist over the next several years. When this ongoing study finishes, researchers will compare influenza-associated illness rates in Temple with those in similarly sized communities without FluMist vaccine. In 2003, researchers conduct data analysis by comparing influenza-associated illness rates in Temple with those in similarly sized communities without FluMist vaccine

(continued)

Table 3.2. (continued)

1998	NIAID's Vaccine Treatment and Evaluation Units begin studies to evaluate the safety of FluMist in HIV-positive adults and children
1997–1998 flu season	The vaccine proves similarly effective in the same children against the influenza strains included in the vaccine. In addition, an unanticipated new influenza strain emerges this season. FluMist proves 86% effective in protecting children against this emergent strain that is not contained in the vaccine. FluMist also provided 94% protection against influenza-related middle-ear infections or otitis media
1996–1997 flu season	NIAID's Vaccine Treatment and Evaluation Units and Aviron perform a pivotal Phase 3 efficacy study that finds the vaccine 93% effective in preventing influenza in children aged 15–71 months
1995	NIAID signs a cooperative research and development agreement with Aviron of Mountain View, California, to continue studying the safety, efficacy, and immunogenicity of FluMist in various populations
1976–1991	NIAID sponsors a series of clinical studies to evaluate the safety, efficacy, and dosage of the live, cold-adapted, attenuated, flu vaccine
Mid–1970s	Brian Murphy, M.D., and other NIAID researchers at the Laboratory of Infectious Diseases take over the lead in developing the live, attenuated flu vaccine
1967	Dr. Hunein Maassab of the University of Michigan develops a live, cold-adapted flu virus for use in a vaccine
1960	The US Army supports research at the University of Michigan to develop a live, attenuated influenza vaccine strategy
1958	A pandemic caused by the H2N2 influenza virus results in more than 69,000 deaths in the United States, underscoring the need for new strategies to prevent the flu

https://www.niaid.nih.gov/topics/Flu/Research/vaccineResearch/Pages/NasalSprayFluVaccine.aspx
http://www.fda.gov/BiologicsBloodVaccines/Vaccines/ApprovedProducts/ucm508761.htm

ACIP Influence on Vaccine Payment

The impact of ACIP recommendations is not limited to medical and public health professional administration practices. The Social Security Act (Section 1928) empowers the ACIP to establish and periodically review and, as appropriate, revise the list of vaccines for administration to children and adolescents eligible to receive vaccines through the Vaccines for Children (VFC) program, along with schedules regarding the appropriate dose and dosing interval and contraindications to administration of the pediatric vaccines [35]. This list is used by CDC Director as delegated by the DHS Secretary to purchase, deliver, and administer pediatric vaccines in the VFC program. The Affordable Care Act (Section 2713 of the Public Health Service Act, as amended) that empowers the ACIP recommendations adopted by the CDC Director must be covered by applicable health plans.

The Affordable Care Act and Immunizations

The Patient Protection and Affordable Care Act (PPACA), commonly called the Affordable Care Act (ACA), is a US federal statute enacted by President Barack Obama on March 23, 2010. The law made prevention, like immunizations, affordable and accessible for all Americans by requiring health plans to cover preventive services and by eliminating cost sharing [36]. Based on the law, regulations were released by HHS, the Department of Labor, and the Treasury that stipulate that if an individual or family enrolls in a new health plan on or after September 23, 2010, that plan will be required to cover recommended preventive services without charging a deductible, co-payment, or coinsurance. These new health plans are required to cover new ACIP recommendations made after September 2009 without cost sharing in the next plan year that occurs 1 year after the date of the recommendation. While many children had access to immunizations under the VFC program, the ACA expanded access for adult immunizations which was previously a notably under covered area of healthcare, especially for those adults without access to health insurance or with limited finances.

The ACA also addressed other barriers to immunization delivery in the United States including providing states the authority to purchase adult vaccines with state funds from federally negotiated contracts. It reauthorized the Section 317 Immunization Grant Program, which makes available federally purchased vaccines and grants to all 50 states, the District of Columbia, five large urban areas, and territories and protectorates, to provide immunization services to priority populations. The ACA also required the General Accountability Office (GAO) to study and report to Congress about Medicare beneficiary access to recommended vaccines under the Medicare Part D benefit.

Vaccines for Children

The VFC program is an entitlement program (a right granted by law) for eligible children, age 18 and younger [35]. It was created under the Omnibus Budget Reconciliation Act (OBRA) passed by Congress on August 10, 1993, in response to a US measles epidemic from 1989 to 1991 during which there were tens of thousands of cases of measles and hundreds of deaths. In the subsequent CDC investigation of the outbreak, it was found that more than half of the children who had measles had not been immunized, even though many of them had seen a healthcare provider.

VFC attempts to remove cost as a barrier to children receiving their recommended vaccination on schedule. The program helps provide vaccines recommended by the ACIP to children whose parents or guardians may not be able to afford them. VFC funding is approved by the Office of Management and Budget

(OMB) and allocated through the Centers for Medicare and Medicaid Services (CMS) to the CDC. CDC buys vaccines at a discount and distributes them to grantees. Grantees typically include state health departments and certain local and territorial public health agencies. The grantees then distribute the vaccines at no charge to private physicians' offices and public health clinics registered as VFC providers for administration to eligible children. VFC program-eligible children are younger than 19 years of age and either Medicaid eligible, uninsured, underinsured, or American Indian or Alaska Native. "Underinsured" children include those children with health insurance, but either their insurance does not cover any or needed vaccines, or the child has exceeded the insurance company's fixed dollar limit or cap allotted for vaccines. Underinsured children are eligible to receive vaccines only at Federally Qualified Health Centers (FQHC), Rural Health Clinics (RHC), or under an approved deputization agreement.

ACIP Membership

While the majority of the 15 voting members of the committee are comprised of experts in medicine and public health, one member is a consumer representative who provides the social and community perspective on the impact of vaccination recommendations [37, 38]. To be appointed, members are nominated after submitting a record demonstrating their personal expertise in vaccinology, immunology, pediatrics, internal medicine, nursing, family medicine, virology, public health, infectious disease and/or preventive medicine, with corroboration of their experience and expertise along with recommendations from the professional scientific community. Nominees are automatically excluded from participation in the ACIP if they are not a US citizen, are employed by the US government, or have certain vaccine-related interests. If an applicant or an immediate family member is directly employed by a vaccine manufacturer (or parent company), holds a patent on a vaccine or vaccine-related product, or serves on a vaccine manufacturer's Board of Directors, she/he is not eligible for appointment. Applicants undergo a formal review process including an interview by the ACIP Steering Committee which includes CDC division members working in vaccine-related areas, an FDA representative, and the ACIP Chair. The top two applicants for each vacant position are presented first to the CDC Director for approval and then forwarded to the DHHS Secretary for final review and appointment. The voting members reflect the diversity of the US population, and attention is paid to trying to balance on the basis of geography, race and ethnicity, sex, and type of expertise when reasonable. Appointments are for 4-year overlapping terms.

Once selected, committee members are asked to recuse themselves during the term of their membership from participating in activities that are or may be construed as a conflict of interest including but not limited to providing advisory or consulting services to a vaccine manufacturer (or its parent company), acceptance of honoraria, or travel reimbursement from a vaccine manufacturer. During their term, ACIP voting members may continue their work on vaccine-related research and studies; however, they are required to declare their conflicts at the start of each meeting and abstain from votes on any recommendations related to vaccines they are studying. For transparency, they are also required to abstain from voting on any other vaccine manufactured by a company funding their research or any vaccine that is similar to the one they are studying. Annually committee members file confidential financial reports with the Office of Government Ethics and disclose publicly all vaccine-related interests and work.

In addition to the 15 appointed voting members of the ACIP, nonvoting liaisons from 8 ex officio organizations and 30 professional organizations (see Table 3.3) attend the meetings and serve on the working groups to provide comment and input from the perspective of groups who will need to implement the guideline recommendations. The current ACIP voting membership roster including the ex officio members and nonvoting liaisons is updated at least annually on the ACIP website.

ACIP Meetings

The full committee, ex officio members, and liaison members meet in person at the Centers for Disease Control and Prevention in Atlanta, Georgia, three times a year typically in February, June, and October. These meetings are open to the public and, for those unable to attend in person, webcast via the Internet. While vaccine manufacturers attend the meeting and are frequently called upon to present data to the ACIP or answer questions about their products, they are not permitted to participate in the committee's deliberations. Members of the general public, including special interest groups, are also permitted to provide written or oral testimony during the public comment periods throughout the public meetings. In addition to the official publication of approved recommendations in the MMWR, a summary of the meeting's minutes, the slide sets presented during the meeting, and archived version of the webcast can be found on the ACIP website within 90 days of the meeting.

ACIP Workgroups

A significant amount of work is required to draft vaccine policy and guidance. It is more work than can be completed during the 6 days of face-to-face meetings. The ACIP uses workgroups to gather, analyze, review, and prepare information for the voting members of the committee to discuss and vote on during the meetings [37, 38, 40]. Each workgroup is chaired by a voting member of the ACIP and at least one additional ACIP member, a CDC subject matter expert, relevant ex officio members, liaison representatives, members of the academic community, and invited consultants. While vaccine manufacturers are often invited to present data on vaccine immunogenicity, effectiveness, and safety to the workgroups, they are not permitted

Table 3.3. Ex officio members and liaison organizations represented at the ACIP [39]

Ex officio members
  Centers for Medicare and Medicaid Services (CMS)
  Department of Defense (DoD)
  Department of Veterans Affairs (DVA)
  Food and Drug Administration (FDA)
  Health Resources and Services Administration (HRSA)
  Indian Health Service (IHS)
  National Vaccine Program Office (NVPO)
  National Institutes of Health (NIH)

Liaison professional organizations
  American Academy of Family Physicians (AAFP)
  American Academy of Pediatrics (AAP)
  American Academy of Physician Assistants (AAPA)
  American College Health Association (ACHA)
  American College of Nurse Midwives (ACNM)
  American College of Obstetricians and Gynecologists (ACOG)
  American College of Physicians (ACP)
  American College of Physicians (ACP) (alternate)
  American Geriatrics Society (AGS)
  America's Health Insurance Plans (AHIP)
  American Medical Association (AMA)
  American Nurses Association (ANA)
  American Osteopathic Association (AOA)
  American Pharmacists Association (APhA)
  Association of Immunization Managers (AIM)
  Association for Prevention Teaching and Research (APTR)
  Association of State and Territorial Health Officials (ASTHO)
  Biotechnology Industry Organization (BIO)
  Council of State and Territorial Epidemiologists (CSTE)
  Canadian National Advisory Committee on Immunization (NACI)
  Infectious Diseases Society of America (IDSA)
  National Association of County and City Health Officials (NACCHO)
  National Association of Pediatric Nurse Practitioners (NAPNAP)
  National Foundation for Infectious Diseases (NFID)
  National Immunization Council and Child Health Program, Mexico
  National Medical Association (NMA)
  National Vaccine Advisory Committee (NVAC)
  Pediatric Infectious Diseases Society (PIDS)
  Pharmaceutical Research and Manufacturers of America (PhRMA)
  Society for Adolescent Health and Medicine (SAHM)
  Society for Healthcare Epidemiology of America (SHEA)

to be a member of a workgroup or to participate in the workgroup deliberations. Unlike the public meetings of the ACIP, workgroup meetings are confidential and not subject to the Federal Advisory Committee Act (FACA) law. Workgroup meetings are subject to Freedom of Information Act (FOIA) requests. The workgroups do not determine ACIP policy; however, they do create and present draft recommendations after careful review of the available evidence to the ACIP members for discussion and vote during the open public ACIP meetings.

Table 3.4 ACIP workgroups (as of August 2016)

	Permanent?	AAFP represented?
Adult immunization	YES	YES
Child/adolescent immunization	YES	YES
General recommendations	YES	YES
Influenza	YES	YES
Anthrax Vaccine	NO	NO
Human papillomavirus vaccines	NO	YES
Meningococcal vaccines	NO	YES
Pneumococcal vaccines	NO	YES
Dengue Vaccine	NO	NO
Herpes zoster vaccine	NO	YES
Japanese encephalitis/yellow fever vaccines	NO	NO
Hexavalent vaccine	NO	YES
Cholera vaccine	NO	YES
RSV vaccine (older adults)	NO	YES
Hepatitis vaccines (older adults)	NO	YES
Evidence-based recommendations	NO	YES

There are four permanent ACIP workgroups: adult immunization, child/adolescent immunization, general recommendations, and influenza. Other workgroups are formed and disbanded as necessary. The complete list of active workgroups is shown in Table 3.4.

Workgroups meet via teleconference/web conference throughout the year as frequently as needed to prepare policy recommendations using the GRADE for consideration at the in-person meetings by the ACIP. Balance of benefits and harms, type or quality of evidence, values and preferences of the people affected, and health economic analyses are all considered in preparing vaccine recommendations.

The GRADE Methodology

The ACIP uses a systematic methodology for evidence review called GRADE or Grading of Recommendations Assessment, Development and Evaluation [41]. The GRADE process provides a standard way of organizing and judging the quality of evidence upon which a recommendation is based. GRADE is a well-respected international guideline process that provides several benefits including a set of explicit and comprehensive criteria for downgrading and upgrading quality of evidence ratings, and provides a clear separation between quality of evidence and strength of recommendations. This includes a transparent process of moving from evidence evaluation to recommendations and clear, pragmatic interpretations of strong versus weak recommendations for clinicians. While use of the GRADE process cannot compensate for missing or poor quality data, it does make it easier to judge the strength of the recommendation being made.

Literature Search Process Using GRADE

In the GRADE process, evidence is gathered related to a specific topic or PICO (population, intervention, comparison, outcome) question [42]. Systematic reviews are utilized first. Further literature is incorporated including randomized control trials, observational studies, etc. The evidence addresses similar populations, interventions, comparisons, and outcomes. The evidence is summarized in tables and a strength of recommendation is assigned [42]. The strength of a recommendation reflects the extent to which one can be confident that desirable effects of an intervention outweigh undesirable effects. GRADE classifies recommendations as strong or weak. Strong recommendations mean that most informed patients would choose the recommended management and that clinicians can structure their interactions with patients accordingly, while weak recommendations mean that patients' choices will vary according to their values and preferences, and clinicians must ensure that patients' care is in keeping with their values and preferences. Ultimately, the strength of recommendation is determined by the balance between desirable and undesirable consequences of alternative management strategies, quality of evidence, variability in values and preferences, and resource use. The ACIP recommendations report strong and weak recommendations as either Category A or Category B. Category A recommendations are made for all persons in an age- or risk-factor-based group, while Category B recommendations are made for individual clinical decision making. ACIP provides evidence tables summarizing the benefits and harms and the strengths and limitations of the body of evidence for review. A summary comparing GRADE and ACIP recommendation terminology is included in Table 3.5.

ACIP Recommendation

Although the workgroup and CDC scientists draft a recommendation, the recommendation is not final until it is both approved by the ACIP by majority vote, and accepted by the Director of the CDC. The overview of steps for final approval is

Table 3.5 Comparison of GRADE and ACIP recommendation categories [43]

GRADE		ACIP	
Strong recommendations	Most informed patients would choose the recommended management clinicians that can structure their interactions with patients accordingly	Category A recommendations	All persons in an age- or risk-factor-based group
Weak recommendations	Patients' choices will vary according to their values and preferences; clinicians must ensure that patients' care is in keeping with their values and preferences	Category B recommendations	Individual clinical decision making

Fig. 3.3 Process of creating an ACIP recommendation

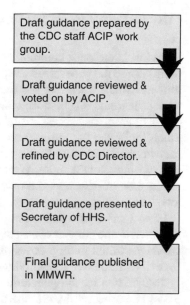

Draft guidance prepared by the CDC staff ACIP work group.

Draft guidance reviewed & voted on by ACIP.

Draft guidance reviewed & refined by CDC Director.

Draft guidance presented to Secretary of HHS.

Final guidance published in MMWR.

shown in Fig. 3.3. At each stage of the process, the recommendation may be edited and revised for clarity. Once it is approved, the final guideline is published in the MMWR and posted on the CDC website. Any subsequent policy update will follow a similar process of being drafted through the workgroup, presented to the ACIP for review and feedback, to final approval from the CDC Director and publication.

Ongoing Monitoring

Post-Licensure Review

Phase IV clinical studies are formal studies that are continued after the vaccine has already been licensed and is on the market. Often these studies are conducted by the manufacturer who is looking to demonstrate the vaccine's success relative to other vaccines on the market, to monitor for long-term protection or impact on the patient's quality of life after receiving the vaccine, or to determine the actual cost-effectiveness after introduction of the vaccine. These additional studies are incredibly important for identifying the less common side effects and adverse events that cannot be seen in the small sample sizes of clinical trials compared to the millions who can be monitored after a vaccine is available to the general population.

Case in Point: Rotavirus Vaccine [44]

Rotavirus is the most common cause of severe diarrhea in infants and young children. Prior to the widespread use of second-generation vaccines in the United States, rotavirus was responsible for nearly 3 million symptomatic gastroenteritis infections and around 60,000 hospitalizations annually. Despite the incredibly large burden of disease, easy access to oral and intravenous rehydration therapy in the United States limits the mortality to under 60 deaths annually [44]. Live attenuated oral rotavirus vaccines were first tested for proof of concept in the early 1980s, and the first vaccine (RotaShield®, Wyeth) was licensed by the FDA on August 31, 1998. At the time of licensure, the risk of intussusception was noted but appeared to be low. The package insert noted that "Intussusception was noted in 5 of 10,054 (0.05%) vaccine recipients compared to 1 of 4,633 (0.02%) placebo recipients." However, as the number of cases of intussusception reached 100 in under a year and within the initial million doses of the licensed vaccine administered in the United States, RotaShield® was withdrawn in 1999.

In 2006 two second-generation rotavirus vaccines were introduced in the United States (Rotarix®, GlaxoSmithKline, and RotaTeq®, Merck), and both remain on the market today. In the past decade, millions of infants in the United States have been safely given the newer rotavirus vaccines. Continued surveillance to monitor for safety signals has carefully tracked both Rotarix® and RotaTeq® for vaccine-attributable intussusception and found a rate of 1:51,000–1:68,000 in the 7 days after dose 1 for both vaccines. Fortunately, this is much less than the vaccine-attributable risk of RotaShield®. Ultimately, CDC and ACIP concluded that the overall benefits of the second-generation rotavirus vaccines outweighed the potential risks and recommend their use.

The rotavirus vaccine is often cited as an example of the post-licensure surveillance working at its best because not only did the concerning safety signals get picked up quickly, but the appropriate agencies were able to respond quickly to update the medical community. Ultimately, a new, safer vaccine was developed to reduce the morbidity and mortality of rotavirus gastroenteritis in infants and children.

Vaccine Adverse Event Reporting System (VAERS)

In addition to the post-licensure studies which are actively studying the vaccines and their impact on health, the United States uses national passive surveillance system called Vaccine Adverse Event Reporting System (VAERS) to track adverse events related to vaccination [45]. The WHO describes a national passive surveillance system as one that relies on healthcare providers in laboratories, hospitals, health facilities, and private practices to report the occurrence of a vaccine-preventable disease to a higher administrative level [46]. US healthcare professionals are asked to submit a report for any adverse event that occurs after the administration of a vaccine licensed in the United States even if they are unsure whether a vaccine caused them.

National Childhood Vaccine Injury Act

The National Childhood Vaccine Injury Act (NCVIA) of 1986 formalized a process for providing financial support to vaccine-injured parties and their families via the federal vaccine injury compensation program and ensuring that vaccine safety protections were maintained in the US mass vaccination system [47]. The law preserved the right for vaccine-injured persons to bring a lawsuit in the court system if federal compensation is denied or is not sufficient. In addition to the financial and legal protections, the law requires healthcare providers to give parents vaccine benefit and risk information before their children are vaccinated, keep written records of vaccine manufacturer names and lot numbers for each vaccination given, enter serious health problems following vaccination into a child's permanent medical record, and report serious health problems following vaccination to VAERS [47]. The NCVIA is the reason why healthcare providers are mandated to provide copies of a designated Vaccine Information Sheet (VIS) before each dose of vaccine is administered. The VIS is a patient education handout created and updated by the Centers for Disease Control and Prevention (CDC) that explains to vaccine recipients, their parents, or their legal representatives both the benefits and risks of a vaccine.

Reporting a Vaccine Adverse Event

Vaccine adverse event reports can be submitted by a patient/parent, by a healthcare professional, or the pharmaceutical company via mail, fax, or online at https://vaers.hhs.gov/esub/index [45]. Vaccine administration errors like giving a live vaccine to an immunocompromised patient or mistimed doses can also be reported to the VAERS for tracking and monitoring. Information is collected about the specific patient including contact information. This data is not accessible to the public; however, the patient/parent or healthcare provider may be contacted for additional information and/or follow-up. The FDA's "Postmarketing Safety Reports for Human Drug and Biologic Products; Electronic Submission Requirements" provides regulations to assist vaccine manufacturers subject to mandatory reporting requirements [48]. It describes the requirements for electronic submission of Individual Case Safety Reports (ICSRs), ICSR attachments, and periodic reports to the FDA by the manufacturer. VAERS reports are taken very seriously, and knowingly filing a false report with the intent to mislead the Department of Health and Human Services is a violation of federal law (18 US Code § 1001) which is punishable by fine and imprisonment.

Surveillance

VAERS is more than a static repository of adverse events; scientists are actively monitoring the reports, tracking trends, identifying new and serious effects, and commissioning additional studies when warranted. If the verified findings suggest that there is any concern for public safety, the CDC, FDA, and vaccine policy makers collaborate to determine if the vaccine's benefits outweigh any potential harms. In the case of mild or newly identified effects, the vaccine may continue to be used but with modifications recommended to the package insert and the VIS. When serious side effects are found and the risk of the vaccine outweighs the benefits, a recommendation to use the vaccine may be withdrawn and the licensure rescinded.

Conclusion

A vaccine's journey from idea through bench and clinical studies, safety monitoring, FDA and CDC review, and ongoing surveillance is painstaking and long. Most vaccines will not make it past the early clinical stages and those that do will undergo ongoing scrutiny through a combination of active and passive surveillance mechanisms for the length of time it is licensed and produced in the United States. Despite the time and care put into protecting the health of the public, at times unexpected adverse events are identified after a vaccine is being used by the public, but there are safeguards in place to not only identify and investigate these warning signals but also to compensate injured parties and limit additional harm to the public. Thanks to the ongoing collaboration of scientists, medical community, public health, government, pharmaceutical industry, and the general public, each year new vaccines are brought to the market, thereby reducing morbidity and mortality from vaccine-preventable diseases and illness.

References

1. Serdobova I, Kieny M-P. Assembling a global vaccine development pipeline for infectious diseases in the developing world. Am J Public Health. 2006;96(9):1554–9.
2. Institute of Medicine (US) Committee on the Evaluation of Vaccine Purchase Financing in the United States. Financing vaccines in the 21st century: assuring access and availability. Washington, DC 2004. Available from: http://www.ncbi.nlm.nih.gov/books/NBK221811/
3. Immunization Action Coalition. Manufacturer. Updated July 30, 2016. Available from: http://www.immunize.org/resources/manufact_vax.asp
4. Services DoHaH. U.S. National vaccine plan. Updated October 4, 2016. Available from: http://www.hhs.gov/nvpo/national-vaccine-plan/index.html#
5. Organization WH. Research and development. Updated 2016. Available from: http://www.who.int/immunization/research/en/
6. Organization WH. Disease-specific areas of work 2016. Updated 2016. Available from: http://www.who.int/immunization/research/development/en/

7. Services USDoHH. National vaccine plan implementation 2010. Available from: http://www.hhs.gov/sites/default/files/nvpo/vacc_plan/2010-2015-Plan/implementationplan.pdf
8. Press TNA. SMART vaccines: strategic multi-attribute ranking tool for vaccines 2015. Available from: https://www.nap.edu/smartvaccines/
9. Anderson KB, Thomas SJ, Endy TP. The emergence of Zika virus a narrative review. Ann Intern Med. 2016;165(3):175–83.
10. National Institute of Allergy and Infectious Disease. Zika virus 2016. Available from: https://www.niaid.nih.gov/topics/zika/Pages/default.aspx
11. Hennessey M, Fischer M, Staples JE. Zika virus spreads to new areas - region of the Americas, may 2015-january 2016. MMWR Morb Mortal Wkly Rep. 2016;65(3):55–8.
12. Disease NIoAaI. NIAID research approach to Zika virus 2016. Available from: https://www.niaid.nih.gov/topics/zika/researchapproach/Pages/default.aspx
13. Disease NIoAaI. Zika virus vaccine research 2016. Available from: https://www.niaid.nih.gov/topics/Zika/ResearchApproach/Pages/vaccineResearch.aspx
14. National Institute of Allergy and Infectious Disease. QUESTIONS AND ANSWERS: Phase 1 clinical trial of the NIAID Zika virus investigational DNA vaccine 2016. Available from: http://www.niaid.nih.gov/news/QA/Pages/Zika-DNA-Vaccine-QA.aspx
15. Food and Drug Administration. About CBER 2016. Updated 5-31-2016. Available from: http://www.fda.gov/AboutFDA/CentersOffices/OfficeofMedicalProductsandTobacco/CBER/ucm123340.htm
16. Administration FaD. Investigational new drug (IND) application 2016. Updated 8-1-2016. Available from: http://www.fda.gov/drugs/developmentapprovalprocess/howdrugsaredeveloped andapproved/approvalapplications/investigationalnewdrugindapplication/default.htm
17. Folaranmi T, Rubin L, Martin SW, Patel M, MacNeil JR. Use of serogroup B meningococcal vaccines in persons aged >/=10 years at increased risk for serogroup B meningococcal disease: recommendations of the advisory committee on immunization practices, 2015. MMWR Morb Mortal Wkly Rept. 2015;64(22):608–12.
18. MacNeil JR, Rubin L, Folaranmi T, Ortega-Sanchez IR, Patel M, Martin SW. Use of serogroup B meningococcal vaccines in adolescents and young adults: recommendations of the advisory committee on immunization practices, 2015. MMWR Morb Mortal Wkly Rept. 2015;64(41):1171–6.
19. Administration FD. First vaccine approved by FDA to prevent serogroup B Meningococcal disease 2014. Updated 10/30/2014. Available from: http://www.fda.gov/NewsEvents/Newsroom/PressAnnouncements/ucm420998.htm
20. Administration FaD. Vaccine product approval process 2015. Updated 8-24-2015. Available from: http://www.fda.gov/biologicsbloodvaccines/developmentapprovalprocess/biologicslicenseapplicationsblaprocess/ucm133096.htm
21. Administration FaD. Vaccines and related biological products advisory committee 2016. Available from: http://www.fda.gov/AdvisoryCommittees/CommitteesMeetingMaterials/BloodVaccinesandOtherBiologics/VaccinesandRelatedBiologicalProductsAdvisoryCommittee/
22. Administration FaD. Guidance for industry: FDA review of vaccine labeling requirements for warnings, use instructions, and precautionary information 2014. Updated 09/15/2014. Available from: http://www.fda.gov/BiologicsBloodVaccines/GuidanceComplianceRegulatoryInformation/Guidances/Vaccines/ucm074845.htm
23. Administration FD. Vaccine product approval process. Updated 08/24/2015. Available from: http://www.fda.gov/BiologicsBloodVaccines/DevelopmentApprovalProcess/BiologicsLicenseApplicationsBLAProcess/ucm133096.htm
24. Petrosky E, Bocchini JA Jr, Hariri S, Chesson H, Curtis CR, Saraiya M, et al. Use of 9-valent human papillomavirus (HPV) vaccine: updated HPV vaccination recommendations of the advisory committee on immunization practices. MMWR Morb Mortal Wkly Rept. 2015;64(11):300–4.
25. Saraiya M, Unger ER, Thompson TD, Lynch CF, Hernandez BY, Lyu CW, et al. US assessment of HPV types in cancers: implications for current and 9-valent HPV vaccines. J Natl Cancer Inst. 2015;107(6):djv086.

26. Josefsberg JO, Buckland B. Vaccine process technology. Biotechnol Bioeng. 2012;109(6): 1443–60.
27. Advisory Committee on Immunization Practices (ACIP). ACIP Charter 2016. Updated April 20, 2016. Available from: http://www.cdc.gov/vaccines/acip/committee/charter.html
28. Grohskopf LA, Sokolow LZ, Olsen SJ, Bresee JS, Broder KR, Karron RA. Prevention and control of influenza with vaccines: recommendations of the advisory committee on immunization practices, United States, 2015-16 influenza season. MMWR Morb Mortal Wkly Rep. 2015;64(30):818–25.
29. Center for Disease Control and Prevention. ACIP votes down use of LAIV for 2016-2017 flu season 2016. Available from: http://www.cdc.gov/media/releases/2016/s0622-laiv-flu.html
30. Carter NJ, Curran MP. Live attenuated influenza vaccine (FluMist(R); Fluenz): a review of its use in the prevention of seasonal influenza in children and adults. Drugs. 2011;71(12):1591–622.
31. Appiah GD, Blanton L, D'Mello T, Kniss K, Smith S, Mustaquim D, et al. Influenza activity - United States, 2014-15 season and composition of the 2015-16 influenza vaccine. MMWR Morb Mortal Wkly Rep. 2015;64(21):583–90.
32. Caspard H, Gaglani M, Clipper L, Belongia EA, McLean HQ, Griffin MR, et al. Effectiveness of live attenuated influenza vaccine and inactivated influenza vaccine in children 2-17 years of age in 2013-2014 in the United States. Vaccine. 2016;34(1):77–82.
33. Food and Drug Administration. FDA information regarding FluMist Quadrivalent vaccine 2016. Updated 06/27/2016. Available from: http://www.fda.gov/BiologicsBloodVaccines/Vaccines/ApprovedProducts/ucm508761.htm
34. Tisa V, Barberis I, Faccio V, Paganino C, Trucchi C, Martini M, et al. Quadrivalent influenza vaccine: a new opportunity to reduce the influenza burden. J Prev Med Hyg. 2016;57(1):E28–33.
35. Center for Disease Control and Prevention. Vaccines for children program 2016. Available from: http://www.cdc.gov/vaccines/programs/vfc/index.html
36. Department of Health and Human Services. Read the Law 2015. Updated August 28, 2015. Available from: http://www.hhs.gov/healthcare/about-the-law/read-the-law/
37. Smith JC. The structure, role, and procedures of the U.S. advisory committee on immunization practices (ACIP). Vaccine. 2010;28(Suppl 1):A68–75.
38. Smith JC, Hinman AR, Pickering LK. History and evolution of the advisory committee on immunization practices--United States, 1964-2014. MMWR Morb Mortal Wkly Rep. 2014;63(42):955–8.
39. Center for Disease Control and Prevention. ACIP Members July 1, 2015 - June 30, 2016. Updated 3-8-2016. Available from: http://www.cdc.gov/vaccines/acip/committee/members.html
40. Smith JC, Snider DE, Pickering LK. Immunization policy development in the United States: the role of the advisory committee on immunization practices. Ann Intern Med. 2009;150(1):45–9.
41. Institute for Clinical Systems Improvement. Reviewing evidence using GRADE 2016. Available from: https://www.icsi.org/_asset/7mtqyr/ReviewingEvidenceUsingGRADE.pdf
42. Guyatt GH, Oxman AD, Kunz R, Falck-Ytter Y, Vist GE, Liberati A, et al. Going from evidence to recommendations. BMJ. 2008;336(7652):1049–51.
43. Centers for Disease Control and Prevention (CDC). New framework (GRADE) for development of evidence-based recommendations by the advisory committee on immunization practices. MMWR Morb Mortal Wkly Rep. 2012;61(18):327.
44. Schwartz JL. The first rotavirus vaccine and the politics of acceptable risk. Milbank Q. 2012;90(2):278–310.
45. Department of Health and Human Services. VAERS: Vaccine Adverse Event Reporting System 2016. Available from: https://vaers.hhs.gov/index
46. Organization WH. National passive surveillance. Available from: http://www.who.int/immunization/monitoring_surveillance/burden/vpd/surveillance_type/passive/en/
47. The National Childhood Vaccine Injury Act of 1986 National Vaccine Information Center. Available from: http://www.nvic.org/injury-compensation/origihanlaw.aspx
48. Federal Drug Administration. Postmarketing safety reporting requirements for drug and biologic products. Updated 03/09/2016. Available from: http://www.fda.gov/Drugs/DrugSafety/ucm299833.htm

Chapter 4
Vaccine-Preventable Diseases and the Vaccines That Prevent Them

Heidi L. Diez, Alexandra Hayward, and Kristi VanDerKolk

Abbreviations

ACIP	Advisory Committee on Immunization Practices
AIDS	Acquired immune deficiency syndrome
B. anthracis	*Bacillus anthracis*
B. pertussis	*Bordetella pertussis*
C. diphtheriae	*Corynebacterium diphtheriae*
C. tetani	*Clostridium tetani*
CDC	Centers for Disease Control and Prevention
CRS	Congenital rubella syndrome
CSF	Cerebrospinal fluid
CVS	Congenital varicella syndrome
DNA	Deoxyribonucleic acid
DT	Diphtheria toxoid and tetanus toxoid
DTaP	Diphtheria toxoid, tetanus toxoid, and acellular pertussis
DTP	Diphtheria toxoid, tetanus toxoid, and whole-cell pertussis
EKG	Electrocardiogram
FDA	Food and Drug Administration

H.L. Diez, PharmD, BCACP (✉)
University of Michigan, College of Pharmacy, Ann Arbor, MI, USA

Family Medicine and Pharmacy Innovations and Partnerships, Michigan Medicine, Ann Arbor, MI, USA
e-mail: hdiez@med.umich.edu

A. Hayward, MPH
Infection Prevention and Epidemiology, Michigan Medicine, Ann Arbor, MI, USA
e-mail: haywarda@med.umich.edu

K. VanDerKolk, MD
Western Michigan University, Homer Stryker MD School of Medicine, Department of Family and Community Medicine, Kalamazoo, MI, USA
e-mail: Kristi.VanDerKolk@med.wmich.edu

© Springer International Publishing AG 2017
P.G. Rockwell (ed.), *Vaccine Science and Immunization Guideline*,
DOI 10.1007/978-3-319-60471-8_4

FUTURE	Females United to Unilaterally Reduce Endo/Ectocervical Disease
H1N1	Hemagglutinin subunit one and neuraminidase subunit one
H3N2	Hemagglutinin subunit three and neuraminidase subunit two
HAV	*Hepatitis A virus*
HBV	*Hepatitis B virus*
HCC	Hepatocellular carcinoma
HepA	Hepatitis A vaccine
HepB	Hepatitis B vaccine
Hib	*Haemophilus influenzae* type b
HIV	Human immunodeficiency virus
HPV	Human papillomavirus
HSCT	Hematopoietic stem cell transplant
IG	Immunoglobulin
IIV3	Trivalent inactivated influenza vaccine
IIV4	Quadrivalent inactivated influenza vaccine
IM	Intramuscular
IPV	Inactivated poliovirus vaccine
IV	Intravenous
LAIV	Live attenuated influenza vaccine
M. tuberculosis	*Mycobacterium tuberculosis*
MMR	Measles, mumps, rubella
MMRV	Measles, mumps, rubella, varicella
MPSV4	Menomune®
MSM	Men who have sex with men
MSW	Men who have sex with women
N. meningitidis	*Neisseria meningitidis*
OPV	Oral poliovirus vaccine
PCV13	Prevnar 13®
PCV7	Prevnar®
PEP	Postexposure prophylaxis
PHN	Postherpetic neuralgia
PPSV23	Pneumovax®
REST	Rotavirus Efficacy and Safety Trial
RNA	Ribonucleic acid
RV1	Rotarix®
RV5	RotaTeq®
S. pneumoniae	*Streptococcus pneumoniae*
S. typhi	*Salmonella typhi*
STD	Sexually transmitted disease
TB	Tuberculosis
Tdap	Tetanus toxoid, diphtheria toxoid, and acellular pertussis
V. cholerae	*Vibrio cholerae*
VZV	Varicella zoster virus

Vaccine-Preventable Diseases and the Vaccines that Prevent Them

In the following section, the 17 vaccine-preventable diseases for which routine immunization is recommended in the USA are discussed. Clinical signs and symptoms of the 17 diseases are reviewed, epidemiology and incidence is discussed, and available vaccines to prevent the 17 diseases are reviewed. The discussion progresses in the order in which the vaccines were developed.

Diphtheria

Prior to the introduction of a vaccine against it, diphtheria was a leading cause of childhood death and a common disease in the USA, with more than 200,000 cases reported during the 1920s. Approximately 5–10% of diphtheria cases were fatal, with the highest case fatality ratios recorded for the very young and the elderly. Today, diphtheria is a rare disease in the USA, primarily because of the high level of vaccination with diphtheria and tetanus toxoid and pertussis vaccine (DTP) among children as well as an apparent reduction in the circulation of toxigenic strains of the bacterium *Corynebacterium diphtheriae* (*C. diphtheriae*) [2]. A three-dose complete vaccination series substantially reduces the risk of developing diphtheria, and those that get the disease get a milder form of it. However, vaccinated persons may continue to be asymptomatic carriers of the bacteria [3]. Waning immunity puts adults at risk for the disease, and travel to endemic areas poses an additional risk factor for travelers.

Disease is caused by the protein synthesis inhibiting exotoxin from *C. diphtheriae* biotype *mitis*, *gravis*, *intermedius*, or *belfanti*. Infection is spread via respiratory droplets, direct contact, and, more rarely, by fomites. Diphtheria may be classified as either *respiratory diphtheria* or *cutaneous diphtheria*. Respiratory diphtheria disease symptoms begin with fever, malaise, and sore throat. The disease incubation period is 2–5 days. The hallmark of respiratory diphtheria is the presence of a white pseudomembrane that develops on the mucous membranes of the tonsils, soft palate, and pharynx as a result of toxin-induced necrosis of tissues. A characteristic "bull neck" from significant cervical soft tissue edema and lymphadenopathy may develop. Untreated, the highly adherent pseudomembrane may progressively extend into the larynx and trachea and cause airway obstruction, resulting in death secondary to membrane aspiration. Additionally, absorption of diphtheria toxin from the site of infection can cause systemic complications including kidney, myocardial, and neurologic damage. Case fatality rate for those infected is ~10%. Cutaneous disease, most common in the tropics, is usually mild, presenting as shallow ulcers, or nondescript sores, and rarely causes toxic complications. Since 1980, cutaneous diphtheria has not been a nationally reportable disease, but respiratory diphtheria remains reportable [4].

The most effective treatment of diphtheria is prompt antitoxin administration, available from CDC on request, and antibiotics with the patient placed in isolation [3]. *CDC Yellow Book* lists the current areas of endemicity around the world in Asia, the South Pacific, the Middle East, Eastern Europe, Haiti, and the Dominican Republic and reports large outbreaks in Indonesia, Thailand, and Laos that have occurred since 2011.

Tetanus

Clostridium tetani (*C. tetani*) is an obligate gram-positive anaerobic bacillus that forms exotoxin-producing spores that cause tetanus, or lockjaw, a life-threatening disease. The *C. tetani* spores are widely distributed in soil and in the intestines and feces of horses, sheep, cattle, dogs, cats, rats, guinea pigs, and chickens. Manure-treated soil may contain large numbers of spores. The spores can also be found in contaminated heroin and on human skin surfaces; a significant number of adults who live in agricultural areas have been found to harbor *C. tetani* [5]. Infection is commonly the result of a puncture wound or cut in the skin, but can occur with any exposure of tetanus-containing soil to an opening in the skin. Mortality rates between 10 and 80% are reported and noted to be highest in affected neonates and the elderly. Reported cases in the USA have declined by greater than 95%, and deaths from tetanus have declined by greater than 99% since 1947, when the disease became reportable nationally [6].

Tetanus is a clinical syndrome lacking confirmatory laboratory tests. It is characterized by generalized rigidity and convulsive spasms of skeletal muscles as disseminated *C. tetani* spores affect the central nervous systems, including peripheral motor end plates, the spinal cord, and the brain, and the sympathetic nervous system. Symptoms are produced when tetanus toxin interferes with release of neurotransmitters, blocking inhibitor impulses, leading to unopposed muscle contractions and spasms. Muscle stiffness usually involves the jaw (lockjaw) and neck and then becomes generalized. The most common form of the disease is generalized tetanus which includes the classic triad of trismus, muscle rigidity, and reflex spasms [7].

With the advent of tetanus toxoid vaccines and the use of tetanus antitoxin for wound management, tetanus is now uncommon in developed countries. There are currently four kinds of vaccines used today to protect against tetanus, all of which are combined with vaccines for other diseases:

- Diphtheria and tetanus (DT) vaccines
- Diphtheria, tetanus, and pertussis (DTaP) vaccines
- Tetanus and diphtheria (Td) vaccines
- Tetanus, diphtheria, and pertussis (Tdap) vaccines

Older adults over 65 years of age are at greater risk for tetanus and fatal disease than younger persons, likely due to inadequate vaccination rather than inadequate response to vaccination. It is established that tetanus immunity wanes following childhood vaccination, leaving many adults susceptible to tetanus [6]. Therefore, continued vaccination is needed throughout the lifespan.

During 2001–2008, a total of 233 cases (an average of 29 cases/year) of tetanus were reported from 45 states with 26 reported fatal outcomes [8]. However, tetanus is still endemic in developing nations and remains an important cause of death globally, with over 250,000 deaths annually in neonates alone.

Pertussis

Whooping cough, or pertussis, is caused by the highly contagious bacteria, *Bordetella pertussis*, and is a nationally notifiable disease. Pertussis is a common, endemic disease in the USA with peaks in reported disease every 3–5 years as well as frequent outbreaks. The incidence rate of pertussis among infants exceeds that of all other age groups. The primary goal of pertussis outbreak control efforts is to decrease morbidity and mortality among infants, with a secondary goal is to decrease morbidity among all others [9].

In the absence of a more likely diagnosis, CDC defines the clinical case definition of pertussis as a cough illness lasting 2 weeks or longer with one of the following symptoms: paroxysm of coughing, inspiratory "whoop," posttussive vomiting, or apnea (with or without cyanosis) in infants aged 1 year or less. The laboratory criteria for diagnosis include the isolation of *Bordetella pertussis* from clinical specimens or positive polymerase chain reaction (PCR) for *B. pertussis*. Symptoms of pertussis usually develop within 5–10 days after exposure, but sometimes not for as long as 3 weeks after exposure.

Classically, pertussis occurs in three distinct phases: the catarrhal phase, the paroxysmal phase, and the convalescent phase. The catarrhal, or prodromal phase, lasts 1–2 weeks and consists of symptoms of typical upper respiratory tract infections, including rhinorrhea, conjunctivitis, mild cough, and low-grade fever. The paroxysmal phase is characterized by paroxysms of cough followed by sudden inspiration against a partially closed glottis. This deep inhalation creates the characteristic "whoop" for which the disease is named. This phase typically lasts 2–4 weeks, but may last up to 20 weeks. While adults may have symptoms of disease ranging from asymptomatic or mild to the typical protracted disease, infants are at high risk of severe complications, including pneumonia, apnea, and death. Severe cough paroxysms may cause sequelae including subconjunctival hemorrhage, cyanosis, hemoptysis, and hernias. Other severe sequelae include bronchopneumonia and neurologic complications. Eventually, in the convalescent stage, cough paroxysms begin to decrease in frequency and severity, though an intermittent cough may persist for months. Treatment does not significantly alter the disease course, but can decrease transmission to others [10].

Prior to vaccination, the USA experienced over 100,000 cases of pertussis annually, with nearly all persons acquiring the disease by the age of 16 (peak incidence from 1 to 4 years of age). Post introduction of the pertussis vaccine, the numbers of annual cases decreased to just over 1000 in the 1970s. The resurgence of pertussis reported in recent years appears to be due to waning immunity. Recent estimates suggest just 10% of children remain immune to pertussis 8.5 years after their final DTaP injection [11]. Infection is primarily seen among adolescents and adults, who transmit the disease to young infants. The majority of infant infections appear to be transmitted from close household contacts, including mothers. For protection of newborns and infants, it is recommended that all pregnant women receive a Tdap booster, preferably between 27 and 36 weeks of gestational age, for transplacental antibody transfer. Additionally, CDC encourages "cocooning" an infant through vaccination of all household or other close contacts of infants with a Tdap booster.

Diphtheria, Tetanus, and Pertussis Vaccine and Vaccine Efficacy

One of the earliest recommended childhood vaccines was the combination vaccine for tetanus, diphtheria, and pertussis developed in the 1940s [12]. Diphtheria toxoid, tetanus toxoid, and whole-cell pertussis (DTP) was licensed in 1949 [13]. The components of the combination vaccines have evolved over time; the most current vaccines protecting against diphtheria toxoid, tetanus toxoid, and pertussis are provided in Table 4.1.

Clinical diphtheria and tetanus efficacy data for both Infanrix® and Daptacel® is limited to immunogenicity studies reported in manufacturer package insert. Immunogenicity demonstrated in separate studies of Infanrix® and Daptacel® was strong, with 100% of sera tested one month after three-dose primary series achieving adequate levels of diphtheria and tetanus antitoxin concentrations [14, 15]. The clinical efficacy of the diphtheria toxoid has been estimated to be 97% [19]. Unfortunately, the duration of immunity provided by primary vaccination antibody titers is thought to decrease after 8 years [20].

Clinical efficacy of DTP varied from 1938 to1983 in the USA, from 54% to 96%. Potential explanations for the wide variance in efficacies were differences in defined protection, standard of clinical diagnostic criteria, vaccine composition, and relationship between serology and protection [21]. Safety concerns with the whole-cell pertussis vaccine (convulsions, hypotonic-hyporesponsive episodes, acute encephalopathy with possible brain damage), though rare, ultimately prompted the development of acellular pertussis vaccines. In 1997, the recommendations changed from DTP (whole cell) to DTaP (acellular) for at least the first three primary doses of routine diphtheria, tetanus, and pertussis. Efficacy for DTaP vs. DTP is difficult to compare in many studies due to differences in study designs, case definitions, and laboratory methods used to confirm the diagnosis of pertussis. The efficacy of three doses of acellular pertussis vaccines was within the range expected for most whole-cell DTP vaccines, ranging from 59% to 89% [22]. Recently, the duration of immunity of DTaP has come into question, and need for earlier or repeated booster doses is under consideration. A study comparing relative risk ratios for pertussis in two

Table 4.1 Diphtheria, tetanus, and pertussis combination vaccines

Vaccine contents/ abbreviation	Trade name	FDA-approved age indication	Year approved	Notes
Diphtheria toxoid, tetanus toxoid, and acellular pertussis (DTaP)	Daptacel®[a]	6 weeks through 6 years	2002	Five-dose series
DTaP	INFANRIX®[b]	6 weeks to 7 years old	1997	
Tetanus toxoid, diphtheria toxoid, and acellular pertussis (Tdap)	Adacel®[c]	10 through 64 years old	2005	
Tdap	Boostrix®[d]	≥10 years and older	2005	
Td	Tenivac®[e]	≥7 years and older	2003	Replaced Decavac, which was discontinued in 2012

Other diphtheria, tetanus, and pertussis combination vaccines

Vaccine contents	Trade name	FDA-approved age indication	Year approved	Notes for use
DT	Generic produced by Sanofi Pasteur[f]	6 weeks through 6 years	1997	five-dose series; pediatric alternative for those that have a contraindication to the pertussis component of DTaP
DTaP + HepB + IPV	Pediarix®[g]	6 weeks through 6 years	2002	three-dose series; combination alternative
DTaP + IPV	Kinrix®[h]	4 to 6 years	2008	Single dose; combination alternative
DTaP + IPV + Hib	Pentacel®[i]	6 weeks through 4 years	2008	four-dose series; combination alternative

[a]Daptacel [Package Insert] [14]
[b]INFANRIX [Package Insert] [15]
[c]Adacel [Package Insert] [16]
[d]BOOSTRIX [Package Insert] [17]
[e]Tenivac [Package Insert] [18]
[f]Diphtheria and Tetanus Toxoids Absorbed [Package Inset] [226]
[g]Pediarix [Package Insert] [317]
[h]Kinrix [Package Insert] [318]
[i]Pentacel [Package Insert] [319]

states, 2 years and 6 years after a five-dose DTaP series, found a 2.5–4-fold increase in relative risk of pertussis 6 years after completion of five-dose DTaP primary series [23]. It is estimated that 90% of children will be susceptible to pertussis 8.5 years after last dose of DTaP series [11].

Both Adacel® and Boostrix® were approved in 2005, as Tdap boosters for adolescents over the age of ten [16, 17]. The estimated efficacy and duration of immunity to Tdap were assessed, with an efficacy of 68.8% after vaccination, declining to 8.9% by 4 or more years [24].

Influenza

Influenza causes millions of illnesses each year in the USA, resulting in thousands of hospitalizations. Depending upon the severity of the influenza season, CDC reports between 3,000 and 49,000 deaths annually from influenza infections. The overall US burden of influenza disease estimated across all age groups during the 2014–2015 season was 40 million flu illnesses, 19 million flu-associated medical visits, and 970,000 flu-associated hospitalizations [25]. Worldwide, seasonal influenza is estimated to cause severe disease in 3–5 million people, leading to 250,000–500,000 deaths annually [26].

There are three antigenic types of influenza: A, B, and C. Influenza A is further subdivided into subtypes by two of its antigenic surface proteins, hemagglutinin and neuraminidase. Influenza A viruses can undergo both antigenic shift and drift, while influenza B viruses only change by antigenic drift [27]. RNA mutations with small antigenic *drifts* occur slowly over time, necessitating the need for an updated annual influenza vaccine. Conversely, antigenic *shift* changes occur abruptly and suddenly, with gene reassortment or exchange resulting in distinct changes to the hemagglutinin and neuraminidase protein antigens. This shift may result in a brand new virulent virus and an influenza epidemic or pandemic. Influenza A is responsible for global influenza pandemics, while influenza B and C are responsible for epidemics of shorter duration. Global pandemics occurred in 1918, 1957, and 2009–2010 (the H1N1, swine flu pandemic), causing millions of deaths; the 1918 influenza A pandemic was responsible for approximately 40–50 million deaths [28].

In the USA, disease caused by influenza typically occurs seasonally, beginning in October, peaking between January and March, and subsiding in early May. In tropical climates, the influenza season may last throughout the year. The influenza virus spreads via large respiratory droplets, primarily through close contact, but the virus can also survive on fomites. The incubation period is 2 days, with a range of 1–4 days. Adults are infectious from 1 day prior to symptom onset through 5–10 days after symptoms begin. Children and immunocompromised hosts have a more prolonged period of continued viral shedding and infectivity. Uncomplicated influenza illness symptoms include abrupt onset of fever, malaise, myalgias, cough, pharyngitis and headache and are typically self-limited, lasting 7–10 days. Presentation may be atypical in children and the elderly. A common complication of influenza infections includes secondary bacterial infections, particularly *Staphylococcus aureus*, *Streptococcus pneumoniae* (*S. pneumoniae*), and *Streptococcus pyogenes*. Other rarer complications include myocarditis, rhabdomyolysis, encephalitis, delirium, and other neuropsychiatric adverse events. In pregnancy, infection can lead to preterm delivery, small-for-gestational-age infants, and fetal death, in addition to maternal complications. Infants, the elderly, and people with chronic conditions are at high risk of influenza-related morbidity and mortality [10].

Influenza Vaccine and Vaccine Efficacy

The first influenza vaccine was approved for military use in the USA in 1945 and civilian use in 1946 [29]. ACIP recommends influenza vaccines for all persons aged 6 months and older. Children under 8 require two doses of influenza vaccine if getting vaccinated for the first time. There are several types of influenza vaccines available. Most are injectable vaccines designed to be injected into the muscle with a needle. There are also injectable vaccines given via a jet injector and intradermal and nasal vaccines. Influenza vaccines are either trivalent (includes two strains of influenza A and one strain influenza B) or quadrivalent (includes two influenza A strains and two influenza B strains). Some vaccines come with adjuvants, and there is one recombinant vaccine that is egg-free. Trivalent vaccines are made to protect against three flu viruses: influenza A H1N1 virus, influenza A H3N2 virus, and one influenza B virus. Quadrivalent vaccines are made to protect against four viruses which include the three viruses found in the trivalent vaccine plus a second influenza B virus [30].

Injectable influenza vaccines include those that are trivalent inactivated vaccines:

- Standard trivalent vaccine for different ages (IIV)

  - One formulation given with a jet injector instead of a needle (for those 18–54)

- High-dose trivalent vaccine (for those 65 and older)
- Recombinant trivalent vaccines (egg-free for those over 18)
- Trivalent made with adjuvant (for those 65 and older)

Injectable influenza vaccines include those that are quadrivalent inactivated vaccines (IIV4):

- Standard quadrivalent vaccine (for different ages)
- An intradermal quadrivalent vaccine (for those 18–64) injected into the skin, not muscle
- Quadrivalent vaccine containing virus grown in cell culture, new 2016 (for those over 4 years)

The quadrivalent nasal spray live attenuated influenza vaccine (LAIV) (for those 2–49 years of age) has been recommended during some flu seasons, but not all.

The influenza vaccine is unique in that it is the only vaccine reformulated annually to confer protection for different viruses each flu season July 1–June 30. Exposure to influenza one season does not confer antibody protection to influenza the following year. In addition to viral changes through antigenic drift and antigenic shift, host factors such as age, medical conditions, prior infections, and prior vaccinations can affect how beneficial the vaccine is to the host [31]. Vaccine effectiveness is measured via the Influenza Vaccine Effectiveness Network, a collaboration among institutions in five geographic locations. Observational studies compare the frequency of influenza illness among vaccinated and unvaccinated people. Patients with respiratory symptoms are tested for influenza, influenza vaccination status is recorded, and vaccine effectiveness is calculated [31]. Influenza vaccine has demonstrated varying degrees of effectiveness year to year. Effectiveness has ranged from 10% to 60% from 2005 through 2016 [32] (Table 4.2).

Table 4.2 Adjusted vaccine effectiveness estimates for influenza seasons from 2005 to 2016

Influenza season[†]	Reference	Study site(s)	No. of patients[‡]	Adjusted overall VE (%)	95% CI
2004–05	[209]	WI	762	10	−36, 40
2005–06	[209]	WI	346	21	−52, 59
2006–07	[209]	WI	871	52	22, 70
2007–08	[210]	WI	1914	37	22, 49
2008–09	Unpublished	WI, MI, NY, TN	6713	41	30, 50
2009–10	[212]	WI, MI, NY, TN	6757	56	23, 75
2010–11	[215]	WI, MI, NY, TN	4757	60	53, 66
2011–12	[214]	WI, MI, PA, TX, WA	4771	47	36, 56
2012–13	[213]	WI, MI, PA, TX, WA	6452	49	43, 55
2013–14	[346]	WI, MI, PA, TX, WA	5999	52	44, 59
2014–15	[347]	WI, MI, PA, TX, WA	9311	19	10, 27
2015–16[a]	ACIP presentation, Flannery [332 kB, 26 pages] [211]	WI, MI, PA, TX, WA	7563	47[a]	39, 53[a]

[a]Estimate from Nov 2, 2015–Apr 15, 2016. http://www.cdc.gov/flu/professionals/vaccination/effectiveness-studies.htm

A high-dose, trivalent, inactivated influenza vaccine was created to improve antibody responses in adults aged 65 and older. Vaccine efficacy studies show that when compared to the standard-dose vaccine, the high-dose vaccine was 24.2% more efficacious than the standard-dose vaccine by inducing a significantly higher antibody response and better protection against laboratory-confirmed influenza [33]. Additional evaluation of this data showed that even when stratifying the efficacy by age, comorbidities, frailty, and the number of conditions, the high-dose vaccine was consistently more efficacious than the standard-dose vaccine irrespective of age and presence/number of comorbid or frailty conditions [34].

Recent studies do not show increased efficacy of the live attenuated influenza vaccine to the inactivated influenza vaccine. No consistent conclusions have been found regarding the use of the live, attenuated influenza vaccine from year to the next [31]. Over the past several years, recommendations to preferentially give the live attenuated vaccine over the killed vaccine to children have been made and retracted, and during the 2016–2017 flu season, no recommendation was made to give live attenuated influenza vaccine.

Polio

Poliomyelitis is a crippling and potentially fatal viral disease caused by three serotypes of the species enterovirus C, of the *Picornaviridae* family. Polio spreads from person to person via the oral-oral or fecal-oral route and replicates in the oral and intestinal mucosa. It has no cure and vaccination is the best protection from the disease. Polio was once considered one of the most feared diseases in the USA: in the early 1950s, polio outbreaks caused more than 15,000 cases of paralysis each year in the USA. After the introduction of the trivalent inactivated poliovirus vaccine (IPV) in 1955 and the trivalent oral poliovirus vaccine (OPV) in 1963, the number of polio cases fell rapidly to less than 100 in the 1960s and fewer than 10 in the 1970s. Since 1979, no cases of polio have originated in the USA, but polio disease has been brought into the country by travelers infected with polio [35].

Most polio disease is asymptomatic: approximately 72 out of 100 infected persons do not have any visible symptoms. The incubation period for the onset of initial symptoms is between 3 and 6 days. Approximately 24% of infected patients experience fever, malaise, nausea and vomiting, sore throat, and headache. Minor illness progresses to severe headache and neck stiffness, typically lasting 2–10 days, and completely resolves. Those that develop more serious symptoms affecting the brain and spinal cord may experience paresthesias, meningitis, and paralysis. Less than 1% of cases of poliomyelitis progress to paralytic polio: when cases do progress, the initial typical mild symptoms appear to resolve before flaccid paralysis rapidly develops. Paralysis can continue to extend for several days, affecting proximal more than distal muscles. In 5–10% of cases of paralytic polio, the respiratory muscles are affected, leading to respiratory insufficiency and death. Some survivors of paralytic polio recover with permanent paralysis, muscle atrophy, and/or skeletal deformities. A noninfectious post-polio syndrome can occur 15–40 years following infection and results in irreversible muscle weakness [35].

Since 1988, the World Health Assembly has been working toward complete eradication of poliovirus from the globe. Recently, worldwide surveillance detected type 1 poliovirus in three countries: Nigeria, Afghanistan, and Pakistan [36]. Until the world is rid of polio, vaccination efforts must continue.

Polio Vaccine and Vaccine Efficacy

The first polio vaccine was created by Dr. Jonas Salk and licensed in 1955. It is an inactivated vaccine, given as an injection, and prevents three strains of polio. The second (live attenuated) polio vaccine licensed for use in the USA was created by Dr. Albert Sabin. It also prevents three strains of polio and is given as an oral vaccine. The Sabin oral poliovirus vaccine (OPV) was given in the USA from 1963 through 2000. Today in the USA, only the Salk inactivated vaccine (IPV) is given, as a four-dose series at 2, 4, and 6–18 months of age and a booster dose at 4–6 years of age. Adult travelers to polio-endemic or high-risk areas of the world are recommended to get a polio booster vaccine. Those persons working in a laboratory and handling specimens that might contain polioviruses and healthcare workers treating patients who could have polio should also be vaccinated. In 1988, study investigators demonstrated at least 99% detectable antibodies to all three types of wild virus following the second dose of the polio vaccine and 99–100% detectable antibody levels after the third dose of IPV [37].

Measles

Measles, also known as morbilli or rubeola, is caused by a single-stranded, enveloped RNA virus with one serotype. Humans are the only natural hosts. Measles is spread by respiratory droplets directly or via aerosolized virus and is one of the most infectious diseases known to man, with 12–18 secondary cases following a single infection. In the decade before the live measles vaccine was licensed in 1963, an average of 549,000 measles cases and 495 measles deaths were reported annually in the USA. As most cases were not reported, it is more likely that an average of 3–4 million people were infected with measles annually during the 1950s. In 2000, measles was declared eliminated from the USA (defined by the absence of endemic measles virus transmission for 12 months or longer). However, measles cases and outbreaks still occur every year in the USA with imported cases of disease affecting susceptible Americans [38]. Healthcare providers should report suspected measles cases to their local health department within 24 h.

Outbreaks of measles virus in temperate regions typically occur in late winter and early spring with epidemics occurring every 2–5 years. Worldwide, prior to routine vaccination, an estimated 130 million cases and 70 million deaths occurred annually secondary to measles. Today, in developed countries, the death rate is less than 0.5% but is nearer 10% in areas with limited healthcare resources. Measles is still endemic in many countries. Of the estimated 20 million people who become infected with measles annually worldwide, over 130,000 people die [38].

The incubation period for measles lasts up to 14 days. After the incubation period, symptoms of fever and the "three C's" (cough, coryza, and conjunctivitis) develop. Pathognomonic small, blue-white lesions of the buccal mucosa known as Koplik's spots appear prior to the onset of rash. The characteristic erythematous, maculopapular rash presents initially on the face and ears and then spreads centrifugally to the trunk and extremities, lasting 3–5 days before becoming confluent prior to resolution. Desquamation may occur. Up to 40% of affected people suffer complications, including diarrhea, secondary viral or bacterial pneumonias, stomatitis, croup, otitis media, keratoconjunctivitis leading to blindness, encephalitis, and death. Infection during pregnancy can lead to severe maternal infection including risk of death, preterm labor, and fetal demise. Subacute sclerosing panencephalitis may present 5–15 years after acute infection in up to 1 in 10,000–100,000 cases, leading to cognitive and motor dysfunction, seizures, and death [10, 39]. Measles can be prevented with measles-containing vaccine administered as the combination measles-mumps-rubella (MMR) vaccine. Vaccination levels of greater than 95% are required to prevent and contain disease outbreaks [39, 40].

Mumps

Mumps, caused by the mumps virus, was once a common childhood condition that is typically self-limited and relatively benign. It is moderately contagious and is spread to the upper respiratory tract through respiratory droplets, direct contact, or fomites and has an incubation period of 15–24 days. Mumps is characterized by unilateral or bilateral non-purulent parotid gland swelling, present in 60–75% of cases. The parotid gland swelling typically occurs after the prodromal phase, characterized by fever, anorexia, malaise, and headache. Central nervous system involvement is common, with over 50% of cases demonstrating elevated white blood cell counts in the cerebrospinal fluid. Between 1 and 10% of patients develop meningitis, which is universally benign and without long-term sequelae. Orchitis is common in postpubertal males with the rare complication of infertility. In pregnancy, especially during the first trimester, spontaneous abortions may occur. Other less common complications of mumps include encephalitis, chronic sensorineural hearing loss, mastitis, pancreatitis, EKG abnormalities, and joint involvement. Prior to routine vaccination, nearly all people were infected with mumps by adolescence, with peak incidences occurring in winter and spring. Vaccination has reduced rates of infection in the USA by 99%. Today, incidences have been reported around 300 per 100,000 annually, but underreporting of infection is suspected. Recent outbreaks have occurred in populations with routine mumps vaccination. Outbreaks are suspected to be secondary to insufficient immunization to reach herd immunity threshold as well as waning immunity of MMR vaccination. Outbreaks typically involve adolescents and adults, who experience higher levels of complications than children [10, 41].

Rubella

Rubella, or German measles, and congenital rubella syndrome (CRS) are caused by the rubella virus, an enveloped, positive-stranded RNA virus classified as a *Rubivirus* in the *Togaviridae* family [42]. There is no treatment to cure rubella. Outbreaks usually occur in the spring, while epidemics occur in cycles ranging from 3 to 9 years. Before the rubella vaccine was licensed in the USA in 1969, rubella was a common disease, occurring primarily among young children. Rubella incidence has decreased by more than 99% from the pre-vaccine era and was deemed eliminated from the USA in 2004 [42].

Rubella is spread via the respiratory route and is moderately contagious. Humans are the only natural hosts. Disease is typically benign and self-limited and most prevalent in children and young adults. Symptoms include a generalized erythematous, maculopapular rash, mild fever, and lymphadenopathy. The average incubation period of rubella virus is 17 days with a range of 12–23 days. People infected with rubella are most contagious when the rash is erupting, but can be contagious from 7 days prior to rash development and up to 7 days after rash development [42]. Rubella complications include arthritis, encephalitis, and thrombocytopenia. CRS is a devastating illness affecting infants exposed to rubella in utero. Maternal viremia leads to placental and fetal infection, and spontaneous abortion may result early in the pregnancy. Clinical sequelae in surviving infants include encephalitis, microcephaly and mental retardation, autism, cochlear deafness, cataracts, and cardiac conditions. Neonates may have characteristic "blueberry muffin" lesions as a result of dermal erythropoiesis, interstitial pneumonitis, and hepatosplenomegaly. Following widespread vaccination in the Americas and Europe, current data suggests less than two cases of CRS per 100,000 live births. Unfortunately, rubella and CRS remain endemic in many areas of the world, with the annual global incidence of CRS of greater than 100,000 [43].

MMR Vaccine and Vaccine Efficacy

The measles, mumps, rubella vaccine (MMR, M-M-R® II,) was licensed in 1971 as a live combination vaccine against measles, mumps, and rubella viruses [52]. Today, the vaccine contains a more attenuated measles virus from Enders' attenuated Edmonston strain [53]. Current ACIP recommendation is a two-dose series MMR for children at 12–15 months of age and at 4–6 years of age (may be given earlier, if at least 28 days after the first dose). Some infants traveling out of the country should get a dose of MMR before 12 months of age, and this dose will not count toward their routine series. Adults born before 1957 are generally considered immune to measles, mumps, and rubella and do need the MMR vaccine. Adults born after 1956 who were never vaccinated, and who never had the three disease, are recommended to get the MMR vaccine. Children between 1 and 12 years of age can get a combination quadrivalent measles, mumps, rubella, and varicella vaccine (MMRV, ProQuad®).

Vaccine effectiveness in the prevention of measles after one dose of MMR vaccine in recipients greater than 1 year of age, ranged from 87% to 97% in studies conducted in the USA from 1972 to 1986 [44]. In 1989, ACIP recommended that the routine vaccination schedule be increased from a one-dose to a two-dose schedule after major measles outbreaks occurred in the previous years (including outbreaks in schools with greater than 98% vaccination rates) [45]. Vaccine effectiveness from a 1994 outbreak at an elementary school was approximated at 92% in those children having received one dose of MMR and 100% in those with two doses [46]. Increased effectiveness of patients receiving two doses versus only one dose has been subsequently proven in other outbreaks [47, 48], and the two-dose MMR series has been shown to maintain protection from measles for up to 10 years after the second dose of MMR [49].

The first single live mumps virus vaccine, Mumpsvax®, containing mumps virus from the Jeryl Lynn™ (B level) strain, was licensed in the USA in 1967. This is still the same viral strain used in the current MMR vaccine [13, 50]. Vaccine efficacy against mumps, based on antibody titers, was 95.6% in 5 months after vaccination [51]. Post initiation of MMR vaccine, incidence of mumps rapidly declined in the USA by 98%, from 152,209 cases in 1968 to 2982 cases in 1985 [52]. Clinical efficacy reported from 1985 to 1988 varied from 70 to 91% during the one-dose MMR era [53–55]. After the ACIP recommendation to increase MMR vaccination to a two-dose series, vaccine effectiveness was calculated using data from a 2005 mumps outbreak: vaccine efficacy was 91.6% for those individuals with two doses of MMR (53%) compared to 79.7% with one dose (32%) [56]. Another study using data from a 2006 mumps outbreak determined vaccine effectiveness to be 76–88% for those with two doses of MMR when compared to those with one dose. Of those individuals who had received a two-dose vaccination series, but still contracted mumps, 74–79% of them had received their second dose greater than 10 years prior [57]. Thus the potential benefit of a third dose of MMR during an outbreak has been investigated: a 75.6% reduction in mumps attack rate was seen in those subjects that received a third dose [58]. It remains to be seen whether mumps booster recommendations will change.

The first single, live rubella virus vaccine, Meruvax® II, containing the Wistar RA 27/3 rubella strain, was licensed in the USA in 1979 and is the same viral strain used in the current MMR vaccine [13, 59]. Vaccine efficacy with monovalent rubella vaccine after one dose of the 27/3 strain was historically high, at greater than 95% [60]. The duration of protection from the 27/3 strain, defined by presence of antibodies, was detected at decreasing levels up to 16 years after vaccination. [61]

WHO cites development of rubella antibodies in 95–100% of susceptible persons aged ≥12 months after a single dose of the MMR vaccine, and in outbreak situations, the effectiveness of different rubella vaccines has been estimated at 90–100% [62].

Hepatitis B

Hepatitis B virus (HBV) causes hepatitis B liver infection, the most common viral infection worldwide. There are an estimated 2 billion people infected with HBV and 350 million chronic carriers of HBV worldwide. Over 500,000 people die each year of hepatitis B or its complications [63]. In the USA, 850,000–2.2 million persons are estimated to be living with HBV infection. HBV is transmitted through percutaneous or mucosal exposure to blood or body fluids of an infected person, such as from an infected mother to her newborn during childbirth, through close personal contact within households, through unscreened blood transfusions or unsafe injections in healthcare settings, through injection drug use, and from sexual contact with an infected person. Adults with diabetes are at an increased risk of acquiring HBV infection if they share diabetes-care equipment such as blood glucose meters, finger-stick devices, syringes, and/or insulin pens [64].

In acute HBV infection, nearly all children and up to 70% of adults are asymptomatic. Some acute infections lead to chronic infections and long-term complications. The risk of progression to chronic HBV infection is inversely proportional to age of disease acquisition. While more than 90% of vertically transmitted perinatal infections lead to a chronic carriage state, more than 90% of infections in adolescence or adulthood resolve spontaneously. Chronic HBV infection may lead to hepatocellular hepatic cirrhosis or hepatocellular carcinoma (HCC). Nearly 25% of people infected in childhood will progress to develop cirrhosis or HCC [10]. Half of the total cases and nearly all childhood cases of HCC are related to chronic HBV infection [65, 66]. Vaccination against HBV has been successful in reducing infection with HBV and its complications, including a significant decline in HCC [67].

When present, symptoms of hepatitis B include anorexia, nausea and vomiting, abdominal pain, malaise, and jaundice, lasting for days to weeks. These may not appear for up to 6 months after the time of infection. Extrahepatic manifestations include arthralgias, macular rashes, and glomerulonephritis. More rarely, fulminant hepatitis may occur with rapidly progressive symptoms and death without immediate interventions.

Unvaccinated adults account for 95% of new HBV infection. Persistent attention to vaccination status of adults, especially those with high-risk behaviors, should remain as an area of focus among healthcare professionals [68, 69]. With the initiation of universal childhood hepatitis B (HepB) vaccination starting in 1991, rates of acute hepatitis B in vaccinated children and adolescents decreased by 94%. Furthermore, infant HepB vaccination decreases perinatal transmission in infants born to HBV-infected mothers. Combined administration of HepB vaccine and hepatitis B immunoglobulin within 12 h of birth provides 94% efficacy in preventing vertical transmission in infants born to HBV-infected mothers. Administration of the complete HepB vaccination series along with immunoglobulin is vital for these infants, as the infection rate is 6.7% among infants with less than three doses of vaccine compared to 1.1% in those with complete series [70].

Hepatitis B Vaccine and Vaccine Efficacy

HepB vaccination is given as three or four doses over a 6-month period and is recommended for:

- All infants, starting with the first dose within 24 h of birth, series completed by 6–18 months of age
- All children and adolescents younger than 19 years old not already vaccinated
- People whose sex partners have hepatitis B
- Sexually active persons not in a long-term, mutually monogamous relationship
- Persons seeking evaluation or treatment of a sexually transmitted disease
- Men who have sex with men
- People who share needles, syringes, or other drug injection equipment
- People in close household contact with someone infected with HBV
- Healthcare workers and public safety workers at risk for exposure to body fluids
- People with end-stage renal disease
- Residents and staff of facilities for the developmentally disabled
- Travelers to regions with moderate or high rates of HBV infection
- People with chronic liver disease or chronic kidney disease
- People with HIV
- People with diabetes ages 19–59, consider for those over 60
- Persons in correctional facilities
- Anyone who wishes to be protected from hepatitis B

The first vaccine to protect against hepatitis B was human plasma derived and licensed in 1981 [71]. However, it was later discontinued due to public concern for potential HIV transmission despite studies verifying the safety of the vaccine and no documented cases of HIV transmission [72]. Recombivax HB® was licensed in 1986 as a genetically engineered recombinant vaccine to satisfy the fears of potential disease transfer from plasma-derived vaccines. A few years later, Engerix-B® was licensed in 1989 for the prevention of infection by all subtypes of HBV [1, 73, 74]. Either recombinant vaccine conveys a 95–100% seroprotective rate in vaccinated children [75]. A three-dose vaccination series is recommended, and efficacy is not altered if vaccine brands are interchanged during the series [76]. A 2009 study found that 60% of individuals had sufficient immunity 22 years after the primary vaccine series [77]. Booster doses after the primary series completion are not currently recommended. Combined hepatitis A (HepA) and HepB vaccines indicate

118

Table 4.3 Available hepatitis B vaccines

Vaccine contents/ abbreviation	Trade name	Year licensed	FDA-approved age indication	Volume of dose (mL)	Dose series
HepB	Engerix-B®[a]	1989	Birth through 19 years	0.5	3 doses: at 0, 1, and 6 months of age
			20 years and older	1	3 doses: at 0, 1, and 6 months of age
HepB	Recombivax HB®[b]	1983	Birth through 19 years	0.5	3 doses: at 0, 1, and 6 months of age
			11 years through 15 years		3 doses: at 0, 1, and 6 months of age
			11 years through 15 years	1	2 doses: at 0, 4–6 months
			20 years and older		3 doses: at 0, 1, and 6 months of age
HepA + HepB	Twinrix®[c]	2001	18 years and older	1	3 doses (standard): at 0, 1, and 6 months of age
					4 doses (accelerated): at 0, 7, and 21–30 days, followed by a booster dose at month 12
DTaP + HepB + IPV	Pediarix®[d]	2002	6 weeks through 6 years	0.5	3 doses: at 2, 4, and 6 months of age

[a]Engerix-B [Package Insert] [1]
[b]RECOMBIVAX HD [Package Insert] [73]
[c]TWINRIX [Package Insert]. [Internet] [110]
[d]Pediarix [Package Inset] [Internet] [317]

similar rates of immune response to both anti-HAV and anti-HBV when compared to monovalent vaccines [78].

The following vaccines are available to protect against hepatitis B (Table 4.3):

• Recombivax HB®, licensed in 1983, and Engerix-B®, licensed in 1989, are recombinant HepB vaccines given as three-dose series, at birth, 1–2 months, and 6–18 months of age.
• Twinrix® is a combined HepA (inactivated) and HepB (recombinant) vaccine licensed in 2001 for persons 18 years and older against disease caused by HAV and HBV given as a three-dose series at 0, 1, and 6 months of age.
• Pediarix® (DTap-IPV-HepB) licensed in 2002 is a combined diphtheria and tetanus toxoids and acellular pertussis adsorbed, recombinant hepatitis B, and inactivated poliovirus vaccine given as a three-dose series at 2, 4, and 6 months of age.

Haemophilus influenzae

Haemophilus influenzae is a type of bacteria that mainly causes illness in infants and young children, and is the leading cause of a variety of invasive infections in children. There are six identifiable types of *H. influenzae* bacteria (a through f) and other non-identifiable (nontypeable) types [79]. Much invasive *H. influenzae* disease is caused by the encapsulated type b serotype (Hib), which can cause ear infections, meningitis, epiglottitis, cellulitis, septic arthritis, pneumonia, and bacteremia. Between 3% and 6% of Hib cases in children are fatal; up to 20% of patients who survive Hib meningitis have permanent hearing loss or other long-term neurological sequelae. Patients 65 years of age and older with invasive Hib disease have higher case fatality ratios than children and young adults [79].

Prior to introduction of Hib vaccination, Hib was a frequent nasopharyngeal colonizer in infants and preschool children, serving as a reservoir for transmission of the disease among children and their daycare or household contacts. Incidence of invasive disease was greater than 300 per 100,000 children, with most invasive disease occurring in children under the age of 5. Today, there are fewer than 1 case per 100,000 children under age 5 in the USA [89, 90].

Haemophilus influenzae *Vaccine and Vaccine Efficacy*

The introduction of conjugate vaccines against Hib in 1988 resulted in a rapid decline of disease over a brief period compared to other vaccines [80]. Several brands of Hib vaccine are available, and depending on which vaccine is used, a child is recommended to receive either three or four doses at 2, 4, and 6 months of age (6-month dose may not be necessary depending on brand of vaccine) and a booster dose at 12–15 months of age. Healthy adults and children over 5 years of age are not recommended to receive the Hib vaccine. However, it is recommended for children and adults with special conditions such as asplenia or sickle cell disease, presurgical splenectomy, following a bone marrow transplant, or for those with HIV.

There are currently three monovalent Hib vaccines available in the USA, differing by the protein conjugate. PedvaxHIB® was the first of the currently available vaccines approved in 1989 and is conjugated to an outer membrane protein complex of the B11 strain of *Neisseria meningitidis* serogroup B [81]. ActHIB® and Hiberix® were approved in 1993 and 2009, respectively, and are conjugated to tetanus toxoid [82, 83]. The antibody response after three doses of PedvaxHIB® or ActHIB® is similar, 88% and 97%, respectively [84]. Hiberix® was initially approved as a booster dose in the Hib series (prior to fifth birthday), after completion of the primary series [85]. Immunogenicity of Hiberix® was established via a noninferiority study, meeting minimal protective antibody levels [83]. The incidence of *Haemophilus influenzae* invasive disease in children under 5 years old decreased by 97% during the decade of 1987–1997 [86].

Varicella Zoster Virus: Chicken Pox

Varicella zoster virus (VZV) is the human herpesvirus responsible for causing the highly contagious disease varicella (chicken pox), as well as herpes zoster (shingles). Varicella results after primary infection with VZV, which then stays in the body in the sensory nerve ganglia as a latent infection. Reactivation of latent infection causes herpes zoster. The incubation period for varicella is 14–16 days after exposure to varicella or a herpes zoster rash, with a range of 10–21 days [87]. VZV is spread primarily through the respiratory route, but can also be contracted through direct contact with skin lesions, or across a mother's placenta. The rash of varicella is generalized and present in varying stages of development progressing from macules to papules to vesicles before crusting. The rash usually appears first on the head, chest, and back and then spreads to the rest of the body. Infection is generally benign and self-limiting. Serious complications include bacterial superinfection, cellulitis, pneumonitis, meningoencephalitis, and stroke. Severe complications are more common when primary infection occurs in adulthood. Congenital varicella syndrome (CVS) is a rare disorder that affects infants born to mothers infected with varicella during the first 20 weeks of pregnancy. Newborns may show skin lesions, limb abnormalities, chorioretinitis, microcephaly, and cognitive impairment. If CVS develops within the final days before delivery, or within a day or two afterward, there is a risk of neonatal varicella, which carries a mortality rate as high as 30% [10, 88].

Prior to the availability of VZV vaccination, mortality rates secondary to varicella infection were 0.41 per 100,000 in the USA, with a hospitalization rate of 2.7 per 100,000. Vaccination has significantly decreased those rates to 0.14 and 0.6, respectively [89]. Additionally, varicella outbreaks confer high financial costs to society with vaccination saving money. Compared to no vaccination program, the US varicella vaccination program results in societal cost savings of over $0.9 billion dollars [90].

Varicella Zoster: Chicken Pox Vaccine and Vaccine Efficacy

Varivax® was licensed in 1995 initially as a single dose, live attenuated varicella virus vaccine [91]. Children who have never had chicken pox are recommended to get two doses of varicella vaccine at 12–15 months of age and again at 4–6 years of age (may be given earlier, if at least 3 months after the first dose). People 13 years of age and older who have never had chicken pox or received the vaccine are recommended to get two doses at least 28 days apart. Varivax® demonstrated 100% efficacy 9 months postvaccination, in healthy naïve recipients aged 1–14 years [92]. Long-term efficacy was demonstrated to be 96% after a second varicella season and 95.1% after 7 years [93]. Since routine varicella vaccination started in the USA, several post licensure efficacy studies have demonstrated varied efficacy. Vaccine effectiveness after one dose varies depending on categorization of varicella severity and clinical or lab diagnosis [94]. A 2004 study reported vaccine efficacy of 97% one year postvaccination, declining to 86% after two years and 81% after eight years [95]. In June 2007, ACIP recommended a second varicella dose between ages 4 and 6 years [96]. Efficacy following two doses of varicella was calculated at 98.3% compared to 86% following one dose of varicella in children 4 years and older [97]. Unfortunately, despite improved vaccine efficacy after two doses, outbreaks are still reported, but with less impact. The impact of the two-dose varicella vaccination program has resulted in a 60% reduction in outpatient visits and a 38% reduction in hospitalizations [98]. MMRV (ProQuad® licensed in 2005), a combination vaccine containing both varicella and MMR vaccines, may be given to persons 12 years of age and younger. MMRV was found to be noninferior to MMR® II and Varivax® [99].

Hepatitis A

The *Hepatitis A virus* (HAV) causes hepatitis A liver infection, an acute, usually self-limited viral illness in children, but a potentially more serious infection in adults. In children under age 6, infection with HAV is usually asymptomatic or produces mild symptoms. Adults may experience more severe symptoms that include fever, malaise, nausea, vomiting, abdominal pain, jaundice, and, rarely, acute fulminant hepatitis. The risk of jaundice and other severe symptoms increases with age. Up to 10% of infected patients may have a relapsing course lasting up to 6 months. Unlike infections with hepatitis B and C, HAV infection does not lead to chronic liver infections. Worldwide, HAV is responsible for over 1 million cases of acute hepatitis annually, leading to 35,000 deaths [10, 100, 101]. In the USA, the number of Hepatitis A cases reported has declined from 1670 reported cases in 2010 to 1239 reported cases in 2014 [102].

HAV is transmitted through the fecal-oral route, through close person-to-person transmission, and during foodborne outbreaks. The average incubation period for hepatitis A is 28 days (range 15–50 days) [103]. In 1996, ACIP recommended HepA vaccination only to those persons at high risk for the disease, but by 1999, the recommendations were expanded to include children living in 11 states with average hepatitis A rates of over 20 cases per 100,000 population. In 2006, ACIP recommendations again expanded to include routine vaccination of all children at 1 year of age and older in all 50 states.

Hepatitis A Vaccine and Vaccine Efficacy

Hep A inactivated vaccine is given as a two-dose series given over 6 months for children and adults. A combined HepA and HepB vaccine is available for adults 18 years of age and older, given in a three-dose series over 6 months. HepA vaccination is recommended for:

- All children aged 12 months or older
- Travelers to certain countries
- Family members or caregivers of a recent adoptee from countries where hepatitis A is common
- Men who have sex with men
- Users of injection and non-injection illegal drugs
- People with chronic liver disease
- People treated with clotting factor concentrates
- People who work with HAV-infected animals or in a HAV research lab

There are currently three vaccines available to immunize against hepatitis A: two inactivated monovalent vaccines and one combination vaccine (Table 4.4).

Havrix® was licensed in 1995 initially for persons 2–18 years of age, and Vaqta® was licensed in 1996 for persons 2–17 years of age for prevention of disease caused by HAV [104, 105]. The two inactivated monovalent HepA vaccines were compared in an open-label randomized trial. They were shown to be similar in rapid serial conversion rates after the primary dose as well as demonstrating equivalent immunogenicity after one booster dose [106]. Two studies examining the vaccine efficacy over time found lasting antibody concentrations 17 years after primary vaccination series and seropositive protection rates greater than 95% after 25 years [107, 108]. Success of the HepA vaccine is illustrated by the 96.6% decrease in reported hepatitis A disease from 1996 to 2011 [109]. With recent increases in hepatitis A cases in adults over the age of 40, future vaccination efforts may need to focus on this older population [109].

Twinrix®, a combined HepA (inactivated) and HepB (recombinant) vaccine, was licensed in 2001 for persons 18 years of age and older against disease caused

Table 4.4 Available hepatitis A vaccines

Vaccine contents/abbreviation	Trade name	FDA-approved age indication	Volume of dose	Number of doses in series
HepA	Havrix®[a]	12 months through 18 years old	0.5 mL	Two
		19 years and older	1 mL	
HepA	Vaqta®[b]	12 months through 18 years old	0.5 mL	Two
		19 years and older	1 mL	
HepB + HepA	Twinrix®[c]	18 years and older	1 mL	Three

[a] Havrix [104]
[b] Vaqta [Package Insert] [105]
[c] TWINRIX [Package Insert]. [Internet] [110]

by HAV and HBV as a three-dose series at 0, 1, and 6 months [110]. Efficacy trials indicate similar rates of immune response to both anti-HAV and anti-HBV when compared to monovalent vaccines [111].

Rotavirus

Rotavirus is a contagious virus that causes acute, severe gastroenteritis and is the leading cause of gastroenteritis in infants and children worldwide. Rotavirus infects the proximal small intestine, producing an enterotoxin that destroys the epithelial surface, resulting in blunted villi, extensive damage, and shedding of massive quantities of virus in the stool. Spread is common within families [112]. Nearly every US child who is not vaccinated against rotavirus as an infant is expected to be infected with rotavirus within the first year of life. In developing countries, rotavirus gastroenteritis is responsible for approximately half a million deaths per year among children less than 5 years of age [113]. During the 1990s and early 2000s, rotavirus resulted in approximately 410,000 physician visits, 205,000–272,000 emergency department visits, and 55,000–70,000 hospitalizations among US infants and children, with total annual direct and indirect costs of approximately $1 billion [112].

Rotavirus is spread through the fecal-oral route, through person-to-person contact, and through fomites [114]. Risk factors associated with increased risk for hospitalization for infants include lack of breastfeeding, low birth weight, daycare attendance, the presence of another child less than 24 months of age in the household, and either having Medicaid insurance or having no medical insurance [115]. The incubation period for rotavirus gastroenteritis is 1–3 days. Reinfection occurs up to five times in the first 2 years of life, but severity of disease decreases with each subsequent infection. Peak incidence of infection occurs at 4–23 months of age. Symptoms include vomiting, followed by profuse and watery diarrhea that may lead to dehydration and electrolyte disturbances. Neurologic symptoms include encephalopathy, encephalitis, or seizures. Without supportive medical treatment, rotavirus can be deadly in children [116].

Since initiating regular vaccination, the USA has seen reductions in rotavirus activity ranging from 50 to 90%. Hospitalizations due to rotavirus acute gastroenteritis have declined by 50–90%, with all-cause acute gastroenteritis hospitalizations decreasing by 30–60% [117].

Rotavirus Vaccine and Vaccine Efficacy

Two rotavirus vaccines currently licensed for use in infants in the USA are recommended for either a two- or three-dose series between the ages of 2 months and 6 months, depending on the brand. Both vaccines are given orally, and the first dose of either vaccine is most effective if given before a infant is 15 weeks of age. All infants should receive all doses of rotavirus vaccine before they turn 8 months old [118].

In 2006, RotaTeq® (RV5) was licensed as a pentavalent, oral, live three-dose vaccine series, and in 2008, Rotarix® (RV1) was licensed as a monovalent, oral, live two-dose vaccine series against rotavirus [13, 119]. The Rotavirus Efficacy and Safety Trial (REST) demonstrated RV5 had 98% efficacy against severe rotavirus gastroenteritis in the first season after immunization and sustained efficacy at 88% after the second rotavirus season, lasting for 3.1 years after the last vaccine dose. An 86% decrease in clinic visits and a 95.8% reduction in hospitalizations due rotavirus gastroenteritis were also shown. An extension trial of REST determined sustained efficacy of RV5 up to 3.1 years after the last dose of vaccine [120, 121]. Another study, the human rotavirus study, revealed RV1 had 84.7% efficacy against severe rotavirus gastroenteritis within the first year of life and hospitalization was avoided in 84% of vaccine recipients [122]. Moreover, RV1 demonstrated 90.4% efficacy against severe episodes after the second consecutive rotavirus season [123]. In addition, it is estimated that the societal cost savings of the complete vaccine series of RotaTeq® and Rotarix® are nearly 60 million dollars [124].

Pneumococcal Infections

Streptococcus pneumoniae (*S. pneumoniae*), or pneumococcus, is a common bacterial cause of otitis media, sinusitis, community-acquired pneumonia, and septicemia. The World Health Organization (WHO) estimates that *S. pneumoniae* kills close to half a million children under 5 years of age worldwide every year, with most deaths occurring in developing countries. Children younger than 2 years old, adults 65 years or older, and adults 19–64 years old with certain medical conditions or risk factors are at increased risk for pneumococcal disease. In the USA, prior to 2000, pneumococcal disease caused more than 700 cases of meningitis, 13,000 cases of septicemia, 5 million ear infections, and 200 deaths in children under the age of 5. Since the advent of a pneumococcal vaccine in 2000, severe pneumococcal disease has fallen by 88% in children [125].

Transmission of pneumococcal bacteria is through direct contact with respiratory secretions like saliva or mucus [126]. Asymptomatic nasopharyngeal carriage of pneumococcal serotypes is common in infants and children, especially in those who attend daycares or are exposed to overcrowded living situations [127]. Adults living with children may also be asymptomatic carriers. Disease is usually episodic, however, person-to-person transmission can occur via respiratory droplets.

The more severe clinical syndromes of pneumococcal disease result in pneumonia, bacteremia, and meningitis. *S. pneumoniae* is the most common clinical presentation of pneumococcal disease among adults and is one of the most frequent causes of community-acquired pneumonia. CDC estimates that as many as 400,000 hospitalizations from pneumococcal pneumonia occur annually in the USA. Bacteremia occurs in up to 25–30% of patients with a case fatality rate of 5–7%, higher among the elderly. Symptoms of pneumococcal pneumonia include an abrupt onset of fever and chills or rigors after a short incubation period of 1–3 days. Typically, there is only a single rigor without repeated shaking chills. Other complications of pneumococcal pneumonia include empyema, pericarditis, and respiratory failure. Children with pneumococcal pneumonia often show tachypnea, retractions, and other symptoms of respiratory distress [128].

Invasive pneumococcal disease can also present initially as bacteremia, sepsis, and meningitis, without pneumonia occurring first. Among children 2 years of age and younger, bacteremia without a known site of infection is the most common invasive clinical presentation of pneumococcal infection, accounting for approximately 70% of invasive disease in this age group [125]. More than 12,000 cases of pneumococcal bacteremia occur each year with an overall case fatality rate of about 20%, or as high as 60% among elderly patients. Patients with asplenia who develop bacteremia may experience a fulminant clinical course. Estimates of invasive pneumococcal disease are 15–30 per 100,000 people per year in developed countries [128].

Furthermore, pneumococci cause over 50% of all cases of bacterial meningitis in the USA with an estimated 3000–6000 cases occurring each year [128]. Meningitis presents classically with fever, headache, and nuchal rigidity and can rapidly progress to obtundation and death. Fatality rates in children are currently less than 10% with appropriate antibiotic therapy, however, long-term sequelae including sensorineural hearing loss, seizures, motor dysfunction, and cognitive impairment occur in 20–50% of survivors. In the USA, invasive disease incidence in children under 5 decreased from 95 per 100,000 to 22–25 per 100,000 between 1999 and 2002, and rates continue to decline [129].

Pneumococcal Vaccines and Their Efficacies

There are currently two types of pneumococcal vaccines: pneumococcal conjugate vaccine (PCV13 or Prevnar 13®) and pneumococcal polysaccharide vaccine (PPSV23 or Pneumovax®). There are age-based as well as disease-based recommendations for the vaccines. (See https://www.cdc.gov/vaccines/vpd/pneumo/hcp/recommendations.html for full dosing recommendations.)

PCV13 is a 13-valent protein conjugate vaccine recommended for all children under 5 years of age, all adults 65 years or older, and people 6 years or older with certain risk factors.

PCV13 vaccine is recommended for:

- Infants and children younger than 2 years old in four-dose series at 2, 4, 6, and 12–15 months.
- Children 2–5 years (to receive one dose) with the following medical conditions such as the following:

  - Sickle cell disease
  - A damaged spleen or no spleen
  - Cochlear implant(s)

- Cerebrospinal fluid (CSF) leaks
- HIV/AIDS or other immunocompromising diseases such as diabetes, cancer, or liver disease
- Chronic heart or lung disease
- Who take medications that affect the immune system such as chemotherapy or steroids

- Adults 19 years or older (to receive one dose) with conditions that weaken the immune system such as HIV infection, organ transplantation, leukemia, lymphoma, and severe kidney disease.
- Children 6–18 years of age (to receive one dose) with certain medical conditions such as sickle cell disease, HIV, other immunocompromising conditions, cochlear implant, or CSF leaks who have not previously received PCV13 regardless of whether they have previously received the PCV7 (Prevnar®) or the PPSV23 should receive one dose PCV13.
- Children who are unvaccinated or have not completed the PCV series should get the vaccine (the number of doses recommended and the intervals between them will depend on the child's age when vaccination begins).
- PCV13 may be given at the same time as other vaccines, but it should not be given with PPSV23 nor with the meningococcal conjugate vaccines.

PPSV23 is a 23-valent polysaccharide vaccine recommended for all adults who are ≥65 years of age and for people 2–64 years of age who are at high risk for pneumococcal disease.

PPSV23 vaccine is recommended for:

- All adults ≥65 years
- Anyone 2–64 years of age or has a long-term health problem such as heart disease, lung disease, sickle cell disease, diabetes, alcoholism, cirrhosis, CSF leaks, or cochlear implant
- Anyone 2–64 years of age who has a disease or condition that lowers the body's resistance to infection such as long-term steroids, certain cancer drugs, and radiation therapy
- Any adult 19–64 years of age who is a smoker or has asthma

The PCV13 vaccine replaced the previously recommended 7-valent Prevnar® vaccine in 2010 [130]. Five additional serotypes added to the 7-valent vaccine provide protection against 61% of invasive pneumococcal disease strains [131]. Four doses of PCV13 are recommended to elicit the greatest antibody response to the greatest number of serotypes [130]. A meta-analysis of pneumococcal vaccination in children less than 24 months demonstrated an efficacy of 63–74% against invasive pneumococcal disease, 29% against otitis media, and 6–7% against clinical pneumonia for all serotypes. Due to the high burden of disease, even a low vaccine efficacy for otitis media and clinical pneumonia can result in a great impact overall [132].

The pneumococcal polysaccharide vaccine (PPV23) contains 23 of the strains that account for 85–90% of invasive pneumococcal disease cases. In studying and evaluating many studies, it is difficult to assess the efficacy and effectiveness of PPV23 due to the low frequency of invasive infection, inaccuracy of diagnostic criteria for pneumococcal pneumonia, and poor study methodologies. CDC reports effectiveness in case-control studies ranging from 56–81% against invasive disease [133].

Meningococcal Infections

Neisseria meningitidis (*N. meningitidis*) is the bacterial pathogen responsible for meningococcal diseases, caused by six of its 12 serogroups: A, B, C, W, X, and Y. Rates of disease range from 0.6 to 34% and are highest in children younger than 1 year and in adolescents and young adults aged 16 through 23 years, especially those living in overcrowded conditions such as military barracks and college dormitories. Approximately 500,000 cases of meningococcal disease occur annually, with the majority in the winter and fall. Serogroups B, C, and Y cause most of the illness seen in the USA, and serogroup A causes disease in developing countries and in what is known as the "meningitis belt" of sub-Saharan Africa. Nearly all invasive *N. meningitidis* organisms are encapsulated by a polysaccharide capsule. Rates of meningococcal disease have been declining in the USA since the late 1990s [134].

Transmission of *N. meningitidis* occurs through respiratory droplets in close person-to-person contact and exchange of respiratory and throat secretions (saliva or spit). About one in ten people are asymptomatic carriers of *N. meningitidis* in their posterior nasopharynx. Without treatment, the case fatality rate of *Neisseria* bacterial meningitis can be as high as 70%, and one in five survivors may be left with permanent sequelae including hearing loss, developmental delay, neurologic disability, and limb amputation [135]. Clinically, after an incubation period of 1–10 days, meningococcal infections have an abrupt onset of nonspecific symptoms including fever, chills, and malaise which can lead to meningococcal meningitis (50% of cases) and septicemia or bacteremia (35–40% of cases). A macular, maculopapular, petechial, or purpuric rash is classically present with meningococcemia. Meningococcal disease is a reportable condition in all states, and state and local health departments will conduct investigations when disease is reported to ensure all close contacts are provided prophylaxis [134].

Meningococcal Vaccines and Vaccine Efficacies

Meningococcal vaccines help protect against all three serogroups of meningococcal disease seen most commonly in the USA: serogroups B, C, and Y. There are three kinds of vaccines available in the USA:

- Meningococcal conjugate vaccine (Menactra®, MenHibrix®, and Menveo®)
- Meningococcal polysaccharide vaccine (Menomune®)
- Serogroup B meningococcal vaccine (Bexsero® and Trumenba®)

All 11–12-year-olds should be vaccinated with a single dose of a quadrivalent meningococcal conjugate vaccine (Menactra® or Menveo®). A booster dose is recommended at age 16.

Teens and young adults (16–23 years of age) may also be vaccinated with a serogroup B meningococcal vaccine (Bexsero® or Trumenba®), preferably at 16–18 years of age. Two-three doses are needed depending on the brand. Preteens, teens, and young adults should be vaccinated with a serogroup B meningococcal vaccine if they are identified as being at increased risk of meningococcal disease with certain medical condition such as asplenia, having complement component deficiency, and being infected with HIV (Table 4.5).

Menomune® (MPSV4) was the first tetravalent (serogroups A, C, Y, W-135) polysaccharide vaccine licensed for use in 1981 [13]. The immunogenicity and clinical efficacy of MPSV4 among the four serogroups varies across ages. In adults, MPSV4 demonstrated seropositive conversion to serogroup A (95%), serogroup C (100%), and serogroup W-135 (93%) [136]. Serogroup C is poorly immunogenic in children under 18–24 months, while serogroup A component elicits a comparable adult-like response by 4–5 years [137].

Vaccine efficacy was demonstrated to be 85% in subjects 2–29 years [138]. Antibody response to serogroup A and C in children quickly declined to near levels of unimmunized children between booster doses up until 66 months of age [139]. In adults, protective antibody concentrations against serogroup A and C lasted for 10 years [140]. The poor immunogenicity and rapid decline of antibody response to MPSV4 led to the development of conjugated polysaccharide vaccines.

Menactra® was the first conjugate tetravalent (serogroups A, C, Y, W-135) polysaccharide vaccine approved in 2005 for use in ages 9 months to 55 years old [141]. Menactra® licensure was granted via demonstration of noninferior immunogenicity as compared to MPSV4 [137]. In subjects aged 2–10 and 11–18 years, the immunogenicity of Menactra® compared to MPSV4 was higher one month after the first vaccination and remained higher three years after primary vaccination [142, 143]. Conversely, in subjects aged 18–55 years, the percentage of subjects with protective antibody levels was higher in the MPSV4 group than the Menactra® group; however, noninferiority was still established [137].

Menveo®, a second conjugate tetravalent polysaccharide vaccine, was approved in 2010, initially for ages 11–55 years old [13]. For subjects aged 11–17 and 19–55, Menveo® had significantly greater antibody levels for all four serogroups compared to MPSV4 one month after vaccination, and higher levels were maintained 12 months after vaccination (exception serogroup A) [144]. Menveo® has also demonstrated to be noninferior to Menactra® across all four serogroups (notably statistically superior for groups C, W, and Y); thus, the age indication was expanded, ultimately to include those 2 months and older [13, 145]. The duration of protective antibody concentration has been demonstrated to be up to 5 years in the adolescent population. In 2010, ACIP recommended a meningococcal booster dose at age 16. More robust studies are needed to examine persistent efficacy after the adolescent

Table 4.5 All available vaccines

Vaccine	US trade name(s)	Infectious agent(s) covered	Vaccine type	Resources
Adenovirus type 4 and type 7	Adenovirus type 4 and type 7	Adenovirus	Live	[216]
Anthrax	BioThrax	B. anthracis	Inactivated	[217]
BCG	BCG Vaccine USP[a]	M. tuberculosis	Live	[218–222]
Cholera	VAXCHORA[b]	V. cholerae	Inactivated	[223, 224, 348]
Dengue	NA[c]	Dengue virus, serotypes 1–4	Live	[225]
Diphtheria and tetanus	Diphtheria and Tetanus Toxoids Adsorbed USP[d]	C. diphtheriae, C. tetani	Toxoid	[226–230]
Diphtheria, tetanus and pertussis (acellular)	DAPTACEL, INFANRIX	C. diphtheriae, C. tetani, B. pertussis	Toxoid, subunit	[14, 15]
Diphtheria, tetanus and pertussis (whole cell)	NA[e]	C. diphtheriae, C. tetani, B. pertussis	Toxoid, inactivated	[234, 235]
Diphtheria, tetanus, pertussis (acellular), hepatitis B and poliovirus	Pediarix	C. diphtheriae, C. tetani, B. perussis, Hepatitis B virus, Poliovirus	Toxoid, subunit	[317]
Diphtheria, tetanus, pertussis (acellular), hepatitis B, poliovirus (inactivated) and Hib	NA[f]	C. diphtheria, C. tetani, B. pertussis, Poliovirus, Hepatitis B virus, Hib	Toxoid, subunit	[237]
Diphtheria, tetanus, pertussis (acellular), poliovirus (inactivated) and Hib	Pentacel	C. diphtheriae, C. tetani, B. perussis, Poliovirus, Hib	Toxoid, inactivated, killed, conjugated	[319]
Diphtheria, tetanus, pertussis (acellular) and poliovirus (inactivated)	Kinrix, Quadracel	C. diphtheriae, C. tetani, B. pertussis, Poliovirus	Toxoid, subunit	[238, 318]
Diphtheria, tetanus, pertussis (whole cell), hepatitis B and Hib	NA[g]	C. diphtheriae, C. tetani, B. pertussis, Hepatitis B virus, Hib	Toxoid, inactivated, subunit	[239–247]
Diphtheria, tetanus, pertussis (whole cell) and hepatitis B	NA[h]	C. diphtheriae, C. tetani, B. perussis, Hepatitis B virus	Toxoid, inactivated, subunit	[248]

(continued)

Table 4.5 (continued)

Vaccine	US trade name(s)	Infectious agent(s) covered	Vaccine type	Resources
Diphtheria, tetanus, pertussis (whole cell) and Hib	NA[i]	*C. diphtheriae, C. tetani, B. pertussis*, Hib	Toxoid, inactivated, subunit	[249, 250]
Enterotoxigenic *Escherichia coli* (ETEC), Cholera	NA[j]	ETEC, *V. cholerae*	Inactivated, subunit	[349]
Hib	ActHIB, HIBERIX, Pedvax HIB[k]	Hib	Subunit	[81–83, 251, 252]
Hepatitis A	HAVRIX, VAQTA	Hepatitis A virus	Killed	[104, 105]
Hepatitis A and Hepatitis B	Twinrix	Hepatitis A virus, Hepatitis B virus	Killed, subunit	[110]
Hepatitis B	ENGERIX-B, RECOMBIVAX HB[l]	Hepatitis B virus	Subunit	[1, 73, 253–258]
Hepatitis E	NA[m]	Hepatitis E virus	Subunit	[259]
HPV Quadrivalent	Gardasil	HPV types 6, 11, 16, and 18	Subunit	[321]
HPV 9-Valent	Gardasil 9	HPV types 6, 11, 16, 18, 31, 33, 45, 52, and 58	Subunit	[162]
Influenza, seasonal, quadrivalent	FLUARIX QUADRIVALENT, FLUCELVAX QUADRIVALENT, FluLaval Quadrivalent, Fluzone high-dose, Fluzone Quadrivalent, Fluzone Quadrivalent Intradermal	Seasonal influenza types A and B	Subunit	[322–324, 326, 327, 329]
Influenza, seasonal, trivalent	AFLURIA, FLUAD, FLUBLOK, FLUVIRIN Fluzone, Fluzone high-dose[n]	Seasonal influenza types A and B	Subunit	[320, 325, 328, 330–333]
Japanese encephalitis	IXIARO, JE-VAX[o]	Japanese encephalitis virus	Killed or live	[260–262, 334, 335]
Measles	NA[p]	Measles virus	Live	[263–265]
Measles and rubella	NA[q]	Measles virus and rubella virus	Live	[266]

Measles, mumps and rubella	MMR-II	Measles virus, mumps virus, rubella virus	Live	[59, 267, 268, 336]
Measles, mumps, rubella and varicella	ProQuad	Measles virus, mumps virus, rubella virus, varicella virus	Live	[269]
Meningococcal group A	NA[s]	N. meningitidis group A	Subunit	[270, 271]
Meningococcal group B	Trumenba; BEXSERO	N. meningitidis group B	Subunit	[149, 150]
Meningococcal groups A and C	NA[t]	N. meningitidis groups A and C	Inactivated	[272, 273]
Meningococcal groups A, C, Y, W-135	Menactra, MENVEO, Menomune	N. meningitidis groups A, C, Y, W-135	Subunit	[141, 274, 350]
Pneumococcal	Prevnar	S. pneumoniae serotypes 4, 6B, 9 V, 14, 18C, 19F, 23F	Subunit	[351]
Pneumococcal	NA[u]	Streptococcus pneumoniae serotypes 1, 4, 5, 6B, 7F, 9 V, 14, 18C, 19F, 23F	Subunit	[275]
Pneumococcal	Prevnar-13	S. pneumoniae serotypes 1, 3, 4, 5, 6A, 6B, 7F, 9 V, 14, 18C, 19A, 19F, 23F	Subunit	[276]
Pneumococcal	Pneumovax23	S.pneumoniae serotypes 1, 2, 3, 4, 5, 6B, 7F, 8, 9N, 9V, 10A, 11A, 12F, 14, 15B, 17F, 18C, 19F, 19A, 20, 22F, 23F, and 33F	Killed	[337]
Poliovirus, inactivated	IPOL[v]	Poliovirus	Killed	[277–281]
Poliovirus, bivalent types 1 and 3, oral	NA[w]	Poliovirus	Live	[282–286]
Poliovirus, monovalent type 1, oral	NA[x]	Poliovirus	Live	[338–340]
Poliovirus, monovalent type 2, oral	NA[y]	Poliovirus	Live	[288, 289]
Poliovirus, monovalent type 3, oral	NA[z]	Poliovirus	Live	[287]

(continued)

Table 4.5 (continued)

Vaccine	US trade name(s)	Infectious agent(s) covered	Vaccine type	Resources
Poliovirus, trivalent, oral	NA[aa]	Poliovirus	Live	[290–293, 341]
Rabies	RabAvert, Imovax Rabies[ab]	Rabies virus	Killed	[294–298]
Rotavirus	ROTARIX, RotaTeq	Rotavirus	Live	[299, 300]
Rubella	NA[ac]	Rubella virus	Live	[301]
Small pox	ACAM2000	Small pox virus	Live	[302]
Tetanus and diphtheria	DECAVAC, TENIVAC, Tetanus and Diphtheria Toxoids, Absorbed[ad]	*C. diphtheriae, C. tetani*	Toxoid	[18, 231, 232, 342, 343]
Tetanus, diphtheria and pertussis (acellular)	Adacel, BOOSTRIX	*C. diphtheriae, C. tetani, B. pertussis*	Toxoid, subunit	[16, 17]
Tetanus	NA[ae]	*C. tetani*	Toxoid	[303–308]
Tick-borne encephalitis	NA[af]	TBE virus	Killed	[309, 344, 345]
Typhoid	Typhim Vi, Vivotif	*S. typhi*	Inactivated or live	[310, 311]
Varicella (chicken pox)	VARIVAX	VZV	Live	[91]
Yellow fever	YF-VAX[ag]	Yellow fever virus	Live	[312–316]
Zoster	ZOSTAVAX	VZV	Live	[172]

[a]BCG freeze-dried glutamate vaccine; BCG vaccine; BCG vaccine (freeze dried) – intradermal; BCG vaccine SSI

[b]Euvichol; Shanchol

[c]Dengvaxia (CYD-TDV)

[d]Adsorbed DT vaccine; Diftet; diphtheria and tetanus vaccine adsorbed, pediatric; DT VAX

[e]Diphtheria-tetanus-pertussis vaccine adsorbed; DTP vaccine

[f]Hexaxim

[g]Diphtheria, tetanus, pertussis, hepatitis B, and Haemophilus influenzae type b conjugate vaccine; diphtheria, tetanus, pertussis, hepatitis B, and Haemophilus influenzae type b conjugate vaccine adsorbed; Euforvac-Hib injection; Eupenta; Easyfive-TT; Pentabio; Quinvaxem; Shan-5; Tritanrix HB + Hib

[h]Diphtheria, tetanus, pertussis, and hepatitis B vaccine adsorbed; DTP-Hep B 5; DTP-Hep B 10

[i]Diphtheria, tetanus, pertussis, and Haemophilus influenzae type b conjugate vaccine; TETRAct-HIB

[j]Dukoral

[k]Haemophilus influenzae type b vaccine; Vaxem HIB

[l]Euvax B; Heberbiovac HB; hepatitis B vaccine recombinant; hepatitis B vaccine (rDNA) (adult); hepatitis B vaccine (rDNA) (Ped); Hepavax; Hepavax-Gene TF; Shanvac-B

[m]Hecolin

[n]GC FLU; influenza vaccine (split virion, inactivated); Nasovac-S; Vaxigrip

[o]JEEV; IMOJEV MD; Japanese encephalitis vaccine live (SA14–14-2)

[p]Measles vaccine; measles vaccine, live, attenuated; ROUVAX

[q]Measles and rubella virus vaccine live

[r]PRIORIX; TRIMOVAX MÉRIEUX

[s]MenAfriVac; MenAfriVac 5 μg

[t]Polysaccharide meningococcal A + C; polysaccharide meningococcal A + C

[u]Synflorix

[v]IMOVAX POLIO; IPV vaccine SSI; poliomyelitis vaccine; Poliorix

[w]BIOPOLIO B1/3; bivalent oral poliomyelitis vaccine type 1 and 3; bivalent type 1 and 3 oral poliomyelitis vaccine, IP; Polio Sabin One and Three; bivalent types 1 and 3 oral polio vaccine for children

[x]Monovalent type 1 oral poliomyelitis vaccine, IP; oral monovalent type 1 poliomyelitis vaccine; Polio Sabin Mono T1

[y]Oral monovalent type 2 poliomyelitis vaccine (nOPV2); Polio Sabin Mono Two (oral)

[z]Oral monovalent type 3 poliomyelitis vaccine; Polio Sabin Mono T3

[aa]BIOPOLIO; OPVERO; oral polio; poliomyelitis vaccine (oral) trivalent types 1, 2 and 3; polioviral vaccine

[ab]Rabies vaccine; Rabipur; VERORAB

[ac]Rubella vaccine, live, attenuated

[ad]IMOVAX dT

[ae]ShanTT; tetanus adsorbed vaccine BP; tetanus toxoid; Tetatox; TETAVAX; TT vaccine

[af]FSME-IMMUN; FSME-IMMUN (Junior); Encepur; Encepur-K; TBE-Moscow; EnceVir

[ag]Stabilized yellow fever vaccine; STAMARIL; yellow fever; yellow fever vaccine, live

booster dose; however, a small study demonstrated a strong antibody response, higher than seen with primary vaccination [146, 147].

In response to college outbreaks of serogroup B meningococcal disease, the Food and Drug Administration (FDA) fast tracked approval of two serogroup B meningococcal vaccines [148]. Trumenba® is a two- or three-dose series and was the first serogroup B meningococcal vaccine licensed in 2014 [149]. One year later, Bexsero® was licensed as a two-dose series against serogroup B vaccine [150]. As with the conjugate meningococcal processors, the serogroup B vaccine efficacy was based on immune response [148]. Trumenba® immunogenicity response was evaluated when given concomitantly with a HPV vaccine versus with placebo. Protective antibody levels following one month after three doses of Trumenba® ranged from 88.5% to 99.4%, depending on heterologous variant of serogroup B strain; the immune response was more robust after three doses compared to two doses [151]. Antibody titers rapidly declined after the three-dose series, but stabilized after 6 months, and antibody titer protection was demonstrated in more than 50% of subjects four years after vaccine series [152]. Following one dose of Bexsero®, protective antibody levels were evident in 92–97% of adolescents, increasing to almost 100% after two doses, and minimal difference was seen when three doses were given [153]. Protective immunogenicity of Bexsero® against three serogroup B strains 18–24 months after a single dose decreased to 62–73%, after two doses to 77–94%, and after three doses to 86–97% [154]. The sustained impact of these fast-tracked vaccines against serogroup B meningococcal disease remains to be seen.

Human Papillomavirus

Human papillomavirus (HPV) is a sexually transmitted small DNA virus with over 100 distinct types, 35–40 of which are known to infect the skin and mucous membranes of the anogenital region. CDC estimates that HPV accounts for the majority of newly acquired sexually transmitted infections in the USA with recent data indicating nearly 80 million new and existing HPV infections. HPV is the most common sexually transmitted infection in the USA [155].

Most HPV infections are asymptomatic and do not progress to disease, as the body's immune system clears approximately 90% of infections within 2 years. Low-risk HPV genotypes can lead to genital warts, whereas persistence of high-risk types can lead to many types of cancer including cervical cancer, other anogenital cancers, and cancers of the head and neck [156].

Based on CDC data from 2008 to 2012, approximately 38,793 HPV-associated cancers occur in the USA annually; 23,000 among women and 15,793 among men. HPV is thought to be responsible for more than 90% of anal and cervical cancers, about 70% of vaginal and vulvar cancers, and more than 60% of penile cancers. Approximately 70% of head and neck cancers may be linked to HPV and may be associated with a combination of tobacco, alcohol, and HPV. In 2015, the prevalence of genital warts reported in patients who presented to sexually transmitted disease (STD) clinics (as reported by the STD Surveillance Network) shows the highest rates of genital warts in men who have sex with women (MSW) 4.3% (range 1.7–8.1), followed by men who have sex with men (MSM) 3.3% (range 1.9–4.6) and women 0.9% (range 0.7–2.2). HPV types 16 and 18 are known to cause the vast majority of disease and have been implicated in approximately 70% of cases of cervical carcinoma. Clearance rates in women in the USA have been cited as high as 70–100% at 2–5 years and are highest in young women and in those with non-oncogenic genotypes. Women of low socioeconomic status and in developing countries are disproportionately affected, likely due to lower screening rates and availability of HPV vaccines. In 2012, over 200,000 women worldwide died of cervical cancer, 85% of them in developing countries. HPV has been detected in 99.7% of cases of cervical carcinoma, approximately 90% of anal cancers, 40% of vulvar and vaginal cancers, 40% of penile cancers, and 25% of cancers of the head and neck [157].

Human Papillomavirus Vaccine and Vaccine Efficacy

HPV vaccine is recommended for preteen boys and girls at age 11 or 12 so they are protected before exposure to the virus. A more robust immune response is seen in younger preteen patients than in older teens and young adults. The HPV vaccine is given in a two- or three-dose series depending on the patients' age. For patients under 15 years of age, the recommendation is for two doses, 6–12 months apart. For patients ≥15 years of age, the recommendation is for three doses at 0, 1–2, and 6 months of age [158].

Gardasil® was licensed in 2006 as a quadrivalent vaccine against HPV types 6, 11, 16, and 18 [13]. The Females United to Unilaterally Reduce Endo/Ectocervical Disease (FUTURE) II trials demonstrated 100% efficacy against anogenital warts and vulvar or vaginal intraepithelial neoplasia or cancer related to HPV types 6, 11, 16, and 18. The FUTURE II trial also demonstrated 98% prevention of cervical intraepithelial neoplasia grade 2 or 3 or cervical adenocarcinoma in situ related to HPV types 16 and 18 related in HPV-naïve females aged 15–26 years after three doses of quadrivalent vaccine with Gardasil® in greater than 95% of subjects [159, 160]. Gardasil® was approved for use in males in 1999. The prevention of external genital warts; penile, perianal, or perineal intraepithelial neoplasia; or penile, peri-anal cancer related to the four types contained in the vaccine of the per-protocol population was 90.4% for males ages 16–26 [161].

In 2014, a 9-valent HPV vaccine, Gardasil®9, was licensed to protect against the same diseases and precancerous or dysplastic lesions as Gardasil®, with expanded coverage of five additional HPV virus types [31, 33, 45, 52, 58, 162]. The addition of these five types could lead to an additional 14.7% protection from invasive cervical cancer [163]. The Broad Spectrum HPV Vaccine Study demonstrated 96.7% risk reduction of high-grade cervical, vulvar, and vaginal disease, caused by HPV types

31, 33, 45, 52, and 58 in HPV-uninfected females aged 16–26 years after three doses of Gardasil®9 within one year of enrollment [164]. Immunobridging studies were utilized to establish Gardasil®9 efficacy via noninferiority in the following groups: adolescent females aged 9–15 years and males aged 16–26 years. Notably, male and female adolescents (aged 9–15 years) had significantly higher antibody titers to Gardasil®9 compared to females aged 16–26 years receiving the 9-valent HPV [165]. Post clinical trial efficacy data is gradually being published. A 6.1% decrease in prevalence of HPV types 6, 11, 16, and 18 in females aged 14–19 years was demonstrated in those having received three doses (62.5%) of Gardasil® [166]. The impact of HPV vaccination on the incidence and mortality rate of cervical cancer has yet to be determined [167].

Varicella Zoster Virus: Shingles

Varicella zoster virus (VZV) not only causes varicella, but also causes herpes zoster (HZ), or shingles. Shingles occurs following reactivation of latent VZV of cranial nerves or dorsal root ganglia. Approximately 1 million cases of HZ occur annually in the USA, and incidence increases with age; 68% of HZ cases occur in persons over age 50. Almost one out of every three people in the USA will develop shingles in their lifetime [168]. Both natural VZV infection and vaccination against VZV with live, attenuated virus result in latent virus acquisition. Those who are immunized against varicella show decreased shingles incidence than those who acquired the disease naturally [169].

Shingles is characterized by a painful maculopapular or vesicular rash, usually unilateral and following one or two adjacent dermatomes. Less commonly the rash can be more widespread and affect three or more dermatomes; this condition is known as disseminated zoster [170]. The most commonly involved dermatomes include V1 of the trigeminal nerve and the thoracic nerves T1–L2. Approximately 1–4% of people who get shingles are hospitalized for complications, and each year there are approximately 96 shingles-related deaths in the USA [171].

Other complications of shingles include secondary bacterial infections, herpes zoster ophthalmicus, a complication that can lead to blindness without appropriate treatment, aseptic meningitis, transverse myelitis, stroke symptoms, and postherpetic neuralgia (PHN). Prevalence of PHN in the USA is estimated at greater than 500,000.

PHN, with pain persisting over the area of the shingles rash for more than 30 days, is one of the most devastating and common sequelae of shingles infection. PHN can significantly affect quality of life and ability to perform activities of daily living. Its incidence increases with age. Approximately 13% of people 60 years of age and older with zoster will get PHN [170].

Varicella Zoster Virus: Shingles Vaccine Efficacy

Zostavax®, the zoster live attenuated virus vaccine licensed in 2006, is indicated for prevention of herpes zoster [172]. It is approved by FDA for people 50 years of age and older but recommended by ACIP for people 60 years of age and older whether or not they report a prior episode of shingles or prior history of chicken pox.

In the Shingles Prevention Study, overall zoster vaccine efficacy of 51.3% was demonstrated against HZ in patients over 60, with the greatest efficacy occurring in patients 60–69 years old (63.9%), declining by roughly 20% each decade thereafter. Vaccine efficacy to reduce the incidence of PHN varied among age groups, with the highest efficacy (55%) in subjects aged 70–79, followed by those greater than 80 years old (26%). The lowest efficacy of PHN was observed in subjects aged 60–69 at 5% [172, 173]. The Zostavax® Efficacy and Safety Trial found subjects aged 50–59 had a vaccine efficacy between 69.8% and 72.4% [174]. Studies assessing the duration of efficacy suggest a decline in protection after 8 years to 21.1% or less [175]. The ACIP recommendation for zoster vaccination 10 years after current FDA-licensed approval age is due to these studies showing waning protection [176]. Despite the herpes zoster vaccine reduction of 50–60% disease incidence and sequelae, further innovation for a more effective herpes zoster vaccine remains to be seen, especially with the expected increase in the geriatric population [177].

Overview of Vaccine Types

The characteristics of the pathogen targeted by a vaccine determine the type of vaccine that can be produced to protect humans from acquiring the targeted disease or illness. There are currently four major types of vaccines: live attenuated, inactivated, toxoid, and subunit vaccines.

Live Attenuated

A live, attenuated vaccine contains a non-virulent, living version of the pathogen against which it protects. These weakened, or attenuated, pathogens have lost the ability to infect or replicate in a human host, but still elicit an immune response. Methods for attenuating pathogens vary, but involve selectively culturing generations of the pathogen with progressively limited ability to replicate in a human host. This is most readily achieved in viruses, with their rapid replication and mutation rates [178–180].

Live, attenuated vaccines elicit a strong immunological response, with typically long-lived protection. However, there are risks to the use of live vaccines. An immunologically incompetent host may have an insufficient immune response to the vaccine to prevent subsequent illness from the attenuated pathogen. Alternatively, as the live pathogens retain the ability to mutate, they may regain their virulence in humans. Additionally, live, attenuated vaccines are the least stable vaccine type, often requiring refrigeration [178–180].

Inactivated

Killed or inactivated vaccines are an alternative to live, attenuated vaccines. (The word *killed* is usually used to refer to bacterial pathogens, while *inactivated* is used to refer to viruses.) Like attenuated vaccines, inactivated vaccines contain the whole disease-causing pathogen or microbe. Killing, or inactivation, is a result of exposure to heat, radiation, or chemicals such as formaldehyde and formalin. The pathogen that remains following inactivation allows for an immunologic response to a wide array of surface antigens [178]. The killed pathogen cannot revert or mutate to a more virulent form and cause illness or disease. However, the immunologic response to killed or inactivated vaccines is less robust and provides a shorter length of duration of protection than the response to live, attenuated vaccines and typically requires multiple doses, boosters, and/or adjuvants to promote a good immunologic response and maintain protection.

Toxoid

A toxoid is a bacterial toxin, usually an exotoxin, whose toxicity has been inactivated or suppressed either by heat or chemicals that can still produce an immunologic response. Toxoid vaccines carry no risk of infection; however, they generally produce a weak immune response, and therefore multiple doses, boosters, and/or adjuvants are typically required to induce immunity [178]. Tetanus and diphtheria vaccines are examples of toxoid vaccines.

Subunit

Subunit vaccines use specific antigens, or epitopes of antigens, of the targeted pathogen to invoke an immune response. Subunit vaccines can be further subdivided into conjugate, recombinant, and viruslike particle vaccines. In conjugate vaccines, a polysaccharide antigen, which typically elicits a weak immune response, is covalently bound to a strongly immunogenic carrier protein. The carrier protein allows for a more efficient immune response to the polysaccharide antigen, conferring immunity to the targeted pathogen [178, 179].

Recombinant vaccines are produced through recombinant DNA technology. They may be classified as either DNA vaccines or recombinant (protein subunit) vaccines. These types of vaccines use genetic material coding protein antigens from a targeted pathogen that stimulates the immune response that are then inserted into microbial DNA cells of the body. As the host cell reproduces, the protein antigen of the pathogen is expressed and can be used to induce an immunologic response to the targeted pathogen. An example of a recombinant protein vaccine is the HepB vaccine.

Viruslike particle vaccines are similarly created with recombinant DNA technology. The selected viral protein antigens of these vaccines mimic the organization and conformation of authentic native viruses, but without the native viral genome, thus prompting an immune response to the expressed protein in a potentially safer and cheaper manner than other subunit vaccines [179–181]. While there is no risk of virulence or illness with subunit vaccines, there are disadvantages to their use. Often subunit vaccines require multiple doses, boosters, and/or adjuvants to produce sufficient immunity. Additionally, local reactions at the site of vaccination are common [178].

Indications for Routine Vaccine Recommendations

CDC has established routine vaccination recommendations for children and adults and recommendations for people with special conditions, for travelers, for those with certain occupations and exposures and during outbreaks.

Pediatric Vaccine Schedule

Presently, vaccines are recommended by ACIP against 13 diseases for all children and adolescents aged 0 through 18 years, in addition to an annual influenza vaccine recommendation. The first dose in the series of the HepB vaccine is the only vaccine given immediately postpartum, before hospital discharge. This early administration ensures that newborns born to mothers unaware they are infected with HBV will be spared severe illness and possible death if the virus is transmitted during delivery [182]. Two additional doses of HepB are recommended to confer full immunity, the second at 1–2 months of age and the third at 6–18 months of age.

Six vaccines are recommended for children at 2 months of age: HepB, rotavirus, DTaP, Hib, pneumococcal conjugate, and inactivated poliovirus. At 4 months of age, second doses of all of the vaccines given at 2 months of age (except for HepB) are recommended [183].

The type of vaccine administered guides the number of doses required. There are two rotavirus vaccines: the RV1 is a two-dose series while the RV5 has an additional third dose that should be given at 6 months of age. Depending upon the brand of Hib vaccine administered, three doses are sufficient at 2, 4, and 6 months, and a forth dose may be needed at 12–18 months of age. There are currently six Hib vaccines approved for use, three of them are combined with vaccines for other diseases and three of them solely confer vaccination against Hib. Each brand of the Hib vaccine needs to be assessed for the number of doses required [183].

Three additional vaccines recommended to be completed by 6 years of age include DTaP, the pneumococcal conjugate, and inactivated poliovirus vaccines. The DTaP vaccine has a recommended total of five doses through age 6. Three doses at 2, 4, and 6 months of age, one dose at 15–18 months of age, and one dose at 4–6 years of age are recommended. Four doses of the pneumococcal conjugate at 2, 4, 6, and 12–18 months are recommended, and inactivated poliovirus vaccine is recommended at 2, 4, and 6–19 months and 4–6 years of age [183].

MMR, VZV, and HepA vaccines are not recommended until after 1 year of age. The first dose of each of these vaccines should be administered at 12–18 months of age. The second doses of MMR and varicella vaccines should be administered at 4–6 years of age. HepA vaccine has a more specific instruction as to when its second dose should be administered; it needs to be 6–18 months after the initial dose [183].

Immunizations for those over age 6 include TdaP, meningococcal, and HPV vaccines.

Tdap is recommended for children aged 7 through 18 years who are not fully vaccinated, preferentially at 11–12 years of age along with meningococcal and HPV vaccines. A booster dose of meningococcal vaccine should be administered at 16 years of age. The meningococcal B vaccine is not routinely recommended, but it is available as a permissive recommendation and can be administered at a clinician's discretion. A two- to three-dose series of HPV vaccine are recommended on a schedule of 0 and 6–12 months to be completed by 13 years of age (up to age 15) and on a schedule of 0, 1–2, and 6 months if the series is started after age 15 [183].

The influenza vaccine is the only vaccine recommended to be given annually to all individuals 6 months of age and older. For each influenza season, there are usually several vaccine types available. Young children under 8 years of age require two doses of the influenza vaccine administered at least 4 weeks apart the first time they are vaccinated against influenza. Note: influenza recommendations are unique to each influenza season, and the annual recommendation should be referenced each year [184].

Adult Vaccine Schedule

The routine adult vaccine schedule includes vaccines against tetanus, diphtheria, pertussis, varicella, zoster, and pneumococcal diseases. Tdap is given once after 19 years of age, and then a Td booster is recommended once every 10 years thereafter. Adults without evidence of immunity to varicella should receive two doses of varicella vaccine. Evidence of immunity includes documentation of two doses of varicella vaccine at least 4 weeks apart, USA born before 1980 (excluding healthcare personnel and pregnant women), history of varicella disease, history of herpes zoster, laboratory evidence of immunity, or laboratory confirmation of disease. The human papillomavirus vaccine is only recommended in adulthood through 26 years of age, if the vaccine series was not completed during adolescence.

In addition to an annual influenza vaccine, adults over the age of 60 years are recommended to receive a single dose of zoster vaccine regardless of whether they have had chicken pox or a prior episode of herpes zoster. All adults over the age of 65 should receive the PCV13 vaccine and at least 1 year later PPSV23 vaccine.

Vaccine Recommendations for Special Populations

Pregnant Women

Pregnant women should receive a Tdap vaccine with each pregnancy during their third trimester. It is also important to vaccinate pregnant women anytime during pregnancy with influenza vaccination [185, 186]. Rubella and varicella immunity should be assessed. Pregnant women without immunity are to be administered needed MMR and varicella vaccines postpartum before discharge from hospital. Second doses of each vaccine are to be given 4 weeks later. The following live vaccines are contraindicated for pregnant women, varicella, zoster, and MMR, because a risk to the fetus cannot be excluded. HPV vaccine is not recommended during pregnancy.

Immunocompromised Patients

Individuals who have HIV infection should receive vaccine recommendations based upon their CD4+ count. Those with a CD4+ count greater than or equal to 200 (cells/microliter) are no longer contraindicated to receiving live vaccines. All immunocompromised patients are recommended to receive the pneumococcal PCV13 and PPV23 vaccines. Individuals who have received a hematopoietic stem cell transplant (HSCT) should receive a three-dose regimen of the Hib vaccine starting at 6–12 months after a successful transplant. The doses should be separated by at least 4 weeks and given regardless of the patient's vaccination history. Of immunocompromised individuals, only HIV-infected individuals are recommended to receive the hepatitis B vaccine (regardless of CD4+ count). It is important to reference CDC recommendations for the most up-to-date and specific information for immunocompromised patients. Immunocompromised individuals should not receive the three live vaccines: varicella, zoster, and MMR [186].

Men Who Have Sex with Men (MSM)

The hepatitis A and B vaccines are recommended for men who have sex with men. Two doses of HepA vaccine should be given 6 months apart, and three doses of HepB or a combination HepA/HepB given at 0, 2, and 6 months are recommended. For MSM younger than 26 years, three doses of HPV vaccine are recommended at 0, 1–2, and 6 months.

Healthcare Personnel

In addition to the normally recommended vaccine schedule, healthcare workers should receive the HBV series as they could potentially be exposed to infectious blood or body fluids. Additional vaccines may be recommended depending upon what type of healthcare work is performed. Measles, mumps, rubella, and varicella immunity should be assessed, and if not present, appropriate immunizations should be given.

Other Medical Conditions/Indications

For persons with unique medical conditions, specific vaccines may be recommended. These conditions include chronic diseases such as diabetes, heart disease, chronic lung disease (including asthma), kidney disease, liver disease, and alcoholism. All persons with the afore-listed conditions and diseases are recommended to receive one PPSV23 vaccine prior to age 65. In addition, diabetics and those with chronic liver or kidney disease are additionally recommended to complete the HBV vaccination series; those with liver disease are recommended to receive the HAV series as well. For those with chronic kidney disease, one dose of PCV13 before age 65 is also indicated. Full recommendations from CDC may be found at: https://www.cdc.gov/vaccines/schedules/hcp/imz/adult-conditions.html.

Contraindications to Vaccines

In addition to the contraindications for specific populations highlighted above, severe allergic reaction (e.g., anaphylaxis) experienced after receiving a vaccine dose or a known anaphylactic allergy to a vaccine component of any vaccine is a contraindication to receiving doses of that vaccine. Based on 2016 CDC recommendations, people with egg allergies no longer need to be observed for an allergic reaction for 30 min after receiving a flu vaccine. There is a common misconception that people with mild to moderate egg allergies should not receive influenza vaccines. Persons with a history of egg allergy who have experienced only hives after exposure to egg should receive flu vaccine: any licensed and recommended flu vaccine (i.e., any form of IIV or RIV) that is otherwise appropriate for the recipient's age and health status may be used. Persons who report having had reactions to egg involving symptoms other than hives such as angioedema, respiratory distress, lightheadedness, or recurrent emesis or who required epinephrine or another emergency medical intervention may similarly receive any licensed and recommended flu vaccine (i.e., any form of IIV or RIV) that is otherwise appropriate for the recipient's age and health status. For those with severe egg allergies, the influenza vaccine should be administered in an inpatient or outpatient medical setting (including but not necessarily limited to hospitals, clinics, health departments, and physician offices). Vaccine administration should be supervised by a healthcare provider who is able to recognize and manage severe allergic conditions [187].

Postexposure Prophylaxis

Postexposure prophylaxis (PEP) is defined as "a preventive measure taken to protect a person or community from harm after contact with disease-causing chemicals, germs, or physical agents." [188] PEP in the form of vaccines or immunoglobulin (IG) is routinely recommended following exposure to many viral and bacterial diseases.

Viral Hepatitides

Hepatitis A

Hepatitis A is spread to others via close personal contact (household and sex contacts), illicit drugs, and food preparation. Recently exposed people who have not been vaccinated previously should be given the HepA vaccine or IG within 2 weeks after exposure. IG is the recommended treatment for people at increased risk of severe HepA infection, such as the elderly and those who are immunocompromised [189].

After exposure to HAV:

- Healthy persons aged 12 months to 40 years should receive the HepA vaccine (preferred) or immunoglobulin (IG) to be administered within 2 weeks of exposure.
- For those over 40 years old, give IG.
- Give IG for children less than 12 months, immunocompromised persons, or those with chronic liver disease [190].

Hepatitis B

Hepatitis B is spread via exposure to blood or body fluids. After exposure to HBV, timely prophylaxis can prevent HPV infection. The mainstay of PEP is HepB vaccine, but in certain circumstances, HepB IG is recommended in addition to vaccination [191].

For an exposure to a known hepatitis B surface antigen (HBsAg)-positive source:

- Persons who have completed the HepB vaccine series but did not receive post-vaccination testing should receive a single vaccine booster dose.

- Persons in the process of being vaccinated but have not completed the series should receive the appropriate dose of HepB IG (HBIG) and complete the vaccine series.
- Unvaccinated persons should receive both HBIG and HepB vaccine as soon as possible after exposure (preferably within 24 h). The vaccine may be administered simultaneously with HBIG in a separate injection site.

For an exposure to a source with unknown HBsAg status:

- Persons with written documentation of a complete HepB vaccine series require no further treatment.
- Persons who are not fully vaccinated should complete the vaccine series.
- Unvaccinated persons should receive the HepB vaccine series with the first dose administered as soon as possible after exposure, preferably within 24 h [192].

Note:

- For one previously vaccinated with adequate response, no PEP is indicated.
- For a person who is vaccinated with the HepB series once, but a non-responder, a single dose of HBIG is recommended within hours of exposure, followed by the vaccine series.
- For one who is vaccinated and a non-responder after two vaccination series, give HBIG twice within 24 h of exposure [193].

Hepatitis C

Hepatitis C is spread via large or repeated percutaneous exposures to infectious blood. This may occur though injection drug use (the most common means of transmission in the USA currently), receipt of donated blood or organ (now rare in the USA since blood screening began in 1992), through needlestick injuries in the healthcare settings, and during childbirth in a hepatitis C-infected mother. Unfortunately, there is no PEP that has been proven useful after a hepatitis C exposure [194, 195]. An experiment with chimpanzees given IG prior to a needlestick with hepatitis C-positive blood did not prevent the transmission of infection. Additional research has similarly shown that no protective antibody response has been induced to prevent infection.

HIV

After exposure to HIV, short-term antiretroviral therapy is indicated. No vaccine is available.

Note: There exists preexposure prophylaxis, or PrEP, to prevent HIV infections for those that are at substantial risk of getting HIV. A daily pill (taken consistently) containing two medications, tenofovir and emtricitabine, has been shown to reduce the risk of HIB infection in people who are at high risk by up to 92% [196, 197].

Influenza

PEP is recommended for people that have a high risk of complications from an influenza infection who have had contact with an ill individual from 1 day prior to influenza symptoms onset until 1 day after defervescence [195]. Those at a high risk might include those unable to receive the vaccine, exposure during the 2 weeks after influenza immunization, and family members or healthcare providers who are unimmunized and likely to have close exposure to unimmunized infants and toddlers. Chemoprophylaxis can be used in addition to immunization in children who may not respond well to the vaccine or in instances when the circulating strains of influenza virus in the community are not well matched with the seasonal influenza vaccine strains [198]. Widespread or routine use of antiviral medications chemoprophylaxis is not recommended as it could encourage the emergence of antiviral resistant viruses. Oseltamivir and zanamivir are the two antiviral medications used for PEP. Oseltamivir is approved for use in children older than 3 months of age, and zanamivir is approved for use in children 5 years of age or older. It is recommended that chemoprophylaxis be given for 7 days after the last known exposure. However, if more than 48 h have elapsed since the initial exposure to the infectious person, antiviral chemoprophylaxis is not generally recommended [199].

Measles

The most vulnerable to a measles exposure include those unvaccinated or under vaccinated, infants under 12 months of age who would have not yet received the vaccine, pregnant women without evidence of immunity, and immunocompromised people.

- If exposed to measles, the MMR vaccine must be administered within 72 h of the exposure to be effective.
- If the timeframe is missed or if a person is unable to receive the vaccine, IG can be given intramuscular (IM) or intravenous (IV) within 6 days of exposure to help prevent or limit measles infection.
- IG IM is the recommended prophylaxis treatment for children under 12 months of age since they cannot receive the MMR vaccine.
- Pregnant women and severely immunocompromised people should receive IG IV since they cannot receive the MMR vaccine [198].

Meningococcal Disease

Whether vaccinated with meningococcal vaccines or not, anyone who has had close contact with an infected individual with meningococcal disease within the 7 days prior to onset of illness should be treated [200]. Antibiotic prophylaxis should be initiated within 24 h after the infectious patient has been identified [201]. Effective antibiotic regimens may include ceftriaxone, rifampin, or ciprofloxacin. Ceftriaxone is the regimen of choice for pregnant women. Azithromycin is not routinely recommended as a treatment choice, but could be used if needed [198].

Pertussis

The CDC recommends targeting postexposure antibiotics against pertussis to high-risk individuals and people who have close contact with high-risk individuals. PEP can be administered to contacts within 21 days of exposure to onset of cough in the index case. People who are at high risk include all household contacts, infants, women in the third trimester of pregnancy, and persons with preexisting health conditions. Asthma or immunocompromised conditions such as moderate-to-severe asthma may be exacerbated by a pertussis infection [198, 202]. Household contacts (including immunized contacts) should be treated because secondary attack rates are high. Extensive contact tracing and broadscale use of postexposure antibiotics are not effective uses of public health resources, and there is no data to indicate that widespread use of PEP among contacts will effectively control or limit the scope of a pertussis outbreak. All unimmunized or under-immunized contacts should be vaccinated [202].

The preferred antibiotic treatment for PEP in persons older than 1 month includes erythromycin, clarithromycin, and azithromycin. For those younger than 1 month, only azithromycin is recommended. An alternative that is available for patients 2 months and older is trimethoprim/sulfamethoxazole [203].

Rabies

Each year approximately 16,000–39,000 people receive rabies PEP after coming into contact with a potentially rabid animal [204]. Indications for rabies PEP include being bitten or scratched by a suspected rabid animal or when a reliable history of exposure cannot be obtained. For example, if a person awakens in a room to find a bat in the room, PEP may be considered, as contact between the bat through the person's mucous membrane (lips) and the bat cannot be excluded. Treatment can be discontinued if a suspected rabid animal is quarantined and remains healthy for 10 days or if the animal is humanely killed and tests negative for rabies [205]. It is important to treat patients exposed to rabies with PEP because treatment of clinical rabies is an extreme challenge and only one person has recovered from rabies without receiving PEP [204].

Wound cleansing is the first step of PEP. It is especially important because wound cleansing alone without any further PEP has shown a marked reduction in the likelihood of rabies. The recommendations for rabies PEP are the following:

- Those who have not previously received the rabies vaccine should be given both passive antibody and vaccine. Unvaccinated individuals should receive rabies vaccine on days 0, 3, 7, and 14 (a fifth dose on day 28 if immunocompromised). Human rabies IG should be administered around the wound if anatomically feasible, with the rest into the gluteal region.
- Those previously vaccinated with rabies vaccine series should only be readministered the vaccine: only two doses of vaccine (days 0 and 3) are necessary if there is evidence of protective neutralizing antibodies [206].

Tetanus

Puncture wounds, compound fractures, burns, unsterile injections, and crush injuries or wounds with potential contamination with dirt or rust are possible indications for tetanus PEP. If a person is uncertain of their vaccination history or did not complete a three-dose primary series of tetanus-containing vaccine, they should receive a tetanus vaccine and a single dose of tetanus IG.

- For minor and clean wounds, a person should receive a tetanus vaccine if their most recent dose was given more than 10 years ago.
- For puncture wounds or wounds contaminated with dirt, a tetanus vaccine is indicated if their most recent dose was more than 5 years ago [195].

Tuberculosis

Tuberculosis (TB) bacteria are put into the air when a person with TB disease of the lungs or throat coughs, speaks, or sings [207]. Anyone nearby could breathe in these bacteria and therefore should receive PEP. Even if a person previously received bacilli Calmette-Guérin (BCG) immunization or has their own tuberculosis history, they should still receive PEP. A tuberculin skin test or interferon gamma release assay should be performed after the exposure, and then again at 8–12 weeks after exposure. If either of these tests were to be positive, treatment with isoniazid plus vitamin B_6 for 9 months should be completed to ensure infectious TB disease does not develop [195].

While the USA has about 10,000 TB cases per year, it is important to keep in mind that one third of the world's population is infected with TB, and in 2014, 9.6 million people around the world had TB disease [207].

Varicella or Herpes Zoster

Vulnerable populations to a varicella zoster exposure include people older than 12 months of age who are unimmunized or immunocompromised children without evidence of immunity. Individuals who have contraindications for vaccination including pregnant women, immunocompromised people, and children less than 12 months of age are recommended to receive varicella zoster IG. Maximum benefit is achieved when PEP is administered as soon as possible after exposure, but may be effective if administered up to 10 days after exposure. Finally, in the absence of availability of IG and contraindications to vaccination, some experts recommend prophylaxis with acyclovir beginning 7–10 days after exposure (administered four times per day for 7 days) [208].

- The varicella vaccine should be administered within 3–5 days of exposure, with a second dose given at the appropriate age interval [198].
- For children under 13 years of age, the minimum interval between doses is 3 months, while for people greater than 13 years of age the minimum interval is 4 weeks [208].

Conclusion

Vaccines represent a large-scale, highly successful public health program that saves lives, reduces morbidity, and saves money. Multiple vaccine types designed to target a substantial variety of pathogens have been developed through rigorous scientific study and research. Vaccination schedules in infancy, childhood, and adulthood are safe and effective in protecting the most vulnerable populations from disease. Diseases once common and devastating in the USA have had substantial decreases in incidence, morbidity, and mortality with the initiation of routine vaccination programs. Worldwide eradication of several vaccine-targeted diseases appears possible. Ongoing research continues to look at improved vaccine efficacy, the longevity of vaccine protection, and special populations requiring enhanced disease protection.

References

1. Engerix-B [Package Insert on the Internet]. Research Triangle Park (NC): GlaxoSmithKline; 2016 [revised 2016 May; cited 2016 Aug 26]. Available from: https://www.gsksource.com/pharma/content/dam/GlaxoSmithKline/US/en/Prescribing_Information/Engerix-B/pdf/ENGERIX- B.PDF.
2. (CDC) C for DC. Diphtheria, tetanus, and pertussis: recommendations for vaccine use and other preventive measures. Recommendations of the Immunization Practices Advisory committee (ACIP). MMWR Recomm Rep [Internet]. 1991;40(Rr-10):1–28. Available from: http://www.cdc.gov/mmwr/preview/mmwrhtml/00041645.htm.
3. Diphtheria I Clinical Features I CDC [Internet]. [cited 2017 Jan 6]. Available from: https://www.cdc.gov/diphtheria/clinicians.html.
4. Surveillance Manual I Diphtheria I Vaccine Preventable Diseases I CDC [Internet]. [cited 2017 Jan 19]. Available from: https://www.cdc.gov/vaccines/pubs/surv-manual/chpt01-dip.html.
5. Pinkbook I Tetanus I Epidemiology of Vaccine Preventable Diseases I CDC [Internet]. [cited 2017 Jan 6]. Available from: https://www.cdc.gov/vaccines/pubs/pinkbook/tetanus.html.

6. (CDC) C for DC and P. Tetanus surveillance – United States, 2001–2008. MMWR Morb Mortal Wkly Rep [Internet]. 2011;60(12):365–9. Available from: http://www.cdc.gov/mmwr/preview/mmwrhtml/mm6012a1.htm.

7. Tetanus | Clinical Information | Lockjaw | CDC [Internet]. [cited 2017 Jan 9]. Available from: https://www.cdc.gov/tetanus/clinicians.html.

8. Tetanus Surveillance – United States, 2001–2008 [Internet]. [cited 2017 Jan 6]. Available from: https://www.cdc.gov/mmwr/preview/mmwrhtml/mm6012a1.htm.

9. Pertussis | Whooping Cough | Outbreaks | Trends | CDC [Internet]. [cited 2017 Jan 6]. Available from: https://www.cdc.gov/pertussis/outbreaks/trends.html.

10. American Academy of Pediatrics. Red Book 2015. In: David W. Kimberlin, Michael T. Brady, Mary Anne Jackson SSL, editors. Red Book: 2015 Report of the Committee on Infectious Diseases [Internet]. 30th ed. Elk Grove Village: American Academy of Pediatrics; 2015 [cited 2016 Oct 25]. p. 225–870. Available from: http://redbook.solutions.aap.org.

11. McGirr A, Fisman DN. Duration of pertussis immunity after DTaP immunization: a meta-analysis. Pediatrics. 2015;135(2):331–43.

12. Vaccines TH. The development of the immunization schedule. Philadelphia: The College of Physicians of Philadelphia.

13. Immunization Action Coalition. Vaccine timeline [Internet]. Saint Paul: Immunization Action Coalition; 2016 [updated 2017 February 16; cited 2016, August 26]. Available from.: http://www.immunize.org/timeline/.

14. Daptacel [Package Insert on the Internet]. Swiftwater (PA): Sanofi Pasteur Inc; 2002 [revised 2016 Sept; cited 2016 Nov 18]. Available from: https://www.vaccineshoppe.com/image.cfm?doc_id=11179&image_type=product_pdf.

15. INFANRIX [Package Insert on the Internet]. Research Triangle Park (NC): GlaxoSmithKline; 2016 [revised 2016 Oct; cited 2016 Nov 18]. Available from: https://www.gsksource.com/pharma/content/dam/GlaxoSmithKline/US/en/Prescribing_Information/Infanrix/pdf/INFANRIX.PDF.

16. Adacel [Package Insert on the Internet]. Swiftwater (PA): Sanofi Pasteur Inc.; 2005 [revised 2014 March; cited 2016 Aug 26]. Available from: https://www.vaccineshoppe.com/image.cfm?doc_id=10438&image_type=product_pdf.

17. BOOSTRIX [Package Insert on the Internet]. Research Triangle Park (NC): GlaxoSmithKline; 2016 [revised 2016 Oct; cited 2016 Nov 18]. Available from: https://www.gsksource.com/pharma/content/dam/GlaxoSmithKline/US/en/Prescribing_Information/Boostrix/pdf/BOOSTRIX.PDF.

18. Tenivac [Package Insert on the Internet]. Swiftwater (PA): Sanofi Pasteur Inc.; 2003 [revised 2013 April; cited 2016 Aug 26]. Available from: https://www.vaccineshoppe.com/image.cfm?doc_id=12609&image_type=product_pdf.

19. Centers for Disease Control and Prevention. In: Hamborsky J, Kroger A, Wolfe S, editors. Epidemiology and prevention of vaccine-preventable diseases. 13th ed. Washington D.C: Public Health Foundation; 2015.

20. Kjeldsen K, Simonsen O, Heron I. Immunity against diphtheria 25–30 years after primary vaccination in childhood. Lancet. 1985;1(8434):900–2.

21. Fine PE, Clarkson JA. Reflections on the efficacy of pertussis vaccines. Rev Infect Dis. 1987;9(5):866–83.

22. (CDC) C for DC and P. Pertussis vaccination: use of acellular pertussis vaccines among infants and young children. Recommendations of the Advisory Committee on Immunization Practices (ACIP). MMWR Recomm Rep [Internet]. 1997;46(Rr-7):1–25. Available from: http://www.cdc.gov/mmwr/PDF/rr/rr4607.pdf.

23. Tartof SY, Lewis M, Kenyon C, White K, Osborn A, Liko J, et al. Waning immunity to pertussis following 5 doses of DTaP. Pediatrics. 2013;131(4):e1047–52.

24. Klein NP, Bartlett J, Fireman B, Baxter R. Waning Tdap Effectiveness in Adolescents. Pediatrics. 2016;137(3):e20153326.

25. Estimated Influenza Illnesses and Hospitalizations Averted by Vaccination — United States, 2014–15 Influenza Season | Seasonal Influenza (Flu) | CDC [Internet]. [cited 2017 Jan 6]. Available from: https://www.cdc.gov/flu/about/disease/2014-15.htm.

26. WHO | Influenza (Seasonal). WHO. World Health Organization. 2016.
27. How the Flu Virus Can Change: "Drift" and "Shift" | Seasonal Influenza (Flu) | CDC [Internet]. Available from: http://www.cdc.gov/flu/about/viruses/change.htm.
28. Taubenberger JK, Morens DM. 1918 Influenza: the Mother of All Pandemics. Emerg Infect Dis [Internet]. 2006;12(1):15–22. [cited 2017 Jan 6]. Available from: http://wwwnc.cdc.gov/eid/article/12/1/05-0979_article.htm.
29. Influenza | History of Vaccines [Internet]. [cited 2017 Jan 6]. Available from: http://www.historyofvaccines.org/content/articles/influenza.
30. Influenza Vaccination: A Summary for Clinicians | Health Professionals | Seasonal Influenza (Flu) [Internet]. [cited 2017 Jan 6]. Available from: https://www.cdc.gov/flu/professionals/vaccination/vax-summary.htm.
31. CDC. Flu Vaccine Effectiveness: Questions and Answers for Health Professionals | Health Professionals | Seasonal Influenza (Flu) [Internet]. Available from: http://www.cdc.gov/flu/professionals/vaccination/effectivenessqa.htm.
32. CDC. Seasonal Influenza Vaccine Effectiveness, 2005–2016 [Internet]. [cited 2016 Aug 24]. Available from: http://www.cdc.gov/flu/professionals/vaccination/effectiveness-studies.htm.
33. DiazGranados CA, Dunning AJ, Kimmel M, Kirby D, Treanor J, Collins A, et al. Efficacy of high-dose versus standard-dose influenza vaccine in older adults. N Engl J Med [Internet]. 2014;371(7):635–45. [cited 2016 Aug 27]. Available from: http://www.ncbi.nlm.nih.gov/pubmed/25119609.
34. DiazGranados CA, Dunning AJ, Robertson CA, Talbot HK, Landolfi V, Greenberg DP. Efficacy and immunogenicity of high-dose influenza vaccine in older adults by age, comorbidities, and frailty. Vaccine. 2015;33(36):4565–71.
35. Polio | U.S. Polio Elimination | CDC [Internet]. [cited 2017 Jan 6]. Available from: https://www.cdc.gov/polio/us/index.html.
36. Initiative GPE. Polio this week as of 24 August 2016 [Internet]. Geneva: Global Polio Eradication Initiative; 2016. Available from: http://www.polioeradication.org/Dataandmonitoring/Poliothisweek.aspx.
37. McBean AM, Thoms ML, Albrecht P, Cuthie JC, Bernier R. Serologic response to oral polio vaccine and enhanced-potency inactivated polio vaccines. Am J Epidemiol. 1988;128(3):615–28.
38. Measles | For Healthcare Professionals | CDC [Internet]. [cited 2017 Jan 6]. Available from: https://www.cdc.gov/measles/hcp/index.html.
39. Moss WJ, Griffin DE. Measles. Lancet (London, England). 2012;379(9811):153–64.
40. Durrheim DN, Crowcroft NS, Strebel PM. Measles – The epidemiology of elimination. Vaccine [Internet]. 2014;32(51):6880–3. [cited 2016 Aug 30]. Available from: http://www.ncbi.nlm.nih.gov/pubmed/25444814.
41. Hviid A, Rubin S, Mühlemann K. Mumps. Lancet (London, England) [Internet]. 2008;371(9616):932–44. [cited 2016 Aug 28]. Available from: http://www.ncbi.nlm.nih.gov/pubmed/18342688.
42. Rubella | For Healthcare Professionals | CDC [Internet]. [cited 2017 Jan 9]. Available from: https://www.cdc.gov/rubella/hcp.html.
43. Vynnycky E, Adams EJ, Cutts FT, Reef SE, Navar AM, Simons E, et al. Using seroprevalence and immunisation coverage data to estimate the global burden of congenital rubella syndrome, 1996–2010: a systematic review. PLoS One [Internet]. 2016;11(3):e0149160. [cited 2016 Aug 25]. Available from: http://www.pubmedcentral.nih.gov/articlerender.fcgi?artid=4786291&tool=pmcentrez&rendertype=abstract.
44. Uzicanin A, Zimmerman L. Field effectiveness of live attenuated measles-containing vaccines: a review of published literature. J Infect Dis. 2011;204(Suppl):S133–48.
45. (CDC) C for DC and P. Measles prevention. MMWR Suppl [Internet]. 1989;38(9):1–18. Available from: http://www.cdc.gov/mmwr/preview/mmwrhtml/00041753.htm.
46. Vitek CR, Aduddell M, Brinton MJ, Hoffman RE, Redd SC. Increased protections during a measles outbreak of children previously vaccinated with a second dose of measles-mumps-rubella vaccine. Pediatr Infect Dis J. 1999;18(7):620–3.

47. Lynn TV, Beller M, Funk EA, Middaugh JP, Ritter D, Rota PA, et al. Incremental effectiveness of 2 doses of measles-containing vaccine compared with 1 dose among high school students during an outbreak. J Infect Dis. 2004;189(Suppl):S86–90.
48. Yeung LF, Lurie P, Dayan G, Eduardo E, Britz PH, Redd SB, et al. A limited measles outbreak in a highly vaccinated US boarding school. Pediatrics. 2005;116(6):1287–91.
49. LeBaron CW, Beeler J, Sullivan BJ, Forghani B, Bi D, Beck C, et al. Persistence of measles antibodies after 2 doses of measles vaccine in a postelimination environment. Arch Pediatr Adolesc Med. 2007;161(3):294–301.
50. (CDC) C for DC and P. Mumps Vaccination [Internet]. Atlanta; 2015. Available from: http://www.cdc.gov/mumps/vaccination.html.
51. Sugg WC, Finger JA, Levine RH, Pagano JS. Field evaluation of live virus mumps vaccine. J Pediatr. 1968;72(4):461–6.
52. (CDC) C for DC and P. Epidemiologic Notes and Reports Mumps DOUBLEHYPHEN United States, 1985–1986 [Internet]. MMWR Morb Mortal Wkly Rep. Atlanta; 1987. Available from: https://www.cdc.gov/mmwr/preview/mmwrhtml/00000890.htm.
53. Kim-Farley R, Bart S, Stetler H, Orenstein W, Bart K, Sullivan K, et al. Clinical mumps vaccine efficacy. Am J Epidemiol. 1985;121(4):593–7.
54. Chaiken BP, Williams NM, Preblud SR, Parkin W, Altman R. The effect of a school entry law on mumps activity in a school district. JAMA. 1987;257(18):2455–8.
55. Wharton M, Cochi SL, Hutcheson RH, Bistowish JM, Schaffner W. A large outbreak of mumps in the postvaccine era. J Infect Dis. 1988;158(6):1253–60.
56. Schaffzin JK, Pollock L, Schulte C, Henry K, Dayan G, Blog D, et al. Effectiveness of previous mumps vaccination during a summer camp outbreak. Pediatrics. 2007;120(4):e862–8.
57. Marin M, Quinlisk P, Shimabukuro T, Sawhney C, Brown C, Lebaron CW. Mumps vaccination coverage and vaccine effectiveness in a large outbreak among college studentsDOUBLEHYPHENIowa, 2006. Vaccine. 2008;26(29–30):3601–7.
58. Ogbuanu IU, Kutty PK, Hudson JM, Blog D, Abedi GR, Goodell S, et al. Impact of a third dose of measles-mumps-rubella vaccine on a mumps outbreak. Pediatrics. 2012;130(6):e1567–74.
59. M-M-R II [Package Insert on the Internet]. Whitehouse Station (NJ): Merck; 2017 [revised 2017 May; cited 2017 June 28]. Available from: https://www.merck.com/product/usa/pi_circulars/m/mmr_ii/mmr_ii_pi.pdf
60. Beasley RP, Detels R, Kim KS, Gale JL, Lin TL, Grayston JT. Prevention of rubella during an epidemic on Taiwan. HPV-77 and RA 27–3 rubella vaccines administered subcutaneously and intranasally HPV-77 vaccine mixed with mumps and-or measles vaccines. Am J Dis Child. 1969;118(2):301–6.
61. Christenson B, Bottiger M. Long-term follow-up study of rubella antibodies in naturally immune and vaccinated young adults. Vaccine. 1994;12(1):41–5.
62. WHO I 1 July 2011, vol. 86, 27 (pp 277–288). WHO. World Health Organization; 2012.
63. Trépo C, Chan HLY, Lok A. Hepatitis B virus infection. Lancet (London, England) [Internet]. 2014;384(9959):2053–63. [cited 2016 Aug 28]. Available from: http://www.ncbi.nlm.nih.gov/pubmed/24954675.
64. Commentary I U.S. 2014 Surveillance Data for Viral Hepatitis I Statistics & Surveillance I Division of Viral Hepatitis I CDC [Internet]. [cited 2017 Jan 6]. Available from: https://www.cdc.gov/hepatitis/statistics/2014surveillance/commentary.htm#bkgrndB.
65. El-Serag HB. Epidemiology of viral hepatitis and hepatocellular carcinoma. Gastroenterology [Internet]. 2012;142(6):1264–73. e1.[cited 2016 Aug 17]. Available from: http://www.pubmedcentral.nih.gov/articlerender.fcgi?artid=3338949&tool=pmcentrez&rendertype=abstract
66. Dionne-Odom J, Tita ATN, Silverman NS. #38: Hepatitis B in pregnancy screening, treatment, and prevention of vertical transmission. Am J Obstet Gynecol [Internet]. 2016;214(1):6–14. [cited 2016 Aug 28]. Available from: http://www.ncbi.nlm.nih.gov/pubmed/26454123
67. Lavanchy D. Viral hepatitis: global goals for vaccination. J Clin Virol [Internet]. 2012;55(4):296–302. [cited 2016 Aug 28]. Available from: http://www.ncbi.nlm.nih.gov/pubmed/22999800.

68. Mast EE, Margolis HS, Fiore AE, Brink EW, Goldstein ST, Wang SA, et al. A comprehensive immunization strategy to eliminate transmission of hepatitis B virus infection in the United States: recommendations of the Advisory Committee on Immunization Practices (ACIP) part 1: immunization of infants, children, and adolescents. MMWR Recomm Rep. 2005;54(Rr-16):1–31.

69. Mast EE, Weinbaum CM, Fiore AE, Alter MJ, Bell BP, Finelli L, et al. A comprehensive immunization strategy to eliminate transmission of hepatitis B virus infection in the United States: recommendations of the Advisory Committee on Immunization Practices (ACIP) Part II: immunization of adults. MMWR Recomm Rep. 2006;55(Rr-16):1–4.

70. Schillie S, Walker T, Veselsky S, Crowley S, Dusek C, Lazaroff J, et al. Outcomes of infants born to women infected with hepatitis B. Pediatrics. 2015;135(5):e1141–7.

71. (CDC) C for DC and P. Protection against viral hepatitis. Recommendations of the Immunization Practices Advisory Committee (ACIP). MMWR Recomm Rep [Internet]. 1990;39(Rr-2):1–26. Available from: http://www.cdc.gov/mmwr/preview/mmwrhtml/00041917.htm.

72. (CDC) C for DC and P. Achievements in Public Health: Hepatitis B Vaccination DOUBLEHYPHEN- United States, 1982DOUBLEHYPHEN2002 [Internet]. MMWR Morb Mortal Wkly Rep. 2002.; Available from: http://www.cdc.gov/mmwr/preview/mmwrhtml/mm5125a3.htm.

73. RECOMBIVAX HB [Package Insert on the Internet]. Whitehouse Station (NJ): Merck & Co; 2014 [revised 2014 Nov; cited 2016 Aug 26]. Available from: https://www.merck.com/product/usa/pi_circulars/r/recombivax_hb/recombivax_pi.pdf.

74. (CDC) C for DC. Hepatitis B virus: a comprehensive strategy for eliminating transmission in the United States through universal childhood vaccination. Recommendations of the Immunization Practices Advisory Committee (ACIP). MMWR Recomm Rep [Internet]. 1991;40(Rr-13):1–19. Available from: http://www.cdc.gov/mmwr/preview/mmwrhtml/00033405.htm.

75. Greenberg DP. Pediatric experience with recombinant hepatitis B vaccines and relevant safety and immunogenicity studies. Pediatr Infect Dis J. 1993;12(5):438–45.

76. Bush LM, Moonsammy GI, Boscia JA. Evaluation of initiating a hepatitis B vaccination schedule with one vaccine and completing it with another. Vaccine. 1991;9(11):807–9.

77. McMahon BJ, Dentinger CM, Bruden D, Zanis C, Peters H, Hurlburt D, et al. Antibody levels and protection after hepatitis B vaccine: results of a 22-year follow-up study and response to a booster dose. J Infect Dis. 2009;200(9):1390–6.

78. Notice to Readers: FDA Approval for a Combined Hepatitis A and B Vaccine [Internet]. [cited 2017 Jan 16]. Available from: https://www.cdc.gov/mmwr/preview/mmwrhtml/mm5037a4.htm.

79. Haemophilus influenzae | Home | Hib | CDC [Internet]. [cited 2017 Jan 6]. Available from: https://www.cdc.gov/hi-disease/

80. Peltola H. Worldwide Haemophilus influenzae type b disease at the beginning of the 21st century: global analysis of the disease burden 25 years after the use of the polysaccharide vaccine and a decade after the advent of conjugates. Clin Microbiol Rev. 2000;13(2):302–17.

81. PedvaxHIB [Package Insert on the Internet]. Whitehouse Station (NJ): Merck; 1998 [revised 2010 Dec; cited 2016 Aug 26]. Available from: https://www.merck.com/product/usa/pi_circulars/p/pedvax_hib/pedvax_pi.pdf.

82. ActHIB [Package Insert on the Internet]. Swiftwater (PA): Sanofi Pasteur Inc.; 1993 [revised 2016 April; cited 2016 Aug 26]. Available from: https://www.vaccineshoppe.com/image.cfm?doc_id=13692&image_type=product_pdf.

83. HIBERIX [Package Insert on the Internet]. Research Triangle Park (NC): GlaxoSmithKline; 2016 [revised 2016 Jan; cited 2016 Aug 26]. Available from: https://gsksource.com/pharma/content/dam/GlaxoSmithKline/US/en/Prescribing_Information/Hiberix/pdf/HIBERIX.PDF.

84. Granoff DM, Anderson EL, Osterholm MT, Holmes SJ, McHugh JE, Belshe RB, et al. Differences in the immunogenicity of three Haemophilus influenzae type b conjugate vaccines in infants. J Pediatr. 1992;121(2):187–94.

85. (CDC) C for DC and P. Licensure of a Haemophilus influenzae type b (Hib) vaccine (Hiberix) and updated recommendations for use of Hib vaccine. MMWR Morb Mortal Wkly Rep [Internet]. 2009;58(36):1008–9. Available from: http://www.cdc.gov/mmwr/preview/mmwrhtml/mm5836a5.htm.

86. (CDC) C for DC and P. Progress toward eliminating Haemophilus influenzae type b disease among infants and childrenDOUBLEHYPHENUnited States, 1987–1997. MMWR Morb Mortal Wkly Rep [Internet]. 1998;47(46):993–8. Available from: http://www.cdc.gov/mmwr/preview/mmwrhtml/00055745.htm.

87. Chickenpox | Clinical Overview | Varicella | CDC [Internet]. [cited 2017 Jan 6]. Available from: https://www.cdc.gov/chickenpox/hcp/clinical-overview.html.

88. Cobelli Kett J. Perinatal varicella. Pediatr Rev [Internet]. 2013;34(1):49–51. [cited 2016 Aug 28]. Available from: http://www.ncbi.nlm.nih.gov/pubmed/23281363.

89. Flatt A, Breuer J. Varicella vaccines. Br Med Bull. 2012;103(1):115–27.

90. Zhou F, Ortega-Sanchez IR, Guris D, Shefer A, Lieu T, Seward JF. An economic analysis of the universal varicella vaccination program in the United States. J Infect Dis [Internet]. Oxford University Press; 2008;197(Supplement 2):S156–S164. [cited 2017 Jan 8]. Available from: http://www.ncbi.nlm.nih.gov/pubmed/18419391.

91. Varivax [Package Insert on the Internet]. Whitehouse Station (NJ): Merck; 1995 [revised 2017 Feb; cited 2017 June 28]. Available from: https://www.merck.com/product/usa/pi_circulars/v/varivax/varivax_pi.pdf.

92. Weibel RE, Neff BJ, Kuter BJ, Guess HA, Rothenberger CA, Fitzgerald AJ, et al. Live attenuated varicella virus vaccine. Efficacy trial in healthy children. N Engl J Med. 1984;310(22):1409–15.

93. Kuter BJ, Weibel RE, Guess HA, Matthews H, Morton DH, Neff BJ, et al. Oka/Merck varicella vaccine in healthy children: final report of a 2-year efficacy study and 7-year follow-up studies. Vaccine. 1991;9(9):643–7.

94. Seward JF, Marin M, Vazquez M. Varicella vaccine effectiveness in the US vaccination program: a review. J Infect Dis. 2008;197(Suppl):S82–9.

95. Vazquez M, LaRussa PS, Gershon AA, Niccolai LM, Muehlenbein CE, Steinberg SP, et al. Effectiveness over time of varicella vaccine. JAMA. 2004;291(7):851–5.

96. Marin M, Guris D, Chaves SS, Schmid S, Seward JF. Prevention of varicella: recommendations of the Advisory Committee on Immunization Practices (ACIP). MMWR Recomm Rep. 2007;56(Rr-4):1–40.

97. Shapiro ED, Vazquez M, Esposito D, Holabird N, Steinberg SP, Dziura J, et al. Effectiveness of 2 doses of varicella vaccine in children. J Infect Dis. 2011;203(3):312–5.

98. Leung J, Harpaz R. Impact of the maturing varicella vaccination program on varicella and related outcomes in the United States: 1994–2012. J Pediatr Infect Dis Soc. 2015;5(4):395–402.

99. Use of Combination Measles, Mumps, Rubella, and Varicella Vaccine [Internet]. [cited 2017 Jan 19]. Available from: https://www.cdc.gov/mmwr/preview/mmwrhtml/rr5903a1.htm.

100. Aggarwal R, Goel A. Hepatitis A: epidemiology in resource-poor countries. Curr Opin Infect Dis [Internet]. 2015;28(5):488–96. [cited 2016 Aug 28]. Available from: http://www.ncbi.nlm.nih.gov/pubmed/26203853.

101. Wu D, Guo C-Y. Epidemiology and prevention of hepatitis A in travelers. J Travel Med [Internet]. 2013;20(6):394–9. [cited 2016 Aug 28]. Available from: http://www.ncbi.nlm.nih.gov/pubmed/24165384.

102. Commentary | U.S. 2014 Surveillance Data for Viral Hepatitis | Statistics & Surveillance | Division of Viral Hepatitis | CDC [Internet]. [cited 2017 Jan 8]. Available from: https://www.cdc.gov/hepatitis/statistics/2014surveillance/commentary.htm#bkgrndA

103. Hepatitis A Questions and Answers for Health Professionals | Division of Viral Hepatitis | CDC [Internet]. [cited 2017 Jan 6]. Available from: https://www.cdc.gov/hepatitis/HAV/HAVfaq.htm#general.

104. Havrix [Package Insert on the Internet]. Research Triangle Park (NC): GlaxoSmithKline; 2016 [revised 2016 May; cited 2016 Aug 26]. Available from: https://www.gsksource.

com/pharma/content/dam/GlaxoSmithKline/US/en/Prescribing_Information/Havrix/pdf/
HAVRIX.PDF.

105. Vaqta [Package Insert on the Internet]. Whitehouse Station (NJ): Merck; 2014 [revised 2014 Feb; cited 2016 Aug 26]. Available from: https://www.merck.com/product/usa/pi_circulars/v/vaqta/vaqta_pi.pdf.

106. Braconier JH, Wennerholm S, Norrby SR. Comparative immunogenicity and tolerance of Vaqta and Havrix. Vaccine. 1999;17(17):2181–4.

107. Van Herck K, Crasta PD, Messier M, Hardt K, Van Damme P. Seventeen-year antibody persistence in adults primed with two doses of an inactivated hepatitis A vaccine. Hum Vaccin Immunother. 2012;8(3):323–7.

108. Hens N, Habteab Ghebretinsae A, Hardt K, Van Damme P, Van Herck K. Model based estimates of long-term persistence of inactivated hepatitis A vaccine-induced antibodies in adults. Vaccine. 2014;32(13):1507–13.

109. Murphy TV, Denniston MM, Hill HA, McDonald M, Klevens MR, Elam-Evans LD, et al. Progress toward eliminating hepatitis A disease in the United States. MMWR Suppl [Internet]. 2016;65(1):29–41. Available from: http://www.cdc.gov/mmwr/volumes/65/su/su6501a6.htm.

110. TWINRIX [Package Insert on the Internet]. Research Triangle Park (NC): GlaxoSmithKline; 2016 [revised 2016 Dec; cited 2017 June 28]. Available from: https://gsksource.com/pharma/content/dam/GlaxoSmithKline/US/en/Prescribing_Information/Twinrix/pdf/TWINRIX.PDF.

111. Notice to Readers: FDA Approval for a Combined Hepatitis A and B Vaccine [Internet]. [cited 2017 Jan 6]. Available from: https://www.cdc.gov/mmwr/preview/mmwrhtml/mm5037a4.htm.

112. Prevention of Rotavirus Gastroenteritis Among Infants and Children Recommendations of the Advisory Committee on Immunization Practices (ACIP) [Internet]. [cited 2017 Jan 8]. Available from: https://www.cdc.gov/mmwr/preview/mmwrhtml/rr5802a1.htm.

113. Surveillance Manual | Rotavirus | Vaccine Preventable Diseases | CDC [Internet]. [cited 2017 Jan 6]. Available from: https://www.cdc.gov/vaccines/pubs/surv-manual/chpt13-rotavirus.html.

114. Butz AM, Fosarelli P, Dick J, Cusack T, Yolken R. Prevalence of rotavirus on high-risk fomites in day-care facilities. Pediatrics [Internet]. 1993 [cited 2017 Jan 6];92(2):202–5. Available from: http://www.ncbi.nlm.nih.gov/pubmed/8393172

115. Dennehy PH, Cortese MM, Bégué RE, Jaeger JL, Roberts NE, Zhang R, et al. A case-control study to determine risk factors for hospitalization for rotavirus gastroenteritis in U.S. Children. Pediatr Infect Dis J [Internet]. 2006;25(12):1123–31. [cited 2017 Jan 8]. Available from: http://www.ncbi.nlm.nih.gov/pubmed/17133157.

116. Parashar UD, Nelson EAS, Kang G. Diagnosis, management, and prevention of rotavirus gastroenteritis in children. BMJ [Internet]. 2013;347:f7204. [cited 2016 Aug 27]. Available from: http://www.ncbi.nlm.nih.gov/pubmed/24379214.

117. Rha B, Tate JE, Payne DC, Cortese MM, Lopman BA, Curns AT, et al. Effectiveness and impact of rotavirus vaccines in the United States – 2006-2012. Expert Rev Vaccines [Internet]. 2014;13(3):365–376. [cited 2016 Aug 27]. Available from: http://www.ncbi.nlm.nih.gov/pubmed/24392657.

118. Rotavirus Vaccination | CDC [Internet]. [cited 2017 Jan 19]. Available from: https://www.cdc.gov/vaccines/vpd/rotavirus/index.html.

119. Cortese MM, Parashar UD. Prevention of rotavirus gastroenteritis among infants and children: recommendations of the Advisory Committee on Immunization Practices (ACIP). MMWR Recomm Rep [Internet]. 2009;58(Rr-2):1–25. Available from: http://www.cdc.gov/mmwr/preview/mmwrhtml/rr5802a1.htm.

120. Vesikari T, Matson DO, Dennehy P, Van Damme P, Santosham M, Rodriguez Z, et al. Safety and efficacy of a pentavalent human-bovine (WC3) reassortant rotavirus vaccine. N Engl J Med. 2006;354(1):23–33.

121. Vesikari T, Karvonen A, Ferrante SA, Kuter BJ, Ciarlet M. Sustained efficacy of the pentavalent rotavirus vaccine, RV5, up to 3.1 years following the last dose of vaccine. Pediatr Infect Dis J. 2010;29(10):957–63.

122. Ruiz-Palacios GM, Perez-Schael I, Velazquez FR, Abate H, Breuer T, Clemens SC, et al. Safety and efficacy of an attenuated vaccine against severe rotavirus gastroenteritis. N Engl J Med. 2006;354(1):11–22.

123. Vesikari T, Karvonen A, Prymula R, Schuster V, Tejedor JC, Cohen R, et al. Efficacy of human rotavirus vaccine against rotavirus gastroenteritis during the first 2 years of life in European infants: randomised, double-blind controlled study. Lancet. 2007;370(9601):1757–63.

124. Krishnarajah G, Duh MS, Korves C, Demissie K. Public health impact of complete and incomplete rotavirus vaccination among commercially and medicaid insured children in the United States. PLoS One. 2016;11(1):e0145977.

125. Pinkbook I Pneumococcal I Epidemiology of Vaccine Preventable Diseases I CDC [Internet]. [cited 2017 Jan 8]. Available from: https://www.cdc.gov/vaccines/pubs/pinkbook/pneumo.html.

126. Pneumococcal Disease I Transmission and Those at High Risk I CDC [Internet]. [cited 2017 Jan 6]. Available from: https://www.cdc.gov/pneumococcal/about/risk-transmission.html.

127. Givon-Lavi N, Dagan R, Fraser D, Yagupsky P, Porat N. Marked differences in pneumococcal carriage and resistance patterns between day care centers located within a small area. Clin Infect Dis [Internet]. 1999;29(5):1274–1280. [cited 2017 Jan 6]. Available from: http://www.ncbi.nlm.nih.gov/pubmed/10524975.

128. Pneumococcal Disease I Clinical I Features I CDC [Internet]. [cited 2017 Jan 8]. Available from: https://www.cdc.gov/pneumococcal/clinicians/clinical-features.html.

129. Maraqa NF. Pneumococcal Infections. Pediatr Rev [Internet]. 2014;35(7):299–310. [cited 2017 Jan 8]. Available from: http://www.ncbi.nlm.nih.gov/pubmed/24986929.

130. CDC. Licensure of a 13-Valent Pneumococcal Conjugate Vaccine (PCV13) and Recommendations for Use Among Children DOUBLEHYPHEN- Advisory Committee on Immunization Practices (ACIP), 2010 [Internet]. Available from: http://www.cdc.gov/mmwR/preview/mmwrhtml/mm5909a2.htm.

131. CDC, Ncird. Immunology and Vaccine-Preventable Diseases – Pink Book – Pneumococcal Disease.

132. Pavia M, Bianco A, Nobile CGA, Marinelli P, Angelillo IF. Efficacy of pneumococcal vaccination in children younger than 24 months: a meta-analysis. Pediatrics [Internet]. American Academy of Pediatrics. 2009;123(6):e1103–10. [cited 2016 Aug 28]. Available from: http://www.ncbi.nlm.nih.gov/pubmed/19482744.

133. Prevention of Pneumococcal Disease: Recommendations of the Advisory Committee on Immunization Practices (ACIP) [Internet]. [cited 2017 Jan 19]. Available from: https://www.cdc.gov/mmwr/preview/mmwrhtml/00047135.htm#00002348.htm

134. Meningococcal I Technical and Clinical Info I CDC [Internet]. [cited 2017 Jan 8]. Available from: https://www.cdc.gov/meningococcal/clinical-info.html.

135. Meningitis I Lab Manual I Epidemiology I CDC [Internet]. [cited 2017 Jan 6]. Available from: https://www.cdc.gov/meningitis/lab-manual/chpt02-epi.html.

136. Armand J, Arminjon F, Mynard MC, Lafaix C. Tetravalent meningococcal polysaccharide vaccine groups A, C, Y, W 135: clinical and serological evaluation. J Biol Stand. 1982/10/01. 1982;10(4):335–9.

137. Bilukha OO, Rosenstein N. Prevention and control of meningococcal disease. Recommendations of the Advisory Committee on Immunization Practices (ACIP). MMWR Recomm Rep [Internet]. 2005/05/27. 2005;54(Rr-7):1–21. Available from: http://www.cdc.gov/mmwr/preview/mmwrhtml/rr5407a1.htm

138. Rosenstein N, Levine O, Taylor JP, Evans D, Plikaytis BD, Wenger JD, et al. Efficacy of meningococcal vaccine and barriers to vaccination. JAMA. 1998/02/18. 1998;279(6):435–9.

139. Gold R, Lepow ML, Goldschneider I, Draper TF, Gotshlich EC. Kinetics of antibody production to group A and group C meningococcal polysaccharide vaccines administered during the first six years of life: prospects for routine immunization of infants and children. J Infect Dis. 1979/11/01. 1979;140(5):690–7.

140. Zangwill KM, Stout RW, Carlone GM, Pais L, Harekeh H, Mitchell S, et al. Duration of anti-body response after meningococcal polysaccharide vaccination in US Air Force personnel. J Infect Dis. 1994/04/01. 1994;169(4):847–52.

141. Menactra [Package Insert on the Internet]. Swiftwater (PA): Sanofi Pasteur Inc; 2005 [revised 2016 Sept; cited 2016 Nov 18]. Available from: https://www.vaccineshoppe.com/image. cfm?doc_id=12580&image_type=product_pdf.

142. Keyserling H, Papa T, Koranyi K, Ryall R, Bassily E, Bybel MJ, et al. Safety, immunogenic-ity, and immune memory of a novel meningococcal (groups A, C, Y, and W-135) polysac-charide diphtheria toxoid conjugate vaccine (MCV-4) in healthy adolescents. Arch Pediatr Adolesc Med. 2005/10/06. 2005;159(10):907–13.

143. Pichichero M, Casey J, Blatter M, Rothstein E, Ryall R, Bybel M, et al. Comparative trial of the safety and immunogenicity of quadrivalent (A, C, Y, W-135) meningococcal polysac-charide-diphtheria conjugate vaccine versus quadrivalent polysaccharide vaccine in two- to ten-year-old children. Pediatr Infect Dis J. 2005/01/25. 2005;24(1):57–62.

144. Jackson LA, Jacobson RM, Reisinger KS, Anemona A, Danzig LE, Dull PM. A randomized trial to determine the tolerability and immunogenicity of a quadrivalent meningococcal glyco-conjugate vaccine in healthy adolescents. Pediatr Infect Dis J. 2009/01/01. 2009;28(2):86–91.

145. Halperin SA, Gupta A, Jeanfreau R, Klein NP, Reisinger K, Walter E, et al. Comparison of the safety and immunogenicity of an investigational and a licensed quadrivalent meningococcal conjugate vaccine in children 2–10 years of age. Vaccine. 2010/10/15. 2010;28(50):7865–72.

146. Jacobson RM, Jackson LA, Reisinger K, Izu A, Odrljin T, Dull PM. Antibody persistence and response to a booster dose of a quadrivalent conjugate vaccine for meningococcal disease in adolescents. Pediatr Infect Dis J. 2012/11/02. 2013;32(4):e170–7.

147. Cohn AC, MacNeil JR, Clark TA, Ortega-Sanchez IR, Briere EZ, Meissner HC, et al. Prevention and control of meningococcal disease: recommendations of the Advisory Committee on Immunization Practices (ACIP). MMWR Recomm Rep [Internet]. 2013/03/22. 2013;62 (Rr-2):1–28. Available from: http://www.cdc.gov/mmwr/preview/mmwrhtml/rr6202a1.htm

148. Folaranmi T, Rubin L, Martin SW, Patel M, MacNeil JR. Use of serogroup B meningococ-cal vaccines in persons aged >/=10 years at increased risk for serogroup B meningococcal disease: recommendations of the Advisory Committee on Immunization Practices, 2015. MMWR Morb Mortal Wkly Rep. 2015/06/13. 2015;64(22):608–12.

149. Trumenba [Package Insert on the Internet]. Philadelphia (PA): Wyeth Pharmaceuticals Inc.; 2014 [revised 2017 March; cited 2017 June 28]. Available from: http://labeling.pfizer.com/ ShowLabeling.aspx?id=1796.

150. Bexsero [Package Insert on the Internet]. Cambridge (MA): Novartis Vaccines and Diagnostics, Inc.; 2015 [revised 2016 Sept; cited 2016 Nov 18]. Available from: https://www. gsksource.com/pharma/content/dam/GlaxoSmithKline/US/en/Prescribing_Information/ Bexsero/pdf/BEXSERO.PDF.

151. Vesikari T, Ostergaard L, Diez-Domingo J, Wysocki J, Flodmark CE, Beeslaar J, et al. Meningococcal serogroup B bivalent rLP2086 vaccine elicits broad and robust serum bactericidal responses in healthy adolescents. J Pediatr Infect Dis Soc. 2015/09/26. 2016;5(2):152–60.

152. MacNeil JR, Rubin L, Folaranmi T, Ortega-Sanchez IR, Patel M, Martin SW. Use of sero-group B meningococcal vaccines in adolescents and young adults: recommendations of the Advisory Committee on Immunization Practices, 2015. MMWR Morb Mortal Wkly Rep. 2015/10/23. 2015;64(41):1171–6.

153. Santolaya ME, O'Ryan ML, Valenzuela MT, Prado V, Vergara R, Munoz A, et al. Immunogenicity and tolerability of a multicomponent meningococcal serogroup B (4CMenB) vaccine in healthy adolescents in Chile: a phase 2b/3 randomised, observer-blind, placebo-controlled study. Lancet. 2012/01/21. 2012;379(9816):617–24.

154. Santolaya ME, O'Ryan M, Valenzuela MT, Prado V, Vergara RF, Munoz A, et al. Persistence of antibodies in adolescents 18–24 months after immunization with one, two, or three doses of 4CMenB meningococcal serogroup B vaccine. Hum Vaccin Immunother. 2013/07/03. 2013;9(11):2304–10.

155. Satterwhite CL, Torrone E, Meites E, Dunne EF, Mahajan R, Ocfemia MCB, et al. Sexually transmitted infections among US women and men. Sex Transm Dis [Internet]. 2013;40(3):187–93. [cited 2017 Jan 8]. Available from: http://www.ncbi.nlm.nih.gov/pubmed/23403598.

156. HPV Statistics I CDC [Internet]. [cited 2017 Jan 8]. Available from: https://www.cdc.gov/std/hpv/stats.htm.

157. CDC – HPV-Associated Cancer Statistics [Internet]. [cited 2017 Jan 8]. Available from: https://www.cdc.gov/cancer/hpv/statistics/.

158. Meites E, Kempe A, Markowitz LE. Use of a 2-Dose Schedule for Human Papillomavirus Vaccination — Updated Recommendations of the Advisory Committee on Immunization Practices. MMWR Morb Mortal Wkly Rep [Internet]. 2016;65(49):1405–8. [cited 2017 Jan 8]. Available from: http://www.cdc.gov/mmwr/volumes/65/wr/mm6549a5.htm

159. de Sanjose S, Quint WG, Alemany L, Geraets DT, Klaustermeier JE, Lloveras B, et al. Human papillomavirus genotype attribution in invasive cervical cancer: a retrospective cross-sectional worldwide study. Lancet Oncol. 2010/10/19. 2010;11(11):1048–56.

160. Garland SM, Hernandez-Avila M, Wheeler CM, Perez G, Harper DM, Leodolter S, et al. Quadrivalent vaccine against human papillomavirus to prevent anogenital diseases. N Engl J Med [Internet]. 2007/05/15. 2007;356(19):1928–43. Available from: http://www.nejm.org/doi/pdf/10.1056/NEJMoa061760

161. Giuliano AR, Palefsky JM, Goldstone S, Moreira Jr. ED, Penny ME, Aranda C, et al. Efficacy of quadrivalent HPV vaccine against HPV Infection and disease in males. N Engl J Med. 2011/02/04. 2011;364(5):401–11.

162. Gardasil 9 [Package Insert from the Internet]. Whitehouse Station (NJ): Merck; 2016 [revised 2017 Jan; cited 2017 June 28]. Available from: https://www.merck.com/product/usa/pi_circulars/g/gardasil_9/gardasil_9_pi.pdf,

163. Saraiya M, Unger ER, Thompson TD, Lynch CF, Hernandez BY, Lyu CW, et al. US assessment of HPV types in cancers: implications for current and 9-valent HPV vaccines. J Natl Cancer Inst. 2015/05/01. 2015;107(6):djv086.

164. Joura EA, Giuliano AR, Iversen OE, Bouchard C, Mao C, Mehlsen J, et al. A 9-valent HPV vaccine against infection and intraepithelial neoplasia in women. N Engl J Med. 2015/02/19. 2015;372(8):711–23.

165. Petrosky E, Bocchini Jr. JA, Hariri S, Chesson H, Curtis CR, Saraiya M, et al. Use of 9-valent human papillomavirus (HPV) vaccine: updated HPV vaccination recommendations of the advisory committee on immunization practices. MMWR Morb Mortal Wkly Rep [Internet]. 2015/03/27. 2015;64(11):300–4. Available from: http://www.cdc.gov/mmwr/preview/mmwrhtml/mm6411a3.htm.

166. Markowitz LE, Hariri S, Lin C, Dunne EF, Steinau M, McQuillan G, et al. Reduction in human papillomavirus (HPV) prevalence among young women following HPV vaccine introduction in the United States, National Health and Nutrition Examination Surveys, 2003–2010. J Infect Dis [Internet]. Oxford University Press; 2013;208(3):385–93. [cited 2016 Oct 24]. Available from: http://www.ncbi.nlm.nih.gov/pubmed/23785124

167. Luckett R, Feldman S. Impact of 2-, 4- and 9-valent HPV vaccines on morbidity and mortality from cervical cancer. Hum Vaccin Immunother. 2015/11/21. 2016;12(6):1332–42.

168. Shingles I Home I Herpes Zoster I CDC [Internet]. [cited 2017 Jan 8]. Available from: https://www.cdc.gov/shingles/

169. Welsby PD. Chickenpox, chickenpox vaccination, and shingles. Postgrad Med J [Internet]. BMJ Group; 2006;82(967):351–2. [cited 2017 Jan 8]. Available from: http://www.ncbi.nlm.nih.gov/pubmed/16679476

170. Shingles Clinical Overview CDC [Internet]. [cited 2017 Jan 8]. Available from: https://www.cdc.gov/shingles/hcp/clinical-overview.html

171. Shingles I Surveillance, Trends, Deaths I Herpes Zoster I CDC [Internet]. [cited 2017 Jan 8]. Available from: https://www.cdc.gov/shingles/surveillance.html

172. Zostavax [Package Insert on the Internet]. Whitehouse Station (NJ): Merck; 2017 [revised 2017 March; cited 2017 June 28]. Available from: https://www.merck.com/product/usa/pi_circulars/z/zostavax/zostavax_pi2.pdf.

173. Oxman MN, Levin MJ, Johnson GR, Schmader KE, Straus SE, Gelb LD, et al. A vaccine to prevent herpes zoster and postherpetic neuralgia in older adults. N Engl J Med. 2005/06/03. 2005;352(22):2271–84.
174. Schmader KE, Oxman MN, Levin MJ, Johnson G, Zhang JH, Betts R, et al. Persistence of the efficacy of zoster vaccine in the shingles prevention study and the short-term persistence substudy. Clin Infect Dis [Internet]. 2012;55(10):1320–8. Available from: http://www.ncbi.nlm.nih.gov/pubmed/22828595
175. Tseng HF, Harpaz R, Luo Y, Hales CM, Sy LS, Tartof SY, et al. Declining effectiveness of herpes zoster vaccine in adults aged >/=60 Years. J Infect Dis. 2016/02/26. 2016;213(12):1872–5.
176. Hales CM, Harpaz R, Ortega-Sanchez I, Bialek SR. Update on recommendations for use of herpes zoster vaccine. MMWR Morb Mortal Wkly Rep. 2014/08/22. 2014;63(33):729–31.
177. Arnold N, Messaoudi I. Herpes zoster and the search for an effective vaccine. Clin Exp Immunol. 2016/05/11. 2016;187(1):82–92.
178. Baxter D. Active and passive immunity, vaccine types, excipients and licensing. Occup Med (Lond) [Internet]. 2007;57(8):552–6. [cited 2016 Aug 25]. Available from: http://occmed.oxfordjournals.org/content/57/8/552
179. Different Types of Vaccines — History of Vaccines.
180. Services USD of H and H. Vaccines.gov. U.S. Department of Health and Human Services; [cited 2016 Aug 24]; Available from: http://www.vaccines.gov/more_info/types/
181. Givon-Lavi N, Dagan R, Fraser D, Yagupsky P, Porat N. Marked differences in pneumococcal carriage and resistance patterns between day care centers located within a small area. Clin Infect Dis [Internet]. 1999;29:1274–80. Available from: http://cid.oxfordjournals.org/content/29/5/1274.full.pdf
182. Hepatitis B Fact Sheet for Parents | CDC [Internet]. Available from: http://www.cdc.gov/vaccines/parents/diseases/child/hepb.html
183. CDC. Birth-18 Years Immunization Schedule | CDC [Internet]. Available from: http://www.cdc.gov/vaccines/schedules/hcp/imz/child-adolescent.html
184. Seasonal Influenza Vaccine Dosage & Administration | Seasonal Influenza (Flu) | CDC [Internet]. Available from: http://www.cdc.gov/flu/about/qa/vaxadmin.htm
185. CDC. Pregnancy and Vaccination | Guidelines and Recommendations by Vaccine | CDC [Internet]. Available from: http://www.cdc.gov/vaccines/pregnancy/hcp/guidelines.html
186. CDC. Adult Immunization Schedule by Vaccine and Age Group | CDC [Internet]. Available from: http://www.cdc.gov/vaccines/schedules/hcp/imz/adult.html
187. Flu Vaccine and People with Egg Allergies | Seasonal Influenza (Flu) | CDC [Internet]. [cited 2017 Jan 6]. Available from: https://www.cdc.gov/flu/protect/vaccine/egg-allergies.htm
188. Medical Dictionary. Postexposure prophylaxis [Internet]. [cited 2016 Aug 28]. Available from: http://medical-dictionary.thefreedictionary.com/postexposure+prophylaxis
189. CDC. Hepatitis A Questions and Answers for Health Professionals | Division of Viral Hepatitis | CDC [Internet]. Available from: http://www.cdc.gov/hepatitis/hav/havfaq.htm#D1
190. Update: Prevention of Hepatitis A After Exposure to Hepatitis A Virus and in International Travelers. Updated Recommendations of the Advisory Committee on Immunization Practices (ACIP) [Internet]. [cited 2017 Jan 8]. Available from: https://www.cdc.gov/mmWr/preview/mmwrhtml/mm5641a3.htm
191. Postexposure Prophylaxis | HBV | Division of Viral Hepatitis | CDC [Internet]. [cited 2017 Jan 8]. Available from: https://www.cdc.gov/hepatitis/hbv/pep.htm
192. Appendix B: Postexposure Prophylaxis to Prevent Hepatitis B Virus Infection [Internet]. [cited 2017 Jan 8]. Available from: https://www.cdc.gov/mmwr/preview/mmwrhtml/rr5516a3.htm?s_cid=rr5516a3_e
193. Pinkbook | Hepatitis B | Epidemiology of Vaccine Preventable Diseases | CDC [Internet]. [cited 2017 Jan 8]. Available from: https://www.cdc.gov/vaccines/pubs/pinkbook/hepb.html
194. CDC. Updated U.S. Public Health Service Guidelines for the Management of Occupational Exposures to HBV, HCV, and HIV and Recommendations for Postexposure Prophylaxis. MMWRMorbity Mortal Wkly Rep [Internet]. 2001; Available from: http://www.cdc.gov/mmwr/preview/mmwrhtml/rr5011a1.htm

195. Bader M, McKinsey D. Postexposure prophylaxis for common infectious diseases. Am Fam Physician. 2013;88(1):25–32.
196. Grant RM, Lama JR, Anderson PL, McMahan V, Liu AY, Vargas L, et al. Preexposure chemoprophylaxis for HIV prevention in men who have sex with men. N Engl J Med [Internet]. 2010;363(27):2587–99. [cited 2017 Jan 15]. Available from: http://www.nejm.org/doi/abs/10.1056/NEJMoa1011205
197. Thigpen MC, Kebaabetswe PM, Paxton LA, Smith DK, Rose CE, Segolodi TM, et al. Antiretroviral preexposure prophylaxis for heterosexual HIV transmission in Botswana. N Engl J Med [Internet]. 2012;367(5):423–34. [cited 2017 Jan 15]. Available from: http://www.nejm.org/doi/abs/10.1056/NEJMoa1110711
198. Woo TM. Postexposure management of vaccine-preventable diseases. J Pediatr Heal Care [Internet]. Elsevier; 2016;30(2):173–82. [cited 2016 Aug 19]. Available from: http://linkinghub.elsevier.com/retrieve/pii/S0891524515004356
199. CDC. Influenza Antiviral Medications: Summary for Clinicians [Internet]. [cited 2016 Aug 20]. Available from: http://www.cdc.gov/flu/professionals/antivirals/summary-clinicians.htm
200. Meningitis I About Bacterial Meningitis Infection I CDC [Internet]. Available from: http://www.cdc.gov/meningitis/bacterial.html
201. MacNeil, Jessica; Meyer S. Meningococcal Disease – Chapter 3–2016 Yellow Book I Travelers' Health I CDC. Available from: http://wwwnc.cdc.gov/travel/yellowbook/2016/infectious-diseases-related-to-travel/meningococcal-disease
202. CDC. Pertussis I Outbreaks I PEP Postexposure Antimicrobial Prophylaxis I CDC [Internet]. Available from: http://www.cdc.gov/pertussis/outbreaks/pep.html
203. Graham L. Practice guidelines: CDC releases guidelines on antimicrobial agents for the treatment and postexposure prophylaxis of pertussis – American Family Physician. Am Fam Physician [Internet]. 2006;74(2):333–6. Available from: http://www.aafp.org/afp/2006/0715/p333.html
204. CDC. Human Rabies Prevention DOUBLEHYPHEN- United States, 2008 Recommendations of the Advisory Committee on Immunization Practices. MMWR Morb Mortal Wkly Rep [Internet]. 2008;57:1–26. Available from: https://www.cdc.gov/mmwr/preview/mmwrhtml/rr57e507a1.htm
205. WHO I Guide for post-exposure prophylaxis. WHO. World Health Organization; 2013.
206. CDC. CDC – Medical Care – Rabies [Internet]. Available from: http://www.cdc.gov/rabies/medical_care/
207. CDC. CDC I TB I Basic TB Facts I How TB Spreads [Internet]. Available from: http://www.cdc.gov/tb/topic/basics/howtbspreads.htm
208. Varicella (Chickenpox) – Chapter 3–2016 Yellow Book I Travelers' Health I CDC [Internet]. Available from: http://wwwnc.cdc.gov/travel/yellowbook/2016/infectious-diseases-related to-travel/varicella-chickenpox
209. Belongia EA, Kieke BA, Donahue JG, et al. Effectiveness of inactivated influenza vaccines varied substantially with antigenic match from the 2004-2005 season to the 2006-2007 season. J Infect Dis. 2009;199(2):159–67. https://doi.org/10.1086/595861. PubMed PMID: 19086915
210. Belongia EA, Kieke BA, Donahue JG, et al. Influenza vaccine effectiveness in Wisconsin during the 2007-08 season: comparison of interim and final results. Vaccine. 2011;29(38):6558–63. https://doi.org/10.1016/j.vaccine.2011.07.002. Epub 2011 Jul 19. PubMed PMID: 21767593
211. Flannery B, Clippard J, Zimmerman RK, Norwalk MP, Jackson ML, Jackson LA, Monto AS, Petrie JG, McLean HQ, Belongia EA, Gaglani M, Berman L, Foust A, Sessions W, Thaker SN, Spencer S, Fry AM. Early estimates of seasonal influenza vaccine effectiveness – United States, January 2015. MMWR Morb Mortal Wkly Rep. 2015;64(1):10–5.
212. Griffin MR, Monto AS, Belongia EA, et al. Effectiveness of non-adjuvanted pandemic influenza a vaccines for preventing pandemic influenza acute respiratory illness visits in 4 U.S. communities. PLoS One. 2011;6(8):e23085. https://doi.org/10.1371/journal.pone.0023085. Epub 2011 Aug 12. PubMed PMID: 21857999

213. McLean HQ, Thompson MG, Sundaram ME, Kieke BA, Gaglani M, Murthy K, Piedra PA, Zimmerman RK, Nowalk MP, Raviotta JM, Jackson ML, Jackson L, Ohmit SE, Petrie JG, Monto AS, Meece JK, Thaker SN, Clippard JR, Spencer SM, Fry AM, Belongia EA. Influenza vaccine effectiveness in the United States during 2012-2013: variable protection by age and virus type. J Infect Dis. 2017;35(20):2685–93. pii: jiu647. [Epub ahead of print] PubMed PMID: 25406334.

214. Ohmit SE, Thompson MG, Petrie JG, et al. Influenza vaccine effectiveness in the 2011-2012 season: protection against each circulating virus and the effect of prior vaccination on estimates. Clin Infect Dis. 2014;58(3):319–27. https://doi.org/10.1093/cid/cit736. Epub 2013 Nov 13

215. Treanor JJ, Talbot HK, Ohmit SE, et al. Effectiveness of seasonal influenza vaccines in the United States during a season with circulation of all three vaccine strains. CID. 2012;55(7):951–9. Epub 2012 Jul 25. PubMed PMID: 22843783

216. Adenovirus Type 4 and Type 7 Vaccine, Live, Oral. [Package Insert on the Internet]. Sellersville (PA): Barr Labs, Inc; 2011 [revised 2014 April; cited 2016 June 7]. Available from: https://www.fda.gov/downloads/biologicsbloodvaccines/vaccines/approvedproducts/ucm247515.pdf

217. BioThrax (Anthrax Vaccine Adsorbed) [Package Insert on the Internet]. Lansing (MI): Emergent BioSolutions; 2015. [cited 206 June 7]. Available from.: https://www.fda.gov/downloads/biologicsbloodvaccines/vaccines/approvedproducts/ucm247515.pdf.

218. BCG Freeze-Dried Glutamate Vaccine [Package Insert on the Internet]. Tokyo (Japan): Japan BCG Laboratory; 1987. [cited 2016 June 7]. Available from: https://extranet.who.int/gavi/PQ_Web/PreviewVaccine.aspx?nav=0&ID=67.

219. BCG Vaccine U.S.P. [Package Insert on the Internet]. Whitehouse Station (NJ): Organon Teknika Corporation LLC; 1989 [revised 2011; cited 2016 June 7]. Available from: https://www.merck.com/product/usa/pi_circulars/b/bcg/bcg_pi.pdf.

220. BCG Vaccine, Freeze-Dried [Package Insert on the Internet]. Hadapsar (India): Serum Institute of India Pvt. Ltd.; 2003 [cited 2017 June 7]. Available from: http://www.who.int/immunization_standards/vaccine_quality/118_bcg.pdf.

221. BCG Vaccine, Freeze-Dried [Package Insert on the Internet]. Toronto (Canada): InterVax, Ltd.; 2012. [cited 2016 June 7]. Available from: https://extranet.who.int/gavi/PQ_Web/PreviewVaccine.aspx?nav=0&ID=74.

222. BCG Vaccine SSI [Package Insert on the Internet]. Copenhagen: Statens Serum Institut; 2007 [cited 2016 June 7]. Available from: https://extranet.who.int/gavi/PQ_Web/PreviewVaccine.aspx?nav=0&ID=164.

223. Euvichol [Package Insert on the Internet]. Jeollanam-do (South Korea): EuBiologics Co., Ltd.; 2016 [cited 2016 June 7]. Available from: http://www.eubiologics.com/en/products/Euvichol_insert.pdf.

224. Shanchol. [Package Insert on the Internet]. Andhra Pradesh (India): Shantha Biotechnics Ltd.; 2011 [cited 2016 June 7]. Available from: http://shanthabiotech.com/wp-content/uploads/2015/05/shanchol-pack-insert.pdf.

225. World Health Organization. Questions and Answers on Dengue Vaccines (Dengvaxia (CYD-TDV)). WHO. World Health Organization; 2016.

226. Diphtheria and Tetanus Toxoids Adsorbed [Package Insert on the Internet]. Swiftwater, PA: Sanofi Pasteur Inc.; 1997 [revised 2013 June; cited 2016 Nov]. Available from: https://www.vaccineshoppe.com/image.cfm?doc_id=12617&image_type=product_pdf.

227. Adsorbed DT Vaccine [Package Insert on the Internet]. Bandung (India): PT Bio Farma (Persero); 2011 [cited 2017 June 7]. Available from: https://extranet.who.int/gavi/PQ_Web/PreviewVaccine.aspx?nav=0&ID=245.

228. Diftet [Package Insert on the Internet]. Toronto (Canada): National Center for Infectious and Parasitic Diseases; 2008 [cited 2016 June 7]. Available from: https://extranet.who.int/gavi/PQ_Web/PreviewVaccine.aspx?nav=0&ID=77.

229. DT Vax [Package Insert on the Internet]. Lyon (France): Sanofi Pasteur SA; 2006 [cited 2016 June 7]. Available from: https://extranet.who.int/gavi/PQ_Web/PreviewVaccine. aspx?nav=0&ID=90.

230. Diphtheria and Tetanus Vaccine Adsorbed (Pediatric) [Package Insert on the Internet]. Hadapsar (India): Serum Institute of India Pvt. Ltd.; 1995 [cited 2016 June 7]. Available from: https://extranet.who.int/gavi/PQ_Web/PreviewVaccine.aspx?nav=0&ID=118.

231. Diphtheria and Tetanus Vaccine Adsorbed for Adults and Adolescents (Td) [Package Insert on the Internet]. Hadapsar (India): Serum Institute of India Pvt. Ltd.; 1995 [cited 2016 June 7]. Available from: https://extranet.who.int/gavi/PQ_Web/PreviewVaccine.aspx? nav=0&ID=121.

232. IMOVAX dT adult [Package Insert on the Internet]. Lyon (France): Sanofi Pasteur SA. 2000 [cited 2016 June 7]. Available from.: https://extranet.who.int/gavi/PQ_Web/PreviewVaccine. aspx?nav=0&ID=92.

233. Weiss BP, Strassburg MA, Feeley JC. Tetanus and diphtheria immunity in an elderly population in Los Angeles County. Am J Public Heal. 1983/07/01. 1983;73(7):802–4.

234. Diptheria-Tetanus-Pertussis Vaccine Adsorbed [Package Insert on the Internet]. Hadapsar (India): Serum Institute of India Pvt. Ltd; 1995 [cited 2016 June 7]. Available from: https:// extranet.who.int/gavi/PQ_Web/PreviewVaccine.aspx?nav=0&ID=124.

235. DTP Vaccine [Package Insert on the Internet]. Bandung (Indonesia); PT Bio Farma (Persero); 2001. Available from.: https://extranet.who.int/gavi/PQ_Web/PreviewVaccine. aspx?nav=0&ID=8.

236. Diphtheria, Tetanus, Pertussis and Hepatitis B Vaccine Adsorbed [Package Insert on the Internet]. Hadapsar (India): Serum Institute of India Pvt. Ltd.; 2006 [cited 2016 June 7]. Available from: https://extranet.who.int/gavi/PQ_Web/PreviewVaccine. aspx?nav=0&ID=127.

237. Hexaxim [Package Insert on the Internet]. Lyon (France): Sanofi Pasteur SA; 2012 [cited 2016 June 7]. Available from.: https://extranet.who.int/gavi/PQ_Web/PreviewVaccine. aspx?nav=0&ID=285.

238. Quadracel [Package Insert on the Internet]. Swiftwater (PA): Sanofi Pasteur Limited; 2015 [cited 2016 June 7]. Available from: https://www.vaccineshoppe.com/image. cfm?doc_id=13791&image_type=product_pdf.

239. Diphtheria, tetanus, pertussis, hepatitis B and haemophilus influenzae type b conjugate vaccine [Package Insert on the Internet]. Hadapsar (India): Serum Institute of India Pvt. Ltd.; 2010 [cited 2016 June 7]. Available from: https://extranet.who.int/gavi/PQ_Web/PreviewVaccine. aspx?nav=0&ID=194.

240. Easyfive-TT [Package Insert on the Internet]. Malpur (India): Panacea Biotec Ltd.; 2013 [cited 2016 June 7]. Available from: https://extranet.who.int/gavi/PQ_Web/PreviewVaccine. aspx?nav=0&ID=87.

241. Euforvac-Hib [Package Insert on the Internet]. Jeollabuk (Republic of Korea): LG Chemical Ltd.; 2013 [revised 2017 January; cited 2017 July 3]. Available from: https://extranet.who. int/gavi/PQ_Web/PreviewVaccine.aspx?nav=0&ID=254.

242. Eupenta [Package Insert on the Internet]. Chungcheongbuk-do (Republic of Korea): LG Chem Ltd.; 2017 [cited 2017 July 3]. Available from: https://extranet.who.int/gavi/PQ_Web/ PreviewVaccine.aspx?nav=0&ID=304.

243. Pentabio [Package Insert on the Internet]. Bandung (Indonesia): PT Bio Farma (Persero); 2015 [cited 2016 June 7]. Available from: https://extranet.who.int/gavi/PQ_Web/PreviewVaccine. aspx?nav=0&ID=309.

244. Quinvaxem [Package Insert on the Internet]. Incheon (Republic of Korea): Janssen Vaccines Corp.; 2016 [cited 2016 June 7]. Available from: https://extranet.who.int/gavi/PQ_Web/ PreviewVaccine.aspx?nav=0&ID=6.

245. Tritanrix HB+Hib [Package Insert on the Internet]. Rixensart (Belgium): GlaxoSmithKline Biologicals; 2009 [cited on 2016 June 7]. Available from: https://extranet.who.int/gavi/PQ_ Web/PreviewVaccine.aspx?nav=0&ID=56.

246. Shan-5 [Package Insert on the Internet]. Andhra Pradesh (India): Shantha Biotechnics Limited; 2014 [cited on 2016 June 7]. Available from: http://shanthabiotech.com/wp-content/uploads/2015/05/shan5-pack-insert.pdf.

247. Diptheria, tetanus, pertussis (whole cell), hepatitis-B (r-DNA) and haemophilus type b conjugate vaccine (adsorbed) [Package Insert on the Internet]. Andhra Pradesh (India): Biological E. Limited; 2012 [cited 2016 June 7]. Available from: https://extranet.who.int/gavi/PQ_Web/PreviewVaccine.aspx?nav=0&ID=274.

248. DTP-Hep B 5 [Package Insert on the Internet]. Bandung (Indonesia): PT Bio Farma (Persero); 2004 [cited on 2016 June 7]. Available from: https://extranet.who.int/gavi/PQ_Web/PreviewVaccine.aspx?nav=0&ID=10.

249. Diphtheria, tetanus, pertussis and Haemophilus influenzae type b conjugate vaccine [Package Insert on the Internet]. Hadapsar (India): Serum Institute of India Pvt. Ltd.; 2010 [cited 2016 June 7]. Available from: https://extranet.who.int/gavi/PQ_Web/PreviewVaccine.aspx?nav=0&ID=216.

250. TETRAct-HIB [Package Insert on the Internet]. Lyon (France): Sanofi Pasteur SA; 2009 [cited on 2016 June 7]. Available from: https://extranet.who.int/gavi/PQ_Web/PreviewVaccine.aspx?nav=0&ID=96.

251. Vaxem HIB [Package Insert on the Internet]. Italy: Novartis Vaccines and Diagnostics; 2009 [cited on 2016 June 7]. Available from: http://www.who.int/immunization_standards/vaccine_quality/VaxemHib_product_insert.pdf?ua=1.

252. Haemophilus influenzae type b Conjugate Vaccine [Package Insert on the Internet]. Hadapsar (India): Serum Institute of India Pvt. Ltd.; 2007 [cited on 2016 June 7]. Available at: https://extranet.who.int/gavi/PQ_Web/PreviewVaccine.aspx?nav=0&ID=185.

253. Euvax B [Package Insert on the Internet]. Jeollabuk-do (Republic of Korea): LG Chem Ltd; 2016 [cited on 2106 June 7]. Available from: https://extranet.who.int/gavi/PQ_Web/PreviewVaccine.aspx?nav=0&ID=68.

254. Hepatitis B Vaccine Recombinant [Package Insert on the Internet]. Bandung Indonesia: PT Bio Farma (Persero); 2004 [cited on 2016 June 7]. Available from: https://extranet.who.int/gavi/PQ_Web/PreviewVaccine.aspx?nav=0&ID=9.

255. Hepavax-Gene inj. [Package Insert on the Internet]. Incheon (Republic of Korea): Janssen Vaccines Corp.; 2016 [cited on 2016 June 7]. Available from: https://extranet.who.int/gavi/PQ_Web/PreviewVaccine.aspx?nav=0&ID=5.

256. Shanvac –B [Package Insert on the Internet]. Andhra Pradesh (India): Shantha Biotechnics Limited; 2005 [cited on 2016 June 7]. Available from: http://shanthabiotech.com/wp-content/uploads/2015/05/shanvac-b-pack-insert.pdf.

257. Hepatitis B Vaccine (rDNA) Paediatric [Package Insert on the Internet]. Hadapsar (India): Serum Institute of India Pvt. Ltd; 2004 [cited on 2016 June 7]. Available at: https://extranet.who.int/gavi/PQ_Web/PreviewVaccine.aspx?nav=0&ID=132.

258. Hepatitis B Vaccine (rDNA) Adult [Package Insert on the Internet]. Hadapsar (India): Serum Institute of India Pvt. Ltd; 2004 [cited on 2016 June 7]. Available from: https://extranet.who.int/gavi/PQ_Web/PreviewVaccine.aspx?nav=0&ID=130.

259. Group HEVW. Hepatitis E Vaccine Working Group. Hepatitis E vaccine: composition, safety, immunogenicity and efficacy.

260. JEEV [Package Insert on the Internet]. Hyderabad (India): Biological E. Limited; 2013 [cited on 2016 June 7]. Available from: https://extranet.who.int/gavi/PQ_Web/PreviewVaccine.aspx?nav=0&ID=263.

261. IMOJEV MD [Package Insert on the Internet]. Bangkok (Thailand): GPO-MPB Co., Ltd.; 2014 [cited on 2016 June 7]. Available from: https://extranet.who.int/gavi/PQ_Web/PreviewVaccine.aspx?nav=0&ID=276.

262. Japanese encephalitis (JE) live vaccine [Package Insert on the Internet]. Chengdu (China): Chengdu Institute of Biological Products Co., Ltd.; 2016 [cited on 2016 June 7]. Available from: https://extranet.who.int/gavi/PQ_Web/PreviewVaccine.aspx?nav=0&ID=272.

263. Measles vaccine live attenuated (Freeze-dried) [Package Insert on the Internet]. Hadapsar (India): Serum Institute of India Pvt. Ltd.; 1993 [cited on 2016 June 7]. Available from: https://extranet.who.int/gavi/PQ_Web/PreviewVaccine.aspx?nav=0&ID=148.

264. Measles vaccine [Package Insert on the Internet]. Bandung (Indonesia): PT Bio Farma (Persero); 2006 [cited on 2016 June 7]. Available from: https://extranet.who.int/gavi/PQ_Web/PreviewVaccine.aspx?nav=0&ID=252.

265. ROUVAX [Package Insert on the Internet]. Lyon (France): Sanofi Pasteur Inc.; 2003 [revised 2007 February; cited 2016 June 7]. Available from: https://extranet.who.int/gavi/PQ_Web/PreviewVaccine.aspx?nav=0&ID=106.

266. Measles and rubella vaccine live, attenuated (Freeze-dried) [Package Insert on the Internet]. Hadapsar (India): Serum Institute of India Pvt. Ltd.; 2000 [cited on 2016 June 7]. Available from; https://extranet.who.int/gavi/PQ_Web/PreviewVaccine.aspx?nav=0&ID=139.

267. TRIMOVAX MÉRIEUX [Package Insert on the Internet]. Lyon (France): Sanofi Pasteur SA; 2002 [revised 2010 July; cited 2016 June 7]. Available from: https://extranet.who.int/gavi/PQ_Web/PreviewVaccine.aspx?nav=0&ID=107.

268. PRIORIX [Package Insert on the Internet]. Rixensart (Belgium): GlaxoSmithKline Biologicals SA; 2011 [cited on 2016 June 7]. Available from: https://extranet.who.int/gavi/PQ_Web/PreviewVaccine.aspx?nav=0&ID=61.

269. ProQuad [Package Insert on the Internet]. Whitehouse Station (NJ): Merck & Co., Inc.; 2005 [revised on 2017 May; cited on 2017 July 3]. Available from: https://www.merck.com/product/usa/pi_circulars/p/proquad/proquad_pi.pdf.

270. MenAfriVac 5 microgram [Package Insert on the Internet]. Hadapsar: Serum Institute of India Pvt. Ltd.; 2014 [cited on 2016 June 7]. Available from: https://extranet.who.int/gavi/PQ_Web/PreviewVaccine.aspx?nav=0&ID=286.

271. MenAfriVac [Package Insert on the Internet]. Hadapsar (India): Serum Institute of India Pvt. Ltd.; 2010 [cited on 2016 June 7]. Available on: https://extranet.who.int/gavi/PQ_Web/PreviewVaccine.aspx?nav=0&ID=196.

272. Polysaccharide Meningococcal A and C Vaccine [Package Insert on the Internet]. Rio de Janeiro (Brazil): Institute of Technology on Biologicals; 2007 [cited on 2016 June 7]. Available on: https://extranet.who.int/gavi/PQ_Web/PreviewVaccine.aspx?nav=0&ID=22.

273. Polysaccharide Meningococcal A+C [Package Insert on the Internet]. Lyon (France): Sonofi Pasteur SA; 2009 [cited on 2016 June 7]. Available from: https://extranet.who.int/gavi/PQ_Web/PreviewVaccine.aspx?nav=0&ID=113.

274. MENVEO [Package Insert on the Internet]. Research Triangle Park (NC): GlaxoSmithKline; 2017 [cited on 2017 July 3]. Available from: https://www.gsksource.com/pharma/content/dam/GlaxoSmithKline/US/en/Prescribing_Information/Menveo/pdf/MENVEO.PDF.

275. Synflorix [Package Insert on the Internet]. Rixensart (Belgium): GlaxoSmithKline Biologicals s.a.; 2010 [cited on 2016 June 7]. Available on: https://extranet.who.int/gavi/PQ_Web/PreviewVaccine.aspx?nav=0&ID=198.

276. Prevnar 13 [Package Insert on the Internet]. Philadelphia (PA): Wyeth Pharmaceuticals Inc. ; 2016 [revised 2017 April; cited on 2017 July 3]. Available on: http://labeling.pfizer.com/show-labeling.aspx?id=501.

277. IPOL Poliovirus Vaccine Inactivated [Package Insert on the Internet]. Swiftwater (PA): Sanofi Pasteur SA; 2015 [cited on 2016 June 7]. Available from: http://eproofing.springer.com/books/index.php?token=rO-hcIe4_7cfP5mH-KloLz2UXrbik8fcVtq1Sfd63xc.

278. IMOVAX POLIO [Package Insert on the Internet]. Toronto (Canada): Sanofi Pasteur SA; 2006 [cited on 2106 June 7]. Available from: https://www.vaccineshoppecanada.com/document.cfm?file=IMOVAX_Polio_E.pdf.

279. IPV Vaccine SSI [Package Insert on the Internet]. Copenhagen (Denmark): AJ Vaccines A/S; 2009 [cited on 2016 June 7]. Available from: https://extranet.who.int/gavi/PQ_Web/PreviewVaccine.aspx?nav=0&ID=231&AspxAutoDetectCookieSupport=1.

280. Poliomyelitis vaccine [Package Insert on the Internet]. Bilthoven (Netherlands): Bilthoven Biologicals B.V.; 2015 [cited on 2016 June 7]. Available from: https://extranet.who.int/gavi/PQ_Web/PreviewVaccine.aspx?nav=0&ID=230.

281. Poliorix [Package Insert on the Internet]. Rixensart Belgium: GlaxoSmithKline SA; 2010 [cited on 2016 June 7]. Available from: http://www.who.int/immunization_standards/vaccine_quality/poliorix_package_insert_en_june10.pdf.

282. BIOPOLIO B1/3 [package insert]. Telangana (India): Bharat Biotech International Ltd.; 2015 [cited on 2016 June 7]. Available from: http://www.who.int/immunization_standards/vaccine_quality/pq_245_bivalent_OPV_1-3_Bharat_PI_Dec2015.pdf.

283. Bivalent OPV (type 1 and 3) [Package Insert on the Internet]. Hadapsar (India): Serum Institute of India Pvt. Ltd.; 2013 [cited 2016 June 7]. Available from: http://www.who.int/immunization_standards/vaccine_quality/pq_262_281_bOPV_SII_PI_20011253-2.pdf?ua=1.

284. Bivalent Oral Poliomyelitis Vaccine Types 1 and 3 (bOPV) [Package Insert on the Internet]. Bandung (Indonesia): PT Bio Farma (Persero); 2015 [cited on 2016 June 7]. Available from: https://extranet.who.int/gavi/PQ_Web/PreviewVaccine.aspx?nav=0&ID=297.

285. Bivalent Types 1 and 3 Oal Polio Vaccine for Children (bOPV) [Package Insert on the Internet]. Parel (Mumbai): Haffkine Bio- Pharmaceutical Corporation Limited; 2010 [cited on 2106 June 7]. Available from: https://extranet.who.int/gavi/PQ_Web/PreviewVaccine.aspx?nav=0&ID=200.

286. Polio Sabin One and Three (oral) [Package Insert on the Internet]. Rixensart: GlaxoSmithKline Biologicals s.a.; 2015 [cited on 2016 June 7]. Available from: http://www.who.int/immunization_standards/vaccine_quality/OPV_bivalent_GSK_WHO_package_insert_text_english.pdf.

287. Oral Monovalent Type 3 Poliomyelitis Vaccine [Package Insert on the Internet]. Lyon (France): Sanofi Pasteur SA; 2015 [cited on 2017 July 3]. Available from: https://extranet.who.int/gavi/PQ_Web/PreviewVaccine.aspx?nav=0&ID=300.

288. Oral monovalent TYPE 2 poliomyelitis vaccine (mOPV) [Package Insert on the Internet]. Lyon (France): Sanofi Pasteur SA; 2016 [cited on 2016 June 7]. Available from: https://extranet.who.int/gavi/PQ_Web/PreviewVaccine.aspx?nav=0&ID=299.

289. Polio Sabin Mono Two (oral) [Package Insert on the Internet]. Rixensart (Belgium): GlaxoSmithKline Biologicals s.a.; 2011 [cited on 2016 June 7]. Available from: https://extranet.who.int/gavi/PQ_Web/PreviewVaccine.aspx?nav=0&ID=235.

290. OPVERO [Package Insert on the Internet]. Lyon (France): Sanofi Pasteur SA; 2010 [cited on 2016 June 7]. Available from: https://extranet.who.int/gavi/PQ_Web/PreviewVaccine.aspx?nav=0&ID=101.

291. Oral polio (OPV) [package insert]. Bandung (Indonesia): PT Bio Farma (Persero); 1997 [revised 2008 February; cited on 2016 June 7]. Available from: https://extranet.who.int/gavi/PQ_Web/PreviewVaccine.aspx?nav=0&ID=12.

292. Poliomyelitis vaccine (Oral), trivalent types 1, 2, 3 [Package Insert on the Internet]. Hadapsar (India): Serum Institute of India Pvt. Ltd.; 2013 [cited on 2016 June 7]. Available from: https://extranet.who.int/gavi/PQ_Web/PreviewVaccine.aspx?nav=0&ID=261.

293. Polioviral vaccine (OPV) [Package Insert on the Internet]. Parel (Mumbai): Haffkine Bio Pharmaceutical Corporation Limited; 2006 [cited on 2016 June 7]. Available from: https://extranet.who.int/gavi/PQ_Web/PreviewVaccine.aspx?nav=0&ID=63.

294. Imovax rabies [Package Insert on the Internet]. Swiftwater (PA): Sanofi Pasteur SA; 2013 [cited on 2016 June 7]. Available from: https://www.vaccineshoppe.com/image.cfm?doc_id=5983&image_type=product_pdf.

295. RabAvert [Package Insert on the Internet]. Research Triangle Park (NC): GSK Vaccines, GmbH; 2016 [cited on 2016 June 7]. Available from: https://www.gsksource.com/pharma/content/dam/GlaxoSmithKline/US/en/Prescribing_Information/Rabavert/pdf/RABAVERT.PDF.

296. VERORAB [Package Insert on the Internet]. Lyon (France): Sanofi Pasteur SA; 2009 [cited on 2016 June 7]. Available from: https://extranet.who.int/gavi/PQ_Web/PreviewVaccine.aspx?nav=0&ID=111.

297. Rabipur [Package Insert on the Internet]. Marburg (Germany): Novartis Vaccines; 2006 [cited on 2016 June 7]. Available from: http://www.who.int/immunization_standards/vaccine_quality/Rabipur_Product_Insert.pdf.

298. Rabipur [Package Insert on the Internet]. Ankleshwar (India): Chiron Behring Vaccines Private Ltd.; 2002 [cited on 2016 June 7]. Available from: https://extranet.who.int/gavi/PQ_Web/PreviewVaccine.aspx?nav=0&ID=27.

299. ROTARIX [Package Insert on the Internet]. Research Triangle Park (NC): GlaxoSmithKline; 2016 [cited on 2016 June 7]. Available from: https://www.gsksource.com/pharma/content/dam/GlaxoSmithKline/US/en/Prescribing_Information/Rotarix/pdf/ROTARIX-PI-PIL.PDF.

300. RotaTeq [Package Insert on the Internet]. Whitehouse Station (NJ): Merck and Co., Inc.; 2017 [cited on 2017 July 3]. Available from: http://www.merck.com/product/usa/pi_circulars/r/rotateq/rotateq_pi.pdf.

301. Rubella vaccine, live, attenuated [Package Insert on the Internet]. Hadapsar (India): Serum Institute of India Pvt. Ltd.; 2006 [cited on 2016 June 7]. Available from: https://extranet.who.int/gavi/PQ_Web/PreviewVaccine.aspx?nav=0&ID=151.

302. ACAM2000 [Package Insert on the Internet]. Cambridge (MA): Sanofi Pasteur Biologics, LLC; 2007 [revised 2017 May; cited on 2017 July 3]. Available from: http://www.sanofi-pasteur.us/sites/www.sanofipasteur.us/files/sites/default/files/pictures/ACAM%202000%20May2017.pdf.

303. Adsorbed Tetanus Vaccine BP [Package Insert on the Internet]. Hyderabad (India): Biological E. Limited; 2012 [cited on 2016 June 7]. Available from: https://extranet.who.int/gavi/PQ_Web/PreviewVaccine.aspx?nav=0&ID=260.

304. Tetanus toxoid [Package Insert on the Internet]. Hadapsar (India): Serum Institue of India Pvt. Ltd.; 1995 [cied on 2016 June 7]. Available from: https://extranet.who.int/gavi/PQ_Web/PreviewVaccine.aspx?nav=0&ID=135.

305. TETAVAX [Package Insert on the Internet]. Lyon (France): Sanofi Pasteur SA; 2002 [cited on 2016 June 7]. Available from: https://extranet.who.int/gavi/PQ_Web/PreviewVaccine.aspx?nav=0&ID=105.

306. ShanTT [Package Insert on the Internet]. Andhra Pradesh (India): Shantha Biotechnics Limited; 2009 [cited on 2016 June 7]. Available from: http://shanthabiotech.com/wp-content/uploads/2015/05/shan-tt-pack-insert.pdf.

307. Tetatox [Package Insert on the Internet]. Markham (Canada): National Center for Infectious and Parasitic Diseases; 2008 [cited on 2016 June 7]. Available from: https://extranet.who.int/gavi/PQ_Web/PreviewVaccine.aspx?nav=0&ID=76.

308. TT vaccine [Package Insert on the Internet]. Bandung (Indonesia): PT Bio Farma (Persero); 2008 [cited on 2016 June 7]. Available from: https://extranet.who.int/gavi/PQ_Web/PreviewVaccine.aspx?nav=0&ID=15.

309. FSME-IMMUN [Package Insert on the Internet]. Vienna (Austria): Baxter Vaccine AG; 2003 [revised 2006 February; cited on 2017 July 3]. Available from: http://www.masta.org/medi-cal-docs/vaccines/FSME_Adult_SPC.pdf.

310. Vivotif [Package Insert on Internet]. Redwood Lakes (CA): PaxVax Berna GmbH; 2015 [cited on 2016 June 7]. Available from: https://www.paxvaxconnect.com/PDF/Vivotif_Prescribing_Information.pdf.

311. Typhim Vi [Package Insert on the Internet]. Swiftwater (PA): Sanofi Pasteur SA; 2014 [cited on 2016 June 7]. Available from: https://www.vaccineshoppe.com/image.cfm?doc_id=9372&image_type=product_pdf.

312. YF-VAX [Package Insert on the Internet]. Swiftwater (PA): Sanofi Pasteur Inc.; 2016 [cited on 2016 June 3]. Available from: https://www.vaccineshoppe.com/image.cfm?doc_id=13708&image_type=product_pdf.

313. Stabilized yellow fever vaccine [Package Insert on the Internet]. Dakar (Senegal): Institut Pasteur De Dekar; 2001 [cited on 2016 June 7]. Available from: https://extranet.who.int/gavi/PQ_Web/PreviewVaccine.aspx?nav=0&ID=66.

314. STAMARIL [Package Insert on the Internet]. Lyon (France): Sanofi Pasteur SA; 2014 [cited on 2016 June 7]. Available from: https://s3.amazonaws.com/filecache.drivetheweb.com/mr5str_sanofipasteur/202281/969800.pdf.

315. Yellow Fever Vaccine [Package Insert on the Internet]. Rio de Janeiro (Brazil): Institute of Technology on Biologicals Bio- Manguinhos/FIOCRUZ; 2001 [cited on 2016 June 7]. Available from: https://extranet.who.int/gavi/PQ_Web/PreviewVaccine.aspx?nav=0&ID=21.

316. Yellow Fever Vaccine, Live Freeze-Dried [Package Insert on the Internet]. Moscow (Russia): Federal State Budgetary Scientific Institution Chumakov Federal Scientific Center for Reserch & Development of Immune-And Biological Products, Russian Academy of

Sciences; 2011 [cited on 2016 June 7]. Available from: https://extranet.who.int/gavi/PQ_Web/PreviewVaccine.aspx?nav=0&ID=177.

317. Pediarix [Package Insert on the Internet]. Research Triangle Park (NC): GlaxoSmithKline Biologicals; 2016 [cited on 2016 June 7]. Available from: https://www.gsksource.com/pharma/content/dam/GlaxoSmithKline/US/en/Prescribing_Information/Pediarix/pdf/PEDIARIX.PDF.

318. Kinrix [Package Insert on the Internet]. Research Triangle Park (NC): GlaxoSmithKline Biologicals; 2016 [cited on 2016 June 7]. Available from: https://www.gsksource.com/pharma/content/dam/GlaxoSmithKline/US/en/Prescribing_Information/Kinrix/pdf/KINRIX.PDF.

319. Pentacel [Package Insert on the Internet]. Swiftwater (PA): Sanofi Pasteur Limited; 2008 [revised 2016 September; cited on 2017 July 3]. Available from: https://www.vaccineshoppe.com/image.cfm?doc_id=13799&image_type=product_pdf.

320. AFLURIA [Package Insert on the Internet]. King of Prussia (PA): Seqirus, Inc.; 2007 [revised 2016 April; cited on 2016 June 7]. Available from: http://labeling.csl.com/PI/US/Afluria/EN/Afluria-Prescribing-Information.pdf.

321. Gardasil [Package Insert on the Internet]. Whitehouse Station (NJ): Merck; 2006 [cited on 2016 June 7]. Available from: http://www.fda.gov/downloads/BiologicsBloodVaccines/Vaccines/ApprovedProducts/UCM111263.pdf.

322. FLUARIX QUADRIVALENT [Package Insert on the Internet]. Research Triangle Park (NC): GlaxoSmithKline; 2016 [cited on 2017 July 3]. Available from: https://www.gsk-source.com/pharma/content/dam/GlaxoSmithKline/US/en/Prescribing_Information/Fluarix_Quadrivalent/pdf/FLUARIX- QUADRIVALENT.PDF.

323. Fluzone Quadrivalent [Package Insert on the Internet]. Swiftwater (PA): Sanofi Pasteur Inc.; 2013 [revised 2016 June; cited on 2016 June 7]. Available from: https://www.vaccineshoppe.com/image.cfm?doc_id=13725&image_type=product_pdf.

324. Fluzone High-Dose [Package Insert on the Internet]. Swiftwater (PA): Sanofi Pasteur Inc.; 2009 [revised 2016 June; cited on 2016 June 7]. Available from: https://www.vaccineshoppe.com/image.cfm?doc_id=13716&image_type=product_pdf.

325. Flublok Quadrivalent [Package Insert on the Internet]. Meriden (CT): Protein Sciences Corporation; 2013 [cited on 2017 October 18]. Available from: https://www.fda.gov/downloads/biologicsbloodvaccines/vaccines/approvedproducts/ucm524684.pdf.

326. Fluzone Quadrivalent Intradermal [Package Insert on Internet]. Swiftwater (PA): Sanofi Pasteur, Inc.; 2004 [revised 2016 June; cited 2016 June 7]. Available from: https://www.vaccineshoppe.com/image.cfm?doc_id=12935&image_type=product_pdf.

327. FLULAVAL Quadrivalent [Package Insert on the Internet]. Research Triangle Park (NC): GlaxoSmithKline Biologicals; 2013 [revised 2016 November; cited 2017 July 3]. Available from: https://www.gsksource.com/pharma/content/dam/GlaxoSmithKline/US/en/Prescribing_Information/Flulaval_Quadrivalent/pdf/FLULAVAL- QUADRIVALENT.PDF.

328. FLUAD (Influenza Vaccine, Adjuvanted) [Package Insert on the Internet]. Holly Springs (NC): Seqirus, Inc.; 2015 [revised 2016 March; cited 2016 June 7]. Available from: http://www.fluad.com/Common/docs/FLUAD_Package_Insert.pdf.

329. FLUCELVAX Quadrivalent [Package Insert on the Internet]. Holly Springs (NC): Seqirus, Inc.; 2016 [cited 2016 June 7]. Available from: http://flu.seqirus.com/files/us_package_insert_flucelvax.pdf.

330. GC FLU [Package Insert on the Internet]. Jeollaman-do (Republic of Korea: Green Cross Corporation; 2011 [revised 2017 February; cited 2107 July 3]. Available from: https://extranet.who.int/gavi/PQ_Web/PreviewVaccine.aspx?nav=0&ID=233.

331. Influenza vaccine (Split Virion), Inactivated [Package Insert on the Internet]. Henan (China): Hualan Biological Bacterin Co., Ltd.; 2008 [revised 2016 March February; cited 2016 June 6]. Available from: https://extranet.who.int/gavi/PQ_Web/PreviewVaccine.aspx?nav=0&ID=292.

332. Nasovac-S Influenza Vaccine, Live Attenuated [Package Insert on the Internet]. Hadapsar (India): Serum Institute of India Pvt. Ltd.; 2015 [cited on 2016 June 7]. Available from: https://extranet.who.int/gavi/PQ_Web/PreviewVaccine.aspx?nav=0&ID=284.
333. VAXIGRIP [Package Insert on the Internet]. Lyon (France): Sanofi Pasteur SA; 2011 [revised 2016 April; cited 2016 June 7]. Available from: https://extranet.who.int/gavi/PQ_Web/PreviewVaccine.aspx?nav=0&ID=238.
334. IXIARO [Package Insert on the Internet]. Gaithersburg (MD): Valneva Scotland Ltd.; 2009 [revised 2015 August; cited on 2016 June 7]. Available from: https://www.fda.gov/downloads/BiologicsBloodVaccines/Vaccines/ApprovedProducts/UCM142569.pdf.
335. JE-VAX [Package Insert on the Internet]. Swiftwater (PA): The Research Foundation for Microbial Diseases of Osaka University;2005 [cited on 2017 July 3]. Available from: https://www.fda.gov/downloads/BiologicsBloodVaccines/Vaccines/ApprovedProducts/UCM123761.pdf.
336. Measles, Mumps and Rubella Vaccine, Live, Attenuated (freeze-dried) [Package Insert on the Internet]. Hadapsar (India): Serum Institute of India Pvt. Ltd.; 2003 [cited on 2016 June 7]. Available from: https://extranet.who.int/gavi/PQ_Web/PreviewVaccine.aspx?nav=0&ID=141.
337. Pneumovax 23 [Package Insert on the Internet]. Whitehouse Station (NJ): Merck and Co., Inc.; 1986 [revised 2015 May; sited 2016 June 7]. Available from: https://www.merck.com/product/usa/pi_circulars/p/pneumovax_23/pneumovax_pi.pdf.
338. Monovalent type 1 Oral Poliomyelitis vaccine, IP [Package Insert on the Internet]. Parel (Mumbai): Haffkine Bio Pharmaceutical Corporation Ltd.; 2009 [cited on 2017 July 3]. Available from: https://extranet.who.int/gavi/PQ_Web/PreviewVaccine.aspx?nav=0&ID=186.
339. Oral Monovalent Type 1 Poliomyelitis Vaccine [Package Insert on the Internet]. Lyon (France): Sanofi Pasteur SA; 2009 [cited on 2017 July 3]. Available from: https://extranet.who.int/gavi/PQ_Web/PreviewVaccine.aspx?nav=0&ID=115.
340. Polio Sabin Mono T1 [Package Insert on the Internet]. Rixensart (Belgium): GlaxoSmithKline Biologicals SA; 2005 [cited on 2017 July 3]. Available from: https://extranet.who.int/gavi/PQ_Web/PreviewVaccine.aspx?nav=0&ID=182.
341. BIOPOLIO [Package Insert on the Internet]. Hyderabad (India): Bharat Biotech International Limited; 2015 [cited on 2016 June 7]. Available from: https://extranet.who.int/gavi/PQ_Web/PreviewVaccine.aspx?nav=0&ID=290.
342. DECAVAC (Package Insert on the Internet]. Swiftwater (PA): Sanofic Pasteur Inc.; 2011 [cited on 2017 July 3]. Available from: https://www.vaccineshoppe.com/assets/pdf/decavac.pdf.
343. Tetanus and Diphtheria Toxoids Adsorbed [Package Insert on the Internet]. Los Angeles (CA): MassBiologics; 2015 [cited on 2017 July 3]. Available from: http://www.umassmed.edu/globalassets/massbiologics-mbl/about/our-products/td-vaccine-grifols-product-insert.pdf.
344. FSME-IMMUN Junior [Package Insert on the Internet]. Vienna (Austria): Baxter Vaccine AG; 2006 [cited on 2017 July 3]. Available from: http://www.masta.org/medical-docs/vaccines/FSME_Junior_SPC.pdf.
345. Vaccines against tick-borne encephalitis-WHO position paper [Internet]. 2011 March 13. Available from: http://www.who.int/immunization/sage/1_TBE_PP_Draft_13_Mar_2011_SAGE_apr_2011.pdf.
346. Gaglani M, Pruszynski J, Murthy K, Clipper L, Robertson A, Reis M, et al. Influenza Vaccine Effectiveness Against 2009 Pandemic Influenza A(H1N1) Virus Differed by Vaccine Type During 2013–2014 in the United States. J Infect Dis. 2016;213(10):1546–56. Available from: http://www.ncbi.nlm.nih.gov/pubmed/26743842
347. Zimmerman RK, Nowalk MP, Chung J, Jackson ML, Jackson LA, Petrie JG, et al. 2014–2015 Influenza Vaccine Effectiveness in the United States by Vaccine Type. Clin Infect Dis. 2016;63(12):1564–73. Available from: http://www.ncbi.nlm.nih.gov/pubmed/27702768.

348. VAXCHORA [Package Insert on the Internet]. Redwood City (CA): PaxVax; 2016 [cited on 2017 October 6]. Available from: https://www.paxvaxconnect.com/PDF/Vaxchora_Prescribing_Information.pdf.
349. DUKORAL [Package Insert on the Internet]. Parkville, VIC, Australia: CSL Limited. 2015 [cited 2017 October 5]. Available from: http://www.seqirus.com.au/docs/999/385/Dukoral_PI_AU.pdf.
350. Menomune [Package Insert on the Internet]. Swiftwater (PA): Sanofi Pasteur Inc; 1981 [revised 2013 April; cited on 2017 October 5]. Available from: https://www.vaccineshoppe.com/image.cfm?doc_id=10447&image_type=product_pdf.
351. Prevnar [Package Insert on the Internet]. Philadelphia (PA): Wyeth Pharmaceuticals Inc; 2009 [cited on 2017 October 5]. Available from: https://dailymed.nlm.nih.gov/dailymed/archives/fdaDrugInfo.cfm?archiveid=11502.

Chapter 5
Vaccine Adverse Effects: Myths and Realities

Jeffrey L. Moore

Introduction

In 1999 the Centers for Disease Control and Prevention (CDC) identified vaccines as the most prominent of the ten most effective public health interventions of the twentieth century [1, 2]. In the case of many of these vaccines, widespread adoption has resulted in dramatic declines in the incidence of the corresponding diseases, and progress continues to be made in the early part of the twenty-first century. Vaccinating an entire population, with the ambitious schedule and array of vaccines that we now have, is a highly complex undertaking with no shortage of challenges.

The particular challenge addressed in this chapter is the issue of public skepticism, hesitation, and even opposition. These anti-vaccine headwinds have been present since the initial public application of vaccine science, evolving over the past two centuries with the times. Popular myths have arisen regarding vaccines throughout their history and have been widely propagated through various means of communication. In our current twenty-first century era, this remains true, and the propagation of these myths has likely been accelerated by the advent of widespread, nearly instant electronic communication. Cultural factors that have helped foster an environment of skepticism in our time include a decline in public science education, a growing suspicion of "Big Pharma," and a widespread mistrust of government. There is suspicion that government-funded public health agencies are in league somehow with the pharmaceutical industry. The myths dealt with in this chapter spring from these and other avenues of mistrust.

This chapter will examine several myths and offer responses to each, but it is important to note that these responses in themselves may not sway people who are

J.L. Moore, MD (✉)
Department of Family Medicine, University of Wisconsin School of Medicine and Public Health. Marshfield Clinic, Merrill Center, 1205 O'Day St, Merrill, WI 54452, USA
e-mail: moore.jeffrey@marshfieldclinic.org

© Springer International Publishing AG 2017
P.G. Rockwell (ed.), *Vaccine Science and Immunization Guideline*,
DOI 10.1007/978-3-319-60471-8_5

hesitant about vaccines. It is intended that discussion of these myths and realities will provide vaccine advocates with some background knowledge and reassurance upon which to build acceptable answers to patients.

Foundations of vaccine safety

"Vaccine safety has not been studied enough"

A mother has her 11-year-old daughter in the clinic for a routine well-adolescent visit, and per current guidelines, you recommend the HPV vaccine. Mom responds, "I don't know, that vaccine is pretty new; I don't think it has been used long enough to consider it safe yet."   She turns to the daughter and asks, "Do you want a shot today?", (One wonders who is the parent here) and eventually declines on her daughter's behalf [author's experience].

The notion that vaccine safety has not been adequately studied has been a popular one in recent years and has been proclaimed by many of the most vocal recent vaccine opponents. There are popular allegations that vaccines have been rushed through the development and approval process, often with the knowing complicity of regulatory agencies in partnership with pharmaceutical companies. The period of time from public awareness of a new vaccine to the recommendation to have it given to one's own child seems uncomfortably brief to many parents. Given the unfamiliarity that most of the public has with the vaccine development process, such a perception can certainly be understood.

A look at the foundations of vaccine safety is in order here. Vaccine safety is critical for at least the following reasons:

- There are ethical obligations upon developers and implementers of immunization strategies to protect the public to the highest possible degree.
- The public is understandably averse to accepting a vaccine with high serious adverse effect rates.
- Some vaccine adverse effects are rare enough to escape detection in the early phases of development but can become evident when the vaccine has been administered to millions of people, requiring that rigorous post-marketing surveillance be in place to detect concerns. Mechanisms for monitoring for hazards are as important as the initial safety measures.

A well-developed structure to assure the safe vaccine development is in place in the United States, the details of which are discussed elsewhere in this book. Agencies playing a major role in the process include the Food and Drug Administration (FDA), which has the authority to approve or deny the marketing and use of any vaccine; the Advisory Committee on Immunization Practices (ACIP), a committee of vaccine experts that advises the CDC on the best implementation of available vaccines; and ACIP work groups which study in detail the various vaccines being considered for public use. Further structures exist to monitor vaccine safety and efficacy once the product has been released for public use. These include ongoing surveillance by the FDA; monitoring by the Vaccine Adverse Event Reporting System (VAERS), operated under the FDA and CDC; the Vaccine Safety Datalink (VSD), a consortium of major private and public health systems across the United States, working in conjunction with the CDC; and the CDC's Clinical Immunization Safety Assessment Project (CISA), a third pillar in the nation's system of post-marketing vaccine surveillance, combining the efforts of the CDC's Immunization Safety Office and seven major medical research institutions across the United States. CISA evaluates and sponsors research into specific vaccine safety concerns and complements the work of VAERS and VSD.

With the above array of safety monitoring and safety assurance mechanisms, it is rare for major safety issues to go undetected. The process works well. The science of vaccine safety is a self-correcting endeavor. Most safety concerns become evident early in the process of development and even rare events can be detected and further studied under these systems.

Dealing with suspicion

"Side effects get swept under the rug"

A 59-year-old man is in the clinic for a recheck on his hypertension. It is November, within the season for administering influenza vaccine. When he is advised of this, however, he replies, "There are more side effects from that vaccine than they let on. I read that the government and the drug companies hide that information."

The man's reply carries a paranoid tone, but it is actually not rare, and it is held by vaccine-resistant people from a variety of educational levels and backgrounds. Others may not sound so obviously distrusting, but the concept of hidden, secret schemes is a popular one.

There are some seemingly obvious points that should address our concerns and hopefully our patients' concerns as well. One immediate thought is, "How could such a vast and disparate array of parties as the government, the world of academics, clinicians, and the pharmaceutical companies so successfully hide adverse information from an unsuspecting populace?" This phenomenon does illustrate, however, that people in the early twenty-first century have a lesser faith in public and private institutions compared to past decades. In the anti-vaccine community, there is a popular notion that government and industry are too close to one another, cooperating in what turns out to be a campaign of deceit and population-wide control [3, 4].

Perhaps the best response to concerns about hidden vaccine adverse effects is to know some counterexamples that illustrate that, in fact, the vaccine safety system works well. Here are four examples:

- Paralytic poliomyelitis was one of the most dreaded diseases of the twentieth century, with communities and families living in fear during every polio season and having little protective recourse available. Every spring and summer saw families keep their children from public gatherings, pools, and parties for fear of the paralyzing disease and its aftermath. The inactivated polio vaccine (IPV) was developed by Dr. Jonas Salk and colleagues and released to the US market in 1955 and was met with widespread relief and hope. It was followed in 1961 by the attenuated oral polio vaccine (OPV) developed by Dr. Albert Sabin. In the United States, the oral vaccine was adopted as the primary polio vaccination and was a critical element in the eradication of polio in the United States in 1979 and in the Western Hemisphere by 1991. The oral vaccine was preferred because it led to more prompt development of immunity compared to the inactivated vaccine, arrested the transmission of wild poliovirus by infected individuals to others, and was logistically easier to manage. It became evident, however, that the attenuated oral vaccine was capable of causing paralytic polio itself in about 1 recipient out of every 760,000 first-time vaccine recipients. By the late 1990s, it was clear that the number of vaccine-associated paralytic polio cases in the United States exceeded the number of cases attributable to wild polio virus (WPV). The decision was then made to discontinue routine oral polio vaccine administration in the United States and transition completely to the inactivated polio vaccine in 1999. OPV remains in use in widespread areas of the developing world because of its advantages with respect to logistics and rapid development of immunity against polio, which is especially critical in areas where wild polio virus still exists. Based on ongoing worldwide monitoring of polio activity, type 2 poliovirus has been dropped from OPV in April 2016, leaving only types 1 and 3 in the vaccine. The World Health Organization (WHO) is making plans for a worldwide transition from OPV to the IPV once the current pockets of WPV have been eradicated [5].

- Pertussis has been a scourge of childhood for many centuries, and it remains a widespread risk to young children to this day. In 1914 the first pertussis vaccination was developed. Widespread use of the vaccine, however, didn't occur until the 1940s. Following the introduction of widespread vaccination, there was a sharp drop in the incidence and death rate from pertussis nationwide. However, the pertussis vaccine (generally given along with diphtheria and tetanus vaccines) was at that time a whole-cell vaccine; the entire Bordetella pertussis organism, including thousands of antigens, was inactivated and included in the vaccine. It was highly reactogenic, frequently causing fevers, sometimes seizures, sometimes other serious reactions, and raising the alarm of many parents and health-care providers alike. While later studies showed that the whole-cell vaccine did not cause permanent brain damage or excess mortality, it was nonetheless felt appropriate to transition to an acellular vaccine. This transition occurred in the 1990s. Today's acellular pertussis vaccines contain several of the pathogenic components of the pertussis organism but not the whole cell. In fact, there are now five antigens in the acellular vaccine compared to the three thousand in the whole-cell product. Local and systemic reactions to the vaccine are now far less common than they were with the whole-cell vaccine. As of 2016 there are concerns that the acellular vaccine may not be as immunogenic as the whole-cell vaccine, and this remains an area of active research [6]. Ongoing surveillance by the established mechanisms now in place has continued to lead to improvements in vaccine safety and tolerability.

- The first commercially available hepatitis B vaccine was released to the market in 1982. The original product was a serum-derived purified dose of hepatitis B surface antigen. It was drawn from individuals who had chronic hepatitis B and had circulating hepatitis B surface antigen in their serum. While numerous studies confirmed the safety of the vaccine, this development took place during the early days of the HIV epidemic, and the concern about blood-borne pathogens was high on the minds of vaccine developers and patients. In order to further assure the safety of hepatitis B vaccine and allay those concerns of the public, manufacturers developed recombinant DNA techniques for production of the vaccine. The serum-derived hepatitis B vaccine was discontinued in 1990 and is no longer available. In the late 1980s, the recombinant vaccine was widely available and is now the only type of hepatitis B vaccine used [7].
- The first vaccine against rotavirus was developed and released to the market under the brand name RotaShield, in 1999. Pre-licensing studies had not shown any increased risk of any specific disease process following immunization. However, within months of the release to widespread use, VAERS data demonstrated a link between receipt of the RotaShield vaccine and development of intussusception in infants. The ACIP recommended discontinuing use of this vaccine pending further study and eventually recommended withdrawal of the vaccine from the routine immunization schedule for infants. The manufacturer withdrew it from the market in 1999. Two second-generation rotavirus vaccines are now available, Rotarix and RotaTeq. A Vaccine Safety Datalink report in 2010 showed no intussusception risk with the use of RotaTeq above the natural background rate [8]. A 2014 report suggested there still is a risk of intussusception occurring with the use of these vaccines, at a rate in the neighborhood of 1.5 excess cases of intussusception per 100,000 vaccine recipients [9], roughly one-tenth of the risk identified with the earlier RotaShield.

Other examples of drawbacks or adverse effects from vaccines could be quoted, but these four cases illustrate this: the current system works. Ongoing post-marketing surveillance and independent studies have demonstrated the capacity to identify problems; producers have been able to improve their product to address safety concerns. Mechanisms are in place that effectively allow the identification and correction of problem issues with current vaccines. The notion that vaccine adverse effects are deliberately suppressed is not supported by a review of history.

Myth: "We don't see those diseases anymore"

Reality: They're just a plane ride away

History has a great way of teaching; each generation can glean and build upon the lessons of previous generations. The mistakes of previous generations can serve as warning signs to current generations. The inspiring examples of history's heroes can serve to motivate for good. History also has a great way of being ignored or forgotten, often at our peril.

History shows that the vast majority of human experience over the millennia has been accompanied by common serious infectious diseases. Epidemics were not uncommon. Diseases like smallpox, measles, tetanus, diphtheria, pertussis, polio, and many others were well known. Our current life expectancy at birth, 79.7 years [10] in the United States, contrasts sharply with that of all human civilization previously. For example, US life expectancy at birth in 1900 was 47.3 years [11]. A major factor in this difference has been in the reduction of childhood mortality due to infectious diseases that are now preventable with immunizations.

Most families today have never seen measles, polio, or Haemophilus influenzae meningitis. Even chickenpox is becoming a novelty. Many of our patients are only vaguely aware of this history. Their conclusion? These vaccines are not that important; we don't see those diseases anymore.

If only it were so. Immunizations have brought about huge reductions in the incidence, morbidity, and mortality of almost every disease targeted so far, but only one, smallpox, has been eradicated to date (polio is close behind). The rest, however, are still present and still capable of afflicting populations and individuals in whom immunity is not adequate. Recent history has seen outbreaks of vaccine-preventable diseases in the United States and many other parts of the world. A number of twenty-first-century developments have contributed to this, including reduced population coverage with vaccines, increased population densities, increased population mobility, war and natural disasters, and possibly climate change.

Several recent outbreaks illustrate the propensity of vaccine-preventable diseases to reemerge when conditions allow:

- From late 2014 into 2015, a multistate outbreak of measles occurred, evidently starting from an imported measles case at Disneyland, in California. By the end of that outbreak, 147 people had developed measles. In all of 2015, 189 people in the United States developed measles and 22 of them were hospitalized. Of the 159 people infected with measles in January through April 2015 (mostly the Disneyland-connected outbreak), 45% were known to be unvaccinated, 38% had unknown vaccination status, and a small percentage were known to be vaccinated [12].
- In 2014 approximately 383 cases of measles erupted in an Amish community in Ohio. This outbreak was also associated with an imported measles case [13] and was able to spread widely due to the low vaccination status of this particular community. That same year, 22 other outbreaks of measles occurred in the United States, all associated with imported cases. The outbreaks together brought the total number of measles cases in the United States in 2014 to 667.
- After the Andrew Wakefield publication in 1998, MMR vaccination coverage in the United Kingdom dropped significantly, from approximately 92 percent before his paper to a low of around 80 percent on the average afterward. Measles began to reoccur in significant numbers beginning within a few years of the Wakefield paper and has only come down to near pre-1988 levels as of 2014

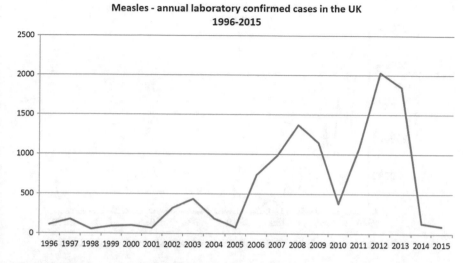

Fig. 5.1 Measles cases in the United Kingdom (*Source*: https://www.gov.uk/government/uploads/system/uploads/attachment_data/file/503791/hpr0816_mmr.pdf)

[Fig. 5.1]. Throughout this past decade, the number of measles cases in the United Kingdom has far outstripped the number in the United States [14].

- A 2016 literature review [15] concluded that a substantial proportion of the US measles cases in the era after elimination were intentionally unvaccinated. ("Elimination" in this case refers to the January 2000 declaration that endemic measles has been eliminated from the United States.) The article further concludes that the phenomenon of vaccine refusal was associated with an increased risk of measles both for people who had refused vaccination and for fully vaccinated individuals.

- Pertussis has seen a resurgence in the past decade [Fig. 5.2] due to a number of factors. It has become well understood that immunity induced by pertussis vaccine fades over a shorter period of time than does immunity with most other vaccines [16]. There is growing recognition that the current acellular vaccine is less immunogenic than the original whole-cell pertussis vaccine. The same study that showed that intentional avoidance of MMR vaccine contributed to the rise in measles incidence in the United States also found that vaccine avoidance was a contributing factor to the rise in pertussis incidence during the same period of time [15] [Fig. 5.2].

- Diphtheria has a history of occurring in cycles of high and low incidence and epidemics. With the advent of effective diphtheria vaccines, however, these epidemics have largely disappeared from North America and most of Europe due to the high acceptance rate of diphtheria vaccines. However, enormous epidemics of diphtheria are still capable of happening; the best illustration is the experience of the former Soviet Union in the 1990s, when over 140,000 cases and 4000 deaths occurred in Russia alone. Multiple factors probably contributed to the incidence

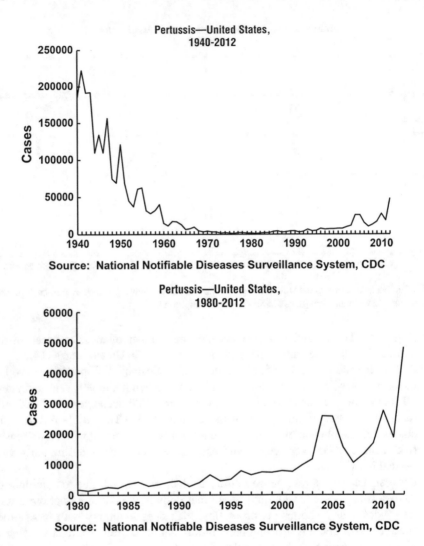

Fig. 5.2 Pertussis resurgence (*Source:* National notifiable diseases surveillance system, CDC)

of diphtheria in that era, and shortage of vaccines in many of the former Soviet States contributed significantly [17]. In 1921, the United States reported 206,000 cases of diphtheria, with 15,520 deaths. In the 1920s, diphtheria incidence dropped precipitously with the introduction of widespread vaccination. Thus, between 2004 and 2015, there were only two cases reported in the United States. In contrast, in 2014, there were 7321 cases of diphtheria reported to the World Health Organization, and it is generally assumed that there were many unreported cases that same year. Given the reservoir of diphtheria cases in scattered areas around the world, high coverage of the US population with diphtheria vaccine is key in preventing a reappearance of the disease in the United States [18].

Other vaccine-preventable diseases have shown the capacity to reoccur in populations with insufficient immunity. Mumps continues to show up in the United States with annual incidences between 200 and 2600 in the past decade. Many of these cases occur in under-immunized individuals, although some can occur in exposed and fully immunized individuals. Polio, on the brink of eradication, still has the capacity to reinfect populations declared free of endemic polio. Examples of this occur in South Asia and in the Middle East. The principle here is that immunizations have eradicated or nearly eradicated many diseases that were once common; however, in all cases except smallpox, the diseases still exist in some parts of the world and can be reintroduced into a population if immunization levels are insufficient. The concept that "We don't see those diseases anymore" is simply not true. Every population needs a sense of vigilance to prevent the resurgence of once vanquished diseases.

Myth: "Natural immunity is better than vaccine induced immunity"

Reality: Encountering the Real Thing can be Devastating

A 61-year-old gentleman at his doctor's office is advised to have a dose of the zoster vaccine. He is of the right age, in otherwise good health, and is an ideal candidate for the vaccine. However, he responds "I don't like putting that artificial stuff in my system." When advised that the vaccine can greatly reduce his risk of acquiring shingles, he replies, "I'd rather take my chances."

The word "natural" carries great weight in the public mind and in marketing in the United States. Labels that reassure the customer that there are no artificial preservatives contained within the package are comforting to the buying public. Tens of millions of people regularly buy and consume multivitamins, herbal products, and other supplements. Among these products, the term "natural" is often the major selling point. As illustrated by the clinical scenario above, the preference for natural products extends into the vaccine world as well. Natural products are assumed by many to be inherently safer than products synthesized in the laboratory or manufacturing facility. For some, the concept of a live virus vaccine, modified in the laboratory to be less virulent, conjures up the same concerns as genetically modified organisms (GMOs) which themselves provoke popular concern. Most communities across the United States have a significant representation of naturopaths, chiropractors, and other alternative health practitioners, among whom vaccination is commonly an objectionable concept.

In a way, the concept of natural immunity being better than vaccine-induced immunity is true. Measles, for example, rarely reoccurs in people who have previously had measles. Second occurrences of chickenpox are uncommon, and when they occur they tend to be very mild. A case of polio leaves the patient immune to that particular strain of the polio virus. People infected with a strain of influenza virus can be found to have some degree of immunity to that strain for decades afterward. Prior to its declared eradication in 1980, smallpox left people with lifelong immunity to the disease – assuming they survived.

By contrast, optimal vaccination against many vaccine-preventable diseases requires multiple doses of the vaccines in question. Measles, mumps, and rubella vaccine is ideally given twice to all children by age 6. Diphtheria, tetanus, and pertussis immunization requires five doses by age 6. Polio vaccine is administered five times by the age of 6, while hepatitis B three times, hepatitis A twice, and rotavirus two or three times. Routine meningococcal vaccination is given to adolescents twice and the human papillomavirus virus vaccine is given in three doses. In the case of each of these vaccines, experience and monitoring have shown that multiple doses are required to achieve adequate immunity. In fact, one could argue that there is nothing quite as effective at inducing immunity as catching the disease itself.

However, not all that is natural is benign. In fact, measles, smallpox, rabies, tetanus, and all the other vaccine-preventable diseases are natural. To deliberately allow infection with the wild type of any vaccine-preventable disease microorganism is to toy with the risk of the complications of such illness. Those risks are present with every one of the currently vaccine-preventable diseases and exceptionally high among some of them. The risk of complications with measles is in the neighborhood of 30 percent [19]. In the United States, the risk of measles mortality during the latter part of the twentieth century was 0.2 percent [19]. The risk of mortality is significantly higher in less developed countries. Prior to varicella immunization, chickenpox carried a mortality of up to 150 children per year in the United States, and 10,000 to 13,000 children were hospitalized for complications of chickenpox annually [20]. Haemophilus influenzae was the most common cause of childhood meningitis and epiglottitis, [21] both of which were commonly fatal among young children.

The advent of immunizations against common diseases has resulted in stunning reductions in the incidence of those diseases. [Table 5.1] A further convincing point is that in every case of the vaccine-preventable diseases mentioned in this section, the complication rate of the disease in question is vastly higher than the rate of complications from the corresponding vaccine. While vaccine complications do occur and while no vaccine is perfect, the numbers are heavily in favor of continuing routine vaccination according to the current schedule. Nature can be nasty; sometimes it's best to outsmart it.

Myth: *"Vaccines cause autism"*

Reality: Multiple Pursuits in Science Answer and Refute the Charge

"Autism has become an epidemic. Twenty-five years ago, 35 years ago, you look at the statistics, not even close. It has gotten totally out of control. … I am totally in favor of vaccines. But I want smaller doses over a longer period of time. Same exact amount, but you take this little beautiful baby, and you pump—I mean, it looks just like it's meant for a horse, not for a child, and we've had so many instances, people that work for me…." Donald Trump in a Republican presidential candidates' debate, September 16, 2015 [23]

The popular concern that vaccines cause autism fueled one of the most intense debates in the recent history of public immunization. The controversy erupted in the 1990s and early 2000s before gradually receding to a degree from the public eye. Fears of autism are not proclaimed as vociferously as in the past but remain a concern among some parents and are still proclaimed by some advocacy groups. The hypothesis arose due to a pair of coincidences:

- The symptoms of autism tend to show up especially prominently among children in the second year of life, around the time that they are receiving a number of vaccines, especially MMR, the vaccine that seems to have drawn the most attention from vaccine opponents.
- The reported incidence of autism has increased in the United States, at least doubling, from the 1980s through the following two decades. This correlates roughly with the increased number of immunizations administered to young children. Certain groups, especially parents of autistic children and autism advocacy groups have assumed, therefore, that the immunizations given to these children are either the sole cause or at least a contributing cause to the development of their autism.

The concept of vaccines causing autism reached a new peak when Andrew Wakefield, a British former surgeon, published his paper, "Ileal-Lymphoid-Nodular Hyperplasia, Nonspecific Colitis, and Pervasive Developmental Disorder in Children" in the Lancet [24] in 1998. Wakefield proposed a mechanism whereby the MMR vaccine could conceivably cause a constellation of neurological symptoms that we generally know as autism. The paper drew tremendous attention and in short order led to a marked decline in the public's willingness to subject their children to the MMR vaccine. (This was followed by a resurgence of measles cases in the United States [25]. The rise in measles cases was even greater in Britain [26].) Autism advocacy groups rallied behind Wakefield and his findings, and celebrities such as Jenny McCarthy and Jim Carrey as well as attorneys such as Robert Kennedy, Jr., vigorously promoted the same claims. Ideas of a link between vaccines and autism have reached nearly the highest echelons of American political life, having provided for example the opening quote above.

The vaccine-autism link has morphed frequently during the debate. Vaccine proponents would say that the skeptics have been moving the goal posts. Hypothetical links have ranged from Dr. Wakefield's original gastrointestinal association with autism, to the thimerosal included in some vaccines, to adjuvants, to the multiplicity of immunizations given at the same time.

The vaccine-autism connection has not held up under scrutiny, however. There are now several lines of evidence, four of which are considered here, to refute the claimed link between vaccines and autism.

Table 5.1. Comparison of twentieth-century annual morbidity and current morbidity: vaccine-preventable diseases

Disease	Twentieth-century annual morbidity	2008 reported cases	Percent decrease (%)
Smallpox	29,005	0	100
Diphtheria	21,053	0	100
Measles	530,217	132	>99
Mumps	162,344	386	>99
Pertussis	200,752	10,007	95
Paralytic polio	16,316	0	100
Rubella	47,745	17	>99
Congenital rubella syndrome	152	0	100
Tetanus	580	15	97
H. influenzae	20,000	219	99

Adapted from American Academy of Family Physicians. Adolescent immunizations and overcoming barriers. CME Bulletin 16(1) Feb 2016
Originally published in [22]

The first line is from Dr. Wakefield's methods. Wakefield's published paper was subjected almost immediately to careful scrutiny, given that no experts in the field had ever previously found evidence to suggest such a connection. The claim was contrary to all previously known science on the issue. Researchers were unable to reproduce Wakefield's published findings. Subsequent investigations found that the laboratory Dr. Wakefield used to substantiate his claims regarding measles vaccine virus and the GI tract was substandard and was biased toward Wakefield's claims. Dr. Wakefield was financially supported by attorneys who were pressing civil claims against vaccine manufacturers, his study subjects were not properly randomized, and it turns out that he had applied for a patent on an alternative measles vaccine prior to publishing his paper. In the end, the Lancet retracted [27] Wakefield's 1998 paper as being fraudulent and the British General Medical Council revoked his privileges to practice medicine in the United Kingdom.

The second major line of evidence is epidemiology, which further undermined the claim of a link between MMR and autism. Very large epidemiologic studies in a number of countries failed to identify any link. A review of autism reports compared with MMR vaccination records over 14 years in California showed no association between MMR vaccine and risk of autism [25]. A very large epidemiologic study in the United Kingdom [28] showed no step-up in autism cases after introduction of MMR vaccine, no difference between vaccinated and unvaccinated children, and no temporal association between MMR administration and a diagnosis of autism. Investigators in Denmark, with its nationwide health database, were similarly unable to find any link whatsoever between the MMR vaccine and autism in a study of over 500,000 children [29]. A 2015 American study of over 95,000 children with older siblings showed that there was no identifiable link between MMR vaccine and autism, even among children with an autism-affected sibling, who would be expected to be at high risk [30].

A third body of evidence comes from the science of toxicology. Mercury, a component of thimerosal, a preservative used in some vaccines, has been cited as a possible cause of neurodevelopmental abnormalities in vaccinated children. Toxicologists, however, point out that in known cases of mercury poisoning there is neurological injury but that the typical pattern is distinctively different from the findings in autistic children. There is also the important distinction between methyl mercury and ethyl mercury, the former being found in contaminated fish, for example, and the latter being the form of mercury found in thimerosal. Ethyl mercury is excreted from the body at a far faster rate than methyl mercury and is considered significantly less toxic. Despite the removal of thimerosal, with its mercury component, from almost all pediatric vaccines, there has been no measurable reduction in the incidence of autism following that change. In fact, a review of all childhood autism cases in Denmark from 1971 through 2000 showed not only that there was no demonstrable association between thimerosal and autism but that the incidence of autism continued to rise after the removal of thimerosal from pediatric vaccine [31]. One of these studies [32] included over 460,000 children.

The final line of evidence supporting the safety of vaccines with respect to neurodevelopmental abnormalities comes from the growing understanding of autism. Autism is a subject of active research and it is now well understood that the roots of autism are prenatal. Manifestations of autism can be identified in children long before their receipt of the MMR vaccine.

Since the controversy of the late 1990s and early 2000s, continued research has given further evidence that there is no identifiable link between vaccines and autism. As the Institute of Medicine states the case in its dry way, "The committee assesses the mechanistic evidence regarding an association between MMR vaccine and autism as lacking," and "The evidence favors rejection of a causal relationship between MMR vaccine and autism" [33]. The question has been settled in Federal Court, specifically in the Office of Special Masters [34], on a number of occasions, and later in federal appeals court. MMR vaccination coverage has been on the increase since its decline in the wake of Dr. Wakefield's paper. Most autism advocacy organizations no longer campaign against immunization [35–37]. Most importantly, immunization providers can confidently continue to provide assurance to those under their care: Vaccines DO NOT cause autism.

Myth: "All these Shots Overwhelm the Immune System"

Reality: A Drop in the Immunological Bucket

The number of immunizations a child now receives according to the current ACIP recommended schedule (2016) is in the neighborhood of 25 shots. This number may vary depending on the combination of vaccines being used but illustrates an important point. Today's children receive immunizations against many more diseases than children of previous generations. One popular assumption as a result of this increased number of vaccinations is that more shots entail a greater number of antigens administered to children. Many people have raised concern that this increased number of vaccines, with the antigen exposure involved, is somehow harmful to the infant immune system; this concern is expressed most vocally by organizations considered in the anti-vaccine camp but is heard often even among those who are more neutral on vaccination in general. Responding to this perception, many people have elected to modify the vaccine schedule in order to "space these shots out" and not allow their children to have the usual number of vaccines per session, thereby reducing their antigen exposure at any given sitting. For example, Dr. Robert W. Sears, a Californian pediatrician, advocates an alternative schedule different from that recommended by the ACIP and the American Academy of Pediatrics, in order to "space out" these vaccines [38].

The reality is considerably different, based on the science of pediatric vaccines. The following paragraphs offer several points of assurance:

- The number of antigens to which a child is now exposed in the routine vaccination schedule has shrunk dramatically in the last 30 years. There were over 3000 different antigens present in the routine vaccine schedule in 1980 and that is now down to around 150. The primary reason for this is the dramatic drop in antigen load that came with the switch from the whole-cell pertussis vaccine to the acellular version. Other vaccines, however, have been further refined to include only those antigens critical for immunogenicity. Compare these numbers to the thousands of antigens to which the infant is exposed immediately at birth and to the millions within a short time thereafter.
- That tiny infant who looks so vulnerable at birth is actually equipped with an incredibly capable immune system. While it is true that there are several pathogens that are particularly virulent in newborns, the vast majority of microorganisms the infant encounters are well within the capability of the innate immune system to manage. In addition a child is born with maternal antibodies which provide a degree of protection for a number of months after birth. It is estimated that any given vaccine administered to an infant "occupies" the attention of less than 0.01 percent of the infant's immune system capacity [39].
- Decades of surveillance have shown that there is no increase in the incidence of immune system failure or autoimmunity in children on today's vaccine schedule compared to the past [40]. In fact, immune suppression is more likely to occur with natural infection with vaccine-preventable diseases than with the vaccine itself. Studies have also shown that vaccinated and unvaccinated children do not differ in their susceptibility to diseases for which there is no vaccine, such as *Candida*, methicillin-resistant *Staphylococcus aureus* (MRSA), or streptococci [41, 42]; i.e., routine immunizations do not suppress general immunity.
- The currently recommended vaccine schedule for the US public is more thoroughly studied and monitored than any other alternative schedule proposed. Alternative schedules created for the sake of limiting simultaneous vaccine antigen exposure have not brought about any reduction in serious adverse effects,

and, in fact, they delay the full immunization of children, increasing the period during which they are vulnerable to vaccine-preventable diseases. Thanks to multi-component vaccines, some of which immunize against five separate illnesses simultaneously, children can be protected from more diseases with fewer injections than just a few years ago. Every one of these multicomponent vaccines has been subjected to rigorous study to prove that the safety equals that of the same vaccines presented separately.

In summary, given the elegant capabilities of the infant and child immune system and the thoroughly vetted safety and efficacy of today's vaccines, parents, physicians, and other providers can be assured that the vaccine schedule presented today is no threat to the immune system of our young patients.

Myth: *"Vaccines are Full of Toxins"*

Reality: Purpose and Safety of Vaccine Components Are Well Established

A mother is in the clinic with her young child, who is due for a number of vaccines by virtue of her age. Mom is very hesitant, however, because "I am concerned about all that mercury in the vaccines." With further inquiry, it becomes evident that mercury is not the only one of her concerns about toxins.

Among concerned parents as well as committed anti-vaccine activists, "toxins" are a major point of focus. It is alleged that there are numerous toxic compounds and elements within our currently used vaccines and that these toxins are responsible for a wide variety of adverse impacts on health. This probably reflects a popular public notion about toxins in general. Alternative health-care literature and web sites refer frequently to toxins in the system and people's needs to detoxify themselves, their livers, their kidneys, their cardiovascular systems, and other organs. The same sentiment has spilled over to affect the vaccine dialogue as well. In addition, there are indeed present within vaccines a number of compounds or elements that in other settings would be considered toxic. There is in the community of vaccine-skeptical people the notion that certain substances are toxic in any quantity, in contrast to the concept of "The dose makes the toxin."

In the CDC's Pink Book, a detailed but publicly understandable compendium of current vaccine knowledge and recommendations, we can find a lengthy list of substances found within vaccine products in the United States [43]. This list includes some substances that are used in the vaccine manufacturing process but largely removed during the final purifying and packaging steps. Other substances are included by design within the final product, primarily to protect the product itself from bacterial contamination, to provide the optimal acid-base balance, to enhance the vaccine's immunogenicity, and to prevent premature chemical breakdown. The following pages list a number of the more common substances contained within our current vaccines, of concern to parents and others.

Mercury

Mercury, specifically contained within a preservative called thimerosal, is present in a number of vaccines, although little or no thimerosal is now included in the routine childhood vaccine schedule. Only the multidose influenza vaccine vial contains thimerosal. All other routine childhood vaccines have had thimerosal removed as a precautionary compromise in 2000. In a sense then, the question should be of considerably less urgency now that there is such limited exposure to thimerosal. However, even beyond that, the reality is that thimerosal has never been shown to cause adverse health events in vaccine recipients. Here are some lines of evidence to allay concerns:

- Thimerosal is a form of ethyl mercury. Ethyl mercury is much more rapidly excreted than the environmentally present methyl mercury, which is present in a variety of foods. Methyl mercury has considerably greater toxicity because it is more likely to penetrate into tissues and is much slower to be excreted.
- Methyl mercury has a known spectrum of toxicities but does not cause autism in well-characterized mercury toxicity cases. Likewise, ethyl mercury has never been shown to cause any toxicity resembling autism.
- Mercury is a common element in the Earth's crust and can be found in infant formula, breast milk, a variety of foods, and even in our atmosphere. All humans are exposed to mercury, although the quantities vary according to local environmental factors and diet. Given that today's pediatric vaccines no longer contain any mercury compounds, vaccines do not play a significant part of children's total mercury exposure.
- Major epidemiologic studies [44], involving hundreds of thousands of children in multiple countries, have shown no association between thimerosal, in any quantity, and autism or even any other consistently demonstrable health problems. The conclusion of the World Health Organization [45] as well as the CDC, the American Academy of Pediatrics [46], and other major bodies is that mercury does not constitute a risk as currently present in our nation's vaccines.

Aluminum

Aluminum is included by design in some of our commonly used vaccines as an adjuvant, a substance added to a vaccine to enhance the immune response. Aluminum hydroxide, for example, is one of those commonly used adjuvants. Adjuvants have been in use in vaccines for over 60 years. As a result of adjuvant use, vaccines can now be used with lower doses of antigen and a smaller number of doses to achieve the same immunogenic response. Aluminum is not without toxicity in some circumstances. The primary example is individuals with severe renal failure, especially those on dialysis, who are at risk of excessive accumulation of aluminum within the body from such sources as foods and especially antacids. In those individuals aluminum can cause neurotoxicity. Various concerned individuals and organizations have raised the question as to whether aluminum in vaccines, particularly when given to infants, can also cause neurotoxicity.

Aluminum is the third most common element in the Earth's crust (behind oxygen and silicon). It is found in measurable quantities in a variety of foods, baking powder (which contains sodium aluminum phosphate), dairy products, infant formula, and even breast milk. Studies of healthy infants show that all infants have detectable levels of aluminum in their blood, whether vaccinated or not. A fully immunized infant by age 6 months receives between 4 and 5 milligrams of aluminum via vaccines. This is in contrast to the approximately 7 milligrams of aluminum ingested by a strictly breastfed infant and over 100 milligrams of aluminum by a formula-fed infant in the first 6 months. An average adult American diet contains 7–9 milligrams of aluminum per day. Measurements of serum aluminum levels in infants before and after vaccination have not shown measurable rises in their aluminum levels [47]. Aluminum compounds are generally excreted by the kidneys, including among infants.

In summary, aluminum salts are a valuable additive to some vaccines to enhance the effectiveness of the vaccine and to optimize the amount of antigen and doses necessary to accomplish the goal of immunization. Normal human physiology as well as calculations and measurements of aluminum dynamics in the body provides ample evidence that the aluminum present in today's vaccines is of negligible health risk to vaccine recipients [48]. Physicians and other health-care providers can be confident in explaining to their patients that aluminum does not pose a risk in the provision of these valuable vaccines.

Formaldehyde

Almost all vaccines require the production and modification of microorganisms, all of which can be harmful to exposed individuals if not somehow modified before formulating the vaccine. A critical step in the manufacturer of many vaccines is to inactivate the live organism that has been cultured for the purpose of developing the vaccine. In many cases an agent used to inactivate these microorganisms is formaldehyde. Formaldehyde is also used in the modification of natural bacteriological toxins to render them biologically harmless while maintaining their antigenic properties; the deadly tetanus toxin, for example, is changed to the harmless but immunogenic tetanus toxoid by treatment with formaldehyde. The final purification processes in manufacturing the vaccine remove all but a trace of formaldehyde, but tiny quantities of formaldehyde can be found in various vaccines. The presence of formaldehyde in a vaccine understandably raises concerns in the public mind, given that formaldehyde is well known as an embalming compound, as well as its known toxicity in certain kinds of exposure. As a result, vaccines have come under question for the inclusion of formaldehyde and the potential vaccine-induced toxicity that may result. Formaldehyde in high concentrations (e.g., in industrial exposures) is known to pose health hazards, and in the same settings, it is considered potentially carcinogenic.

However, the following points can be raised by way of reassurance in the context of vaccine applications:

- Formaldehyde is a naturally existing compound that is actually produced in the human body and used naturally for a number of critically important functions, such as the production of DNA and amino acids. As a result, individuals without any vaccine history or exposure to industrial or environmental formaldehyde still have measurable serum levels of formaldehyde.
- The total amount of formaldehyde to which a child is exposed through vaccination during their entire childhood is dwarfed by the naturally produced formaldehyde in their own body as well as exogenous sources such as food, housing materials, smoke, and others.
- Injected formaldehyde is quickly dispersed from the injection site and metabolized to formic acid, which is promptly excreted in the urine.

There is no evidence that formaldehyde poses a risk to vaccine recipients [49].

Human Tissue

A perusal of all of the ingredients present in certain vaccines (particularly hepatitis A, rabies, and varicella/zoster) shows that these vaccines contain trace amounts of proteins from cell vulture lines MRC-5 and WI-38. MRC-5 and WI-38 are both laboratory-grown tissue cultures that have their ultimate origin from two fetuses that were aborted in the 1960s. Neither one of these fetuses was aborted with research or vaccine production in mind. These tissue cultures are used in the production of the viruses contained in the abovementioned vaccines, as no ideal alternative has been identified as a substitute. The cells used today for vaccine virus production are actually descendants of the original fetal cells, now separated by many generations of cell division and proliferation.

This issue has posed two problems: One is that some vaccines may contain residual quantities of human proteins and DNA or other compounds. The second is that some vaccines have a remote past connection to a pair of abortions.

To answer the second objection first, the National Catholic Bioethics Center has publicly [50] issued the statement that receipt of a vaccine with a historical connection to abortion is permissible. The stated grounds for this position is that the cell lines now used in vaccine production are many generations derived from the original aborted tissue and there is no tissue that was originally part of the involved fetus present in the laboratory tissue used for vaccine production. The second point raised by the Center is that the good of benefiting and protecting human life by these vaccines is felt to outweigh the significance of the original cell line development, especially since the abortions were not carried out with the specific intent of benefiting research.

To address the concern about possible reactions to human-derived substances in the vaccine, the following points can be made:

- The process of vaccine purification prior to packaging removes the great majority of tissue-derived substances.
- No significant reactions have been identified among people receiving a vaccine derived from MRC-5 or WI-38 sources. Incidents of anaphylaxis (a rare but known complication of vaccination [51, 52]) have not conclusively been tracked back to MRC-5 or WI-38 derivatives. Although over 70 million doses of MMR vaccine were distributed in the United States from 1990 (when VAERS was implemented) through 1996, only 33 cases of anaphylactic reactions after MMR vaccination were reported [53].

Other Toxicity Questions

Numerous other components can be found in various vaccines in current common use. Probably all of these substances have been subjected to scrutiny and concern about their potential for causing adverse health effects among vaccine recipients; at the same time, all of these components have also been found through multiple channels to be sufficiently safe for inclusion in our currently available vaccines. Another principle is "the dose makes the toxin," the observation that substances typically considered toxic have no measurable adverse effect on humans when given in the tiny quantities present in today's vaccines. (Conversely, substances that are widely regarded as safe and essential for human life can also be toxic when taken in excessive quantities.) In the case of vaccine components, all of these components are present in quantities of micrograms or at most milligrams. The likelihood of toxicity in quantities such as these is very remote, as the discussions above illustrate. Despite some vocal public concerns, the supposed toxicities of today's vaccines cannot be substantiated; Vaccines are safe, and have been of tremendous public benefit for generations.

Influenza Vaccine Myths

Influenza is the most common of the illnesses for which we use routine immunizations, and it is far and away the most commonly recommended immunization, in that it is recommended for all individuals over the age of 6 months, annually. In this section we will use the word influenza for the technically defined illness caused by one or another strain of the influenza virus. We will use the word "flu" for the much more variably defined and colloquial term for a wide variety of illnesses. Influenza is an illness which occurs in annual epidemics, typically with a high incidence, in the fall or winter season, with a surprisingly high rate of complications requiring medical intervention in the inpatient or outpatient setting, and some risk of mortality, especially in certain risk groups [54, 55]. Those higher-risk groups include infants and young children; people with immune-compromising conditions; pregnant women; people with diabetes, lung disease, heart disease, and chronic kidney disease; and people over 65 years of age.

"I don't need that vaccine, I never get the flu"

This, along with other influenza vaccine myths, is heard very frequently in clinical practice and other venues where immunizations are administered. It is probably common to encounter people who truly have had relatively little personal experience with influenza virus, but it is the exception rather than the norm for our population. A 2007 paper [56] estimated that in 2003 there were 31 million outpatient visits because of influenza, 3.1 million hospital days, and over 610,000 life years lost to influenza. The CDC's Pink Book [19] reports annual US influenza-related deaths vary between 3000 and over 40,000, depending on the population's prior experience with the subtype and the virulence of the strain. The average annual US death rate attributable to influenza, albeit with a very wide year-to-year variation, is over 20,000. An estimated 15 to 42 percent of American children contract influenza in any given epidemic (which is an annual event). In pandemic years, the incidence and rate of complications both tend to be higher. In view of these statistics, it is likely that those who report having never had influenza are perhaps thinking of other illnesses (viral gastroenteritis, colds, and ill-defined viral syndromes are often mistaken for influenza), may not have been diagnosed with influenza, or may have had a relatively mild case. Influenza is, in fact, a very common illness and has an annual incidence rate far above any other currently vaccine-preventable illness.

"The flu isn't really that serious"

Influenza, being as common as it is, breeds a sense of familiarity and complacency. It is difficult for people to grasp that influenza could possibly be a serious illness. Invasive meningococcal infections are very rare in the United States, with annual incidence rates in the neighborhood of 1 per 100,000 population. Influenza, on the other hand, takes thousands of American lives per year. In spite of this, it is often easier to convince people of the wisdom of the meningococcal vaccine than of the influenza vaccine. Furthermore, the vaccine skeptics have this on their side: influenza, for most people in most cases, turns out not to be very serious. Vaccine skeptics, however, underestimate the impact of influenza with respect to its capacity to put people in hospitals, to cause lethal complications, and to cause pediatric deaths due to influenza including among previously normal, healthy children. In addition, the economic impact of annual influenza epidemics is measured in the billions of dollars both in lost work time and in direct medical expenses [56].

"When I get the flu vaccine, I get really sick"

This is perhaps the most common myth expressed in clinical practice [author's experience]. People's perception is that the vaccine can cause influenza or illnesses like it. At least some of these claims have a bit of truth to them, in that the influenza vaccine is capable of causing adverse effects, even though the incidence of serious adverse effects is extremely low. In fact, in randomized placebo-controlled studies, only injection site redness and soreness occur more frequently than with placebo (saline only) [57]. A more plausible explanation is that the influenza vaccine is not perfect at preventing influenza. Some people every year who receive the influenza vaccine will nonetheless contract influenza sometime during the same season, occasionally even within the 2 weeks lag time between the injection and development of immunity. People in that situation can mistakenly equate association with causation. The influenza vaccine does not, in fact, cause influenza, though it is perceived by some as doing so.

Other likely explanations for this perception include the fact that influenza vaccine is given during the fall and winter seasons, when a variety of other respiratory viruses are circulating and people again attribute those illnesses to having received the vaccine. If we assume that the average adult experiences two to four colds per year [58] (more in children), each lasting an average of 10 days and most occurring during the fall and winter months, then there is a high likelihood that some of those illnesses will happen by coincidence within a few days of a dose of influenza vaccine. Again, people are inclined to believe that correlation equals causation. These and other even less plausible reports of adverse events are extremely common in practice.

Another observation is that while claims that "the vaccine makes me sick" are extremely common, it is actually very uncommon for vaccine recipients to return to the clinic in the short term with adverse vaccine effects. People's perception of vaccine-induced harm can be magnified with the passage of time.

The great majority of influenza vaccine doses are the inactivated (killed) version, so there is no plausible means by which the vaccine can cause actual influenza. Finally, the live attenuated influenza vaccine has been shown not to cause influenza [59].

"Nah, that vaccine doesn't work"

Vaccine skeptics have a point here in that the influenza vaccine is admittedly not perfect. According to the US Flu Vaccine Effectiveness (VE) Network, influenza vaccine efficacy from 2004 through 2015 has varied between 10 percent and 60 percent. The majority of those years have had vaccine efficacies between 40 and 60 percent [60], indicating that influenza vaccine can reduce the incidence of "medically attended influenza" by roughly half. This leaves a substantial percentage of the vaccinated public still vulnerable to influenza, at least partially. During years in which the vaccine/wild virus match is poor, much of the population is aware of it, as it is usually widely publicized. Many people assume that the same flaw is common each year. In fact, the influenza vaccine is effective. It does protect from influenza. We would all like it to be 100 percent effective in doing so, but that is not a current reality. Influenza vaccine has been demonstrated to reduce pediatric ICU admissions in the neighborhood of 75 percent during influenza epidemics [61]. The vaccine, when studied in a school-based trial, was shown to provide efficacy at protecting vaccinated children but also offered herd protection even for unvaccinated children [62].

In summary, the influenza vaccine, contrary to widespread public misperception, is a safe and effective means of protection from influenza, which itself is a potentially high-risk illness with major medical and socioeconomic consequences for our society.

HPV Vaccine Myths

Human papillomavirus (HPV) vaccine, first licensed in 2006, was initially available in a quadrivalent formulation. It has proven to be highly effective, with efficacies over 99% against the four strains represented in the vaccine. Given its efficacy in preventing infection with the most oncogenic strains of HPV, the HPV4 vaccine is anticipated to reduce cervical cancer risk by approximately 70 percent and the HPV9 vaccine, approved in December 2014 [63], by up to 90 percent. Given the role that oncogenic strains of HPV play in the genesis of several other cancers, both in males and females, it is expected that HPV vaccination will similarly reduce the incidence of a number of other HPV-related cancers.

A number of myths and misunderstandings have grown up around the phenomenon of HPV vaccination and are dealt with below.

"The vaccine is too new"

The concept that a vaccine is "too new" implies that it has not had adequate preclinical and clinical usage to assure that it is truly safe. HPV vaccine, however, went through several years of preclinical development and testing, similar to other vaccines, before FDA approval and ACIP recommendation. It has now been in widespread clinical use since 2006. Worldwide over 170 million people have received the vaccine by 2014. In the United States, adverse effects of HPV vaccines have been monitored under the VAERS and other mechanisms since 2006. According to the 2012 report of the Institute of Medicine (IOM), the only serious adverse effects of the HPV vaccines are a risk of fainting after injection and an extremely small risk of anaphylaxis [64]. The IOM found insufficient evidence to support a causative role in any other serious adverse effect.

"She doesn't need that vaccine; she is not sexually active"

The majority of parents prefer that their sons and daughters not initiate sexual intercourse during their adolescence. However, National Health and Nutrition Examination Survey (NHANES) surveys generally show that nearly half of American adolescents have their first sexual intercourse prior to completing high school [65]. Actually, administering the vaccine prior to the onset of sexual activity is the perfect time to start, just as the ideal time to fasten a seatbelt is sometime before the first car accident. HPV vaccines are highly immunogenic, but it is strictly *preventive*. It is not effective as a *treatment* for an HPV infection already established. Waiting until after the sexual debut risks allowing exposure to the wild-type virus before the individual has had the chance to develop vaccine-induced immunity.

"I don't want a vaccine to give my kid any ideas"

There is a legitimate concern that early sexual activity in adolescents is fraught with risks. Delaying sexual activity onset is associated with reduced risk of sexually transmitted infections, reduced risk of adolescent pregnancy, and improved academic outcomes, including completion of school. It is not a surprise then that parents have concerns that perhaps an immunized child might consider the vaccine a license to engage in sexual activity. However, a number of reports, including large studies in the United States [66] and Ontario [67], show no difference between vaccinated and unvaccinated females with respect to sexual activity, either by self-report or by medical records review for sexual activity-related concerns. No study has demonstrated any increased participation in high-risk sexual behavior as a result of HPV vaccine administration.

"He doesn't need it. He doesn't have a cervix." (Stated to the author by the mother of an adolescent boy in the Clinic.)

The original ACIP recommendations for the use of HPV4 vaccine were to routinely administer the vaccine to females. The primary aim was to reduce the incidence of cervical dysplasia and cervical cancer. Later ACIP recommendations would add routine administration to males as well, reflecting the growing recognition that HPV plays an important role in a number of other cancers aside from cervical cancer. Much of the public, however, has not become as aware of the HPV connection to other cancers, and many do not see the importance of immunizing males against HPV. Immunization of males, however, has become an increasingly important facet of the overall HPV control strategy. Males are the primary source of HPV infection for females but – even more directly pertinent to males – roughly 37% of HPV-related cancers are experienced by males. The current estimate is that there are about 30,700 total HPV-attributable cancers in the United States annually, 11,600 of them in males, including anal, penile, and oropharyngeal cancers [68, 69]. In view of these developments, the current ACIP recommendation for HPV immunization of males is as strong as the recommendation for females.

"I heard that the vaccine causes ovarian failure"

Primary ovarian insufficiency (POI), defined as cessation of ovarian function prior to the age of 40, occurs in approximately 1% of females. The cause is usually unknown. It is estimated that around 4% of these cases are attributed to autoimmune factors, the ultimate cause of which remains obscure. Among adolescents, there is more likely to be an identifiable background etiology, including such entities such as Turner syndrome, Fragile X syndrome, hyperprolactinemia, a history of cancer treatment, and possibly infections or autoimmunity [70]. Because some cases have occurred among girls who had previously received the HPV vaccine, the concept that the vaccine can cause ovarian failure has gained some traction in the more vaccine-skeptical population. To address this, we need to consider the following points:

- POI occurs naturally with a measurable background rate, including among adolescents. The fact that some cases have been found after HPV immunization (anywhere from months to years) does not specifically imply causation.
- There has been no plausible biological mechanism yet proposed for a causative link between HPV vaccine and POI.
- No evidence of autoimmunity has been found in recipients of the HPV vaccine outside of the natural background rate [71].

HPV vaccine has a well-proven record of safety, tolerability, and efficacy and deserves to be included among the routine immunizations given to adolescents and young adults. HPV vaccine is unique among vaccines in that it is designed and administered to reduce the incidence of certain cancers. The vaccine's safety and efficacy are well established, and it deserves an important role in adolescent and young adult health.

Perspectives

What Works

As the majority of this chapter has demonstrated, there is a host of myths and concerns about immunizations that a sizable minority of the population holds to, causing them to question, if not outright refuse immunization. Ideally, the science that can answer those objections can also provide confidence to the health-care personnel who are providing immunization services. Lest we think, however, that our mastery of technically sophisticated arguments in defense of vaccines will reliably win the day by itself, we must consider elements of an immunization program that really work. If the question is, "What will enhance the acceptance of vaccines by the public?", some attempts at answers are given below:

- **Physician recommendation**. Surveys show that the most trusted source of information about vaccines is the primary care physician. A large European study showed that primary care physicians were the most trusted source of information, followed in varying order (depending on locations) by primary care nurses, public health physicians and nurses, pharmacists, the media, and informational pamphlets [72]. Primary care physicians, nurses, and other providers are likely to be in the best position to offer sound advice about immunization. The established relationship of a primary care setting engenders the trust that makes sound advice acceptable to patients.
- **Caring, non-argumentative advice.** Usually the health-care personnel who are administering vaccines know a great deal more of the science about those vaccines than the people who are receiving them. Depending on the competitiveness of the health-care provider advocating for immunization, it can be tempting to bowl people over with facts. It even becomes tempting to employ argument and debate (author's experience). The problem is that argument and debate rarely work with most patients. An argumentative approach prompts a defensive response, and defensiveness is a powerful force. A gentle, caring, and personal recommendation from a trusted health-care provider is much less likely to prompt such defensiveness [73]. Rigorous scientific studies are critical in building the knowledge base of the immunization provider, but the facts and statistics that impress most of us carry much less weight for most of the public. We will not win over everybody; some people are quite steadfast in their refusal. However, a kind and measured approach leaves the door open for the patient to return later on.
- **Standing orders**. The use of standing orders authorizes supervised health-care staff to administer vaccines in a variety of settings including clinic, hospital, public health facilities, and outreach programs. The use of standing orders has been demonstrated to help smooth patient flow through immunization facilities [74, 75], as well as to increase immunization rates in the populations served. Templates for standing orders can be obtained through the Immunization Action

Coalition (immunize.org). Individual practices can also develop these standing orders of their own.

- **Vaccine information statements**. By federal law a Vaccine Information Statement (VIS) must be provided along with the vaccine. These are required to be the most current copies. In addition to being required with the administration of a vaccine, the VIS can also be a useful source of information to patients who may be hesitant about receiving the vaccine in question. They are written at a level suitable for the general reader, and they provide accurate and timely information about the vaccines as well as adverse effects. Patients can be offered the VIS to take home and consider in a less pressured environment and will sometimes be sufficiently reassured to return for the vaccines. VISs can be obtained through immunize.org as well as directly from the CDC.

- **Immunization information systems**. Also known as an immunization registry, an immunization information system (IIS) is a state-sponsored program by which immunizations provided throughout the state by various physicians and other providers in private and public sectors can be registered securely at a state-operated database. IISs are now operating in all American states and territories, at various degrees of development. Experience has shown that the IIS, especially when integrated with a provider's electronic medical record system, can reduce duplication of immunizations to individuals, provide alerts to immunization staff that a given patient is due for updates, and can provide a portable record of immunizations for people who are away from their medical home or change immunization providers.

- **State mandates**. All states in the United States have mandated immunization programs, most commonly linked to admission to public schools. Some states allow exemption from these mandates only for medical contraindications. Other states allow exemptions for religious reasons and yet others allow for exemption by personal conviction as well. Experience has shown that immunization rates in states that allow exemption based on personal conviction tend to be somewhat lower than in states that do not have such an allowance [76, 77]. Mandates are established through state legislative processes.

Even when the above recommendations are fully in place, not all individuals will accept the immunizations being offered; we won't win everyone over. However, a well-informed health-care work force, practicing in a caring and non-argumentative fashion, can have a major impact on immunization rates and thereby on the control of immunization-preventable disease. Ultimately our goal is the protection of the populations we serve.

References

1. http://www.cdc.gov/about/history/tengpha.htm
2. Centers for Disease Control and Prevention. Achievements in Public Health. Impact of vaccines universally recommended for children -- United States, 1990-1998. MMWR. 1999;48(12):243–8.

3. http://www.nvic.org/NVIC-Vaccine-News/July-2015/21st-century-cures-act-eliminates-good-science.aspx
4. http://themillenniumreport.com/2016/06/the-vaccine-conspiracy-u-s-government-colludes-with-big-pharma-to-poison-the-america-people-2/
5. Patel M, Orenstein W. A world free of polio — the final steps. N Engl J Med. 2016 Feb 11;374:501–3.
6. Klein N, Bartlett J, Fireman B, Rowhani-Rahbar A, Baxter R. Comparative effectiveness of acellular versus whole-cell pertussis vaccines in teenagers. Pediatrics. 2013;131(6):e1716.
7. CDC. Achievements in Public Health. Hepatitis B vaccination --- United States, 1982--2002. MMWR Morb Mortal Wkly Rep. 2002;51(25):549–52.
8. Belongia EA, Irving SA, Shui IM, Kulldorf M, Lewis E, Yin R, et al. Real-time surveillance to assess risk of intussusception and other adverse events after pentavalent, bovine-derived rotavirus vaccine. Pediatr Infect Dis J. 2010;29(1):1–5.
9. Yih WK, Lieu TA, Kulldorf M, Martin D, McMahill-Walraven CN, Platt R, et al. Intussusception risk after rotavirus vaccination in U.S. infants. N Engl J Med. 2014;370:503–12.
10. https://www.cia.gov/library/publications/the-world-factbook/rankorder/2012rank.html
11. http://demog.berkeley.edu/~andrew/1918/figure2.html
12. Majumder MS, Cohn EL, Mekaru SR, Huston JE, Brownstein JS. Substandard vaccination compliance and the 2015 measles outbreak. JAMA Pediatr. 2015;169(5):494–5.
13. Measles Cases and Outbreaks. http://www.cdc.gov/measles/cases-outbreaks.html
14. Oxford Vaccine Group. Vaccine knowledge project http://www.cdc.gov/measles/cases-outbreaks.html
15. Phadke VK, Bednarczyk RA, Salmon DA, Omer SB. Association between vaccine refusal and vaccine-preventable diseases in the United States. JAMA. 2016;315(11):1149–58.
16. Misegades LK, Winter K, Harriman K, Talarico J, Messonnier NE, Clark TA, et al. Association of childhood pertussis with receipt of 5 doses of pertussis vaccine by time since last vaccine dose, California, 2010. JAMA. 2012;308(20):2126–32.
17. Vitek CR, Wharton M. Diphtheria in the former Soviet union: reemergence of a pandemic disease. Emerg Infect Diseases. 1998; 4(4): 539–50. http://wwwnc.cdc.gov/eid/article/4/4/98-0404_article
18. CDC. Diphtheria. http://www.cdc.gov/diphtheria/clinicians.html
19. Centers for Disease Control and Prevention. Epidemiology and prevention of vaccine-preventable diseases. In: Atkinson W, Hamborsky J, Wolfe S, editors. 12th ed., second printing. Washington DC: Public Health Foundation; 2012.
20. CDC. Monitoring the Impact of Varicella Vaccination. http://www.cdc.gov/chickenpox/hcp/monitoring-varicella.html.Updated Jul 1, 2016.
21. Elizabeth C, Briere EC, Rubin L, Moro PL, Cohn A, Clark T, et al. Prevention and control of haemophilus influenzae type b disease: recommendations of the advisory committee on immunization practices (ACIP). CDC MMWR Recomm Rep. 2014;63(RR01):1–14.
22. Hinman AR, Orenstein WA, Schuchat A. CDC. Vaccine-preventable diseases, immunizations, and MMWR Surveill Summ. 2011;60 Suppl 4:49–57.
23. http://www.businessinsider.com/donald-trump-vaccines-autism-2015-9. Accessed 8 Aug 2016.
24. Wakefield AJ, Murch SH, Anthony A, Linnell J, Casson DM, Malik M, et al. Ileal-lymphoid-nodular hyperplasia, non-specific colitis, and pervasive developmental disorder in children. Lancet. 1998;28:351.
25. Dales L, Hammer SJ, Smith NJ. Time trends in autism and in MMR immunization coverage in California. JAMA. 2001;285(9):1183–5.
26. http://www.bbc.com/news/health-22277186
27. Retraction—Ileal-lymphoid-nodular hyperplasia, non-specific colitis, and pervasive developmental disorder in children. Lancet. 2010;375:445.

28. Taylor B, Miller E, Farrington CP, Petropoulos MC, Favot-Mayaud I, Li J, et al. Autism and measles, mumps, and rubella vaccine: no epidemiological evidence for a causal association. Lancet. 1999;353(9169):2026–9.
29. Madsen KM, Hviid A, Vestergaard M, Schendel D, Wohlfahrt J, Thorsen P, et al. A population-based study of measles, mumps, and rubella vaccination and autism. N Engl J Med. 2002;347(19):1477–82.
30. Jain A, Marshall J, Buikema A, Bancroft T, Kelly JP, Newschaffer CJ. Autism occurrence by MMR vaccine status among US children with older siblings with and without autism. JAMA. 2015;313(15):1534–40.
31. Madsen KM, Lauritsen MB, Pedersen CB, Thorsen P, Plesner A, Andersen PH, et al. Thimerosal and the occurrence of autism: negative ecological evidence from Danish population-based data. Pediatrics. 2003;112:604–6.
32. Hviid A, Stellfeld M, Wohlfahrt J, Melbye M. Association between thimerosal-containing aaccine and autism. JAMA. 2003;290(13):1763–6.
33. IOM (Institute of Medicine). Adverse effects of vaccines: evidence and causality. Washington, DC: The National Academies Press; 2012. p. 153.
34. http://www.uscfc.uscourts.gov/sites/default/files/vaccine_files/Vowell.Snyder.pdf
35. http://leftbrainrightbrain.co.uk/2015/07/15/jim-carrey-you-are-part-of-the-problem-for-us-in-the-autism-community/. Accessed 18 June 2016.
36. http://autisticadvocacy.org/2015/09/asan-statement-on-gop-primary-debate-comments-on-autism-and-vaccination/. Accessed 18 June 2016.
37. http://theautismresearchfoundation.org/measles-surge-in-britain-after-autism-related-vaccine-scare/. Accessed 18 June 2016.
38. Sears RW. The vaccine book. New York: Little, Brown & Co.; 2011.
39. King GE, Hadler SC. Simultaneous administration of childhood vaccines: an important public health policy that is safe and efficacious. Pediatr Infect Dis J. 1994;13:394–407.
40. Davidson M, Letson GW, Ward JI, Ball A, Bulkow L, Christenson P, et al. DTP immunization and susceptibility to infectious diseases. Is there a relationship? Am J Dis Child. 1991;145(7):750.
41. Black SB, Cherry JD, Shinefield HR, Fireman B, Christenson P, Lampert D, et al. Apparent decreased risk of invasive bacterial disease after heterologous childhood immunization. Am J Dis Child. 1991;145(7):746.
42. Storsaeter J, Olin P, Renemar B, Lagergård T, Norberg R, Romanus V, et al. Mortality and morbidity from invasive bacterial infections during a clinical trial of acellular pertussis vaccines in Sweden. Pediatr Infect Dis J. 1988;7(9):637.
43. Centers for Disease Control and Prevention. Epidemiology and prevention of vaccine-preventable diseases. In: Atkinson W, Hamborsky J, Wolfe S, editors. 12th ed., second printing. Washington DC: Public Health Foundation; 2012. Appendix B. http://www.cdc.gov/vaccines/pubs/pinkbook/downloads/appendices/B/excipient-table-2.pdf
44. Hurley AM, Tadrous M, Miller ES. Thimerosal-containing vaccines and autism: a review of recent epidemiologic studies. J Pediatr Pharmacol Ther. 2010; 15(3):173–181. (Also accessible through http://www.ncbi.nlm.nih.gov/pmc/articles/PMC3018252/).
45. http://www.who.int/vaccine_safety/committee/topics/thiomersal/statement_jul2006/en/
46. Heron J, Golding J, ALSPAC Study Team. Thimerosal exposure in infants and developmental disorders: a prospective cohort study in the United Kingdom does not show a causal association. Pediatrics. 2004;114:577–83.
47. http://www.publichealth.org/public-awareness/understanding-vaccines/goes-vaccine/
48. Mitkus RJ, King DB, Hess MA, Forshee RA, Walderhaug MO. Office of biostatistics and epidemiology, and office of vaccines research and review, food and drug administration, center for biologics evaluation and research, Rockville, MD. Study Reports Aluminum in Vaccines Poses Extremely Low Risk to Infants. http://www.fda.gov/BiologicsBloodVaccines/ScienceResearch/ucm284520.htm

49. U.S. Food and Drug Administration. FDA study reinforces no safety concerns from residual formaldehyde in some infant vaccines http://www.fda.gov/BiologicsBloodVaccines/ScienceResearch/ucm349473.htm. Accessed 21 June 2016.
50. National Catholic Bioethics Center. FAQ on vaccines. 2006. Available at: http://www.ncbcenter.org/page.aspx?pid=1284.
51. McNeil MM, Weintraub ES, Duffy J, et al. Risk of anaphylaxis after vaccination in children and adults. J Allergy Clin Immunol doi:10.1016/j.jaci.2015.07.048. Also accessed at http://www.ncbi.nlm.nih.gov/pubmed/26452420
52. http://www.fda.gov/downloads/BiologicsBloodVaccines/Vaccines/ApprovedProducts/UCM123789.pdf
53. CDC. MMWR Recommendations and Reports. Sept 6, 1996 / 45(RR-12); 1-35. https://www.cdc.gov/mmwr/preview/mmwrhtml/00046738.htm
54. Biggerstaff M, Jhung MA, Reed C, Fry AM, Balluz L, Finelli L. Influenza-like illness, the time to seek healthcare, and influenza antiviral receipt during the 2010-2011 influenza season-United States. J Infect Dis. 2014;210(4):535.
55. Poehling KA, Edwards KM, et al. New vaccine surveillance network. The underrecognized burden of influenza in young children. N Engl J Med. 2006;355(1):31.
56. Molinari N-A M, Ismael R, Ortega-Sanchez IR. The annual impact of seasonal influenza in the US: measuring disease burden and costs. Vaccine. 2007;25:5086–96. https://www.researchgate.net/profile/Noelle-Angelique_Molinari/publication/6292605_The_annual_impact_of_seasonal_influenza_in_the_US_measuring_disease_burden_and_costs/links/0046352711898ecad6000000.pdf
57. Centers for Disease Control and Prevention. Misconceptions about seasonal flu and flu vaccines. www.cdc.gov/flu/about/qa/misconceptions.htm
58. Mossad SB. Upper respiratory tract infections. http://www.clevelandclinicmeded.com/medicalpubs/diseasemanagement/infectious-disease/upper-respiratory-tract-infection/   August 2013.
59. Tosh PK, Boyce TG, Poland GA. Flu myths: dispelling the myths associated with live attenuated influenza vaccine. Mayo Clin Proc. 2008;83(1):77–84. doi:10.4065/83.1.77.
60. http://www.cdc.gov/flu/professionals/vaccination/effectiveness-studies.htm
61. Ferdinands JM, Olsho LE, Agan AA, Bhat N, Sullivan RM, Hall M, Mourani PM, Thompson M, Randolph AG. Pediatric acute lung injury and sepsis investigators (PALISI) network. Effectiveness of influenza vaccine against life-threatening RT-PCR-confirmed influenza illness in US children, 2010–2012. J Infect Dis. 2014;210(5):674. http://www.ncbi.nlm.nih.gov/pubmed/24676207
62. Glezen WP, Gaglani MJ, Kozinetz CA, Piedra PA. Direct and indirect effectiveness of influenza vaccination delivered to children at school preceding an epidemic caused by 3 new influenza virus variants. J Infect Dis. 2010;202(11):1626. http://www.ncbi.nlm.nih.gov/pmc/articles/mid/NIHMS233190/
63. http://www.fda.gov/NewsEvents/Newsroom/PressAnnouncements/ucm426485.htm
64. IOM (Institute of Medicine). Adverse effects of vaccines: evidence and causality. Washington, DC: The National Academies Press; 2012. p. 521.
65. CDC. Sexual risk behaviors: HIV, STD, & teen pregnancy prevention. http://www.cdc.gov/HealthyYouth/sexualbehaviors/index.htm
66. Bednarczyk RA, Davis R, Ault K, Orenstein W, Omer SB. Sexual activity–related outcomes after human papillomavirus vaccination of 11- to 12-year-olds. Pediatrics. 2012;130(5):798. http://www.ncbi.nlm.nih.gov/pubmed/23071201
67. Smith LM, Strumpf EC, Levesque LE. Effect of human papillomavirus (HPV) vaccination on clinical indicators of sexual behaviour among adolescent girls: the Ontario grade 8 HPV vaccine cohort study. CMAJ. 2014, 2015;187(2) doi:10.1503/cmaj.140900.
68. CDC. How many cancers are linked with HPV each year? http://www.cdc.gov/cancer/hpv/statistics/cases.htm

69. Viens LJ, Henley SJ, Watson M, et al. Human papillomavirus–associated cancers — United States, 2008–2012. MMWR Morb Mortal Wkly Rep. 2016;65:661–6. doi:10.15585/mmwr. mm6526a1.
70. Primary ovarian insufficiency in adolescents and young women. Committee opinion no. 605. American College of Obstetricians and Gynecologists. Obstet Gynecol 2014;123:193–7.
71. Arnheim-Dahlström L, Pasternak B, Svanström H, Sparén P, Hviid A. Autoimmune, neurological, and venous thromboembolic adverse events after immunisation of adolescent girls with quadrivalent human papillomavirus vaccine in Denmark and Sweden: cohort study. BMJ. 2013;347 doi:10.1136/bmj.f5906.
72. Stefanoff P, Mamelund S, Robinson M, et al. Tracking parental attitudes on vaccination across European countries: the vaccine safety, attitudes, training and communication project (VACSATC). Vaccine. 2010;28(35):5731–7.
73. Healy CM, Pickering LK. How to communicate with vaccine-hesitant parents. Pediatrics. 2011;127(Supplement 1):S127.
74. Guide to Community Preventive Services. Increasing appropriate vaccination: standing orders. www.thecommunityguide.org/vaccines/standingorders.html. Accessed 21 June 2016.
75. Modlin JF et al. Advisory committee for immunization practices. MMWR Recommendations and Reports. Use of standing orders programs to increase adult vaccination rates. 2000; 49 (RR01); 15–26.
76. Lee C, Robinson J. Systematic review of the effect of immunization mandates on uptake of routine childhood immunizations. J Infect. 2016;72(6):659–66.
77. Omer SB, Salmon DA, Orenstein WA, de Hart MP, Halsey N. Vaccine refusal, mandatory immunization, and the risks of vaccine-preventable diseases. N Engl J Med. 2009;360:1981–8. doi:10.1056/NEJMsa0806477.

Chapter 6
Barriers to Improved Immunization Rates and Ways to Overcome Them

Pamela G. Rockwell and Paul Hunter

Introduction

Infectious diseases were prevalent and had great impact on the health and welfare of the population in the United States (US) from the country's beginning through the early twentieth century. Though the smallpox vaccine was developed in 1796 and four other vaccines against rabies, typhoid, cholera, and plague were developed by late in the nineteenth century, no vaccines were widely used during the nineteenth century. During the twentieth century, great strides occurred in the control of many vaccine-preventable diseases (VPDs) [1], and reduction of VPDs continues to be ranked by public health experts as one of the top ten public health achievements in the twenty-first century [2]. Both the addition of newly developed vaccines to universally recommended immunization guidelines and the increased numbers of vaccinated persons contribute to this achievement. However, the rates of increases in vaccination coverage seen in children have slowed or even reversed in the past several years [2a] (Fig. 6.1). The preservation of herd immunity by way of maintaining high immunization rates is an important public health concern. Though US vaccination rates remain high enough overall to maintain herd immunity for most common

P.G. Rockwell, DO
Department of Family Medicine, University of Michigan Medical School,
3039 Overridge Drive, Ann Arbor, MI 48104, USA
e-mail: prockwel@med.umich.edu

P. Hunter, MD (✉)
Department of Family Medicine and Community Health, School of Medicine
and Public Health, University of Wisconsin, Madison, WI, USA

City of Milwaukee Health Department, 841 N Broadway Street #315,
Milwaukee, WI 53202, USA
e-mail: phunte@milwaukee.gov

© Springer International Publishing AG 2017
P.G. Rockwell (ed.), *Vaccine Science and Immunization Guideline*,
DOI 10.1007/978-3-319-60471-8_6

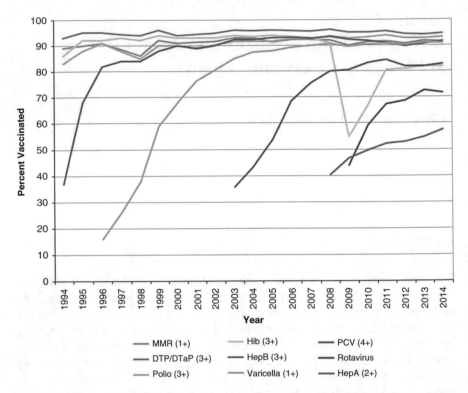

Fig. 6.1 Vaccine-specific coverage among children 19–35 months, National Immunization Survey, 1994–2014 [2a]

VPDs, conditions which may undermine herd immunity exist, posing a practical concern for clinicians, public health officials, and the public at large. Poor patient acceptance of vaccines, the import of VPDs from other countries, and vaccine composition changes that alter vaccine effectiveness may all affect herd immunity. The change from whole cell to acellular composition for the pertussis vaccine (made to address vaccine safety concerns) [3] during the 1990s requires a higher rate of vaccination to achieve herd immunity. An example of an imported case of measles causing a US outbreak of the disease was seen in 2014–2015. Centers for Disease Control and Prevention (CDC) linked this measles outbreak to a traveler who became infected with measles overseas and then visited Disneyland in California. The resulting measles outbreak affected 111 persons, the majority of whom were not previously vaccinated against measles, and spread the disease from California over several states, affecting poorly vaccinated subpopulations [4].

Family physicians strive to improve immunization rates in accordance with American Academy of Family Physicians (AAFP) policy vaccine recommendations. These recommendations follow the evidence-based, graded Advisory Committee on Immunization Practices (ACIP) recommendations on vaccines. The Office of Disease Prevention and Health Promotion (ODPHP) strives to improve the health of all Americans and has put together objectives for the Healthy People 2020 campaign which include goals to reduce, eliminate, or maintain elimination of cases of 17 VPDs across the lifespan [5]. There are several common barriers to improving immunization rates that merit discussion. Some barriers require the development and implementation of clinical protocols into healthcare systems to overcome them. Other barriers require education of the public as well as physicians and other professionals. With improved understanding of these barriers, physicians can better work with their clinic managers and staff, healthcare system administrators, community, local health departments, and politicians to make necessary changes to improve immunization rates. This chapter will identify several common barriers to improved immunization rates and explore ways to overcome them.

Commonly cited barriers to improved vaccine uptake in adults [6, 6a] and children include:

1. Lack of community demand for vaccination
2. Lack of physician knowledge on vaccine recommendations
3. Lack of regular assessment of vaccine status/missed opportunities for vaccination
4. Poor patient access to vaccinations
5. Complex vaccination schedules
6. Health system barriers
7. Financial disincentives for vaccination
8. Limited use of electronic records, tools, and immunization registries
9. Patient hesitancy and vaccine refusal
10. Poor physician communication regarding vaccine recommendations

These barriers will be broadly discussed, and when possible, evidence-based-proven methods to overcome these barriers will be outlined. Expert opinion will be offered when evidence is lacking. Some barriers may not have obvious solutions but may benefit from a discussion around the contributing circumstances that created them. Communication tips to more effectively talk to patients when recommending vaccines will be presented.

The next chapter (Chap. 8) will discuss overcoming immunization barriers differently, through a discussion of systems-based changes to immunization barriers and use of the 4 pillars model to improve vaccination rates.

Barrier Lack of Community Demand for Vaccination

A commitment to immunization is a global and national priority to ensure public health and good economic fiscal responsibility. Individuals and communities must understand the value of vaccines and demand immunization as both their right and responsibility. The public's understanding of vaccine importance for both children and adults is variable and requires ongoing education. The Guide to Community Preventive Services (The Community Guide) [106] identifies lack of community demand as a barrier to improving immunization rates and improving public health. The National Vaccine Program, run through the Department of Health and Human Services, lists *Increase Community Demand for Adult Immunizations* as its third of ten priorities of the implementation of the National Adult Immunization Plan [107].

Most adults understand that there are many recommended childhood vaccinations and that children are recommended to receive vaccinations to attend daycares and schools. Many adults, however, are not aware of what vaccines are recommended routinely for them and do not know what vaccines they may be missing. Overall, the prevalence of illness attributable to VPDs is greater among adults than among children. Despite longstanding recommendations for many adult vaccines, vaccination coverage among US adults is low, ranging from 20% coverage for Tdap in all adults over 19 years of age to 61.3% for pneumococcal coverage in adults aged 65 years or more [7]. Among those adults 65 and older, the failure to be vaccinated with the pneumococcal vaccine is directly associated with their lack of knowledge about the vaccine [8]. The older adult population clearly needs education in an ongoing fashion regarding the availability of vaccinations recommended to maintain good health [9].

Misinformation regarding vaccines may further contribute to lack of community demand for vaccinations. There exist three common themes of vaccine misinformation. These include misinformation around the adverse effects of vaccines, the lack of understanding of vaccine-preventable disease severity, and the fear of disease development after the administration of vaccines. Deficiencies in parents' knowledge about the adverse effects and contraindications of vaccines often lead to under immunization of children [10]. Many parents mistakenly fear that vaccination overwhelms their child's immune system, especially when more than one vaccine is given at the same visit. Current studies do not support this hypothesis. Although we now give children more vaccines than we have in the past, the actual number of antigens they receive has declined over the past generation. Previously, one vaccine against smallpox contained about 200 proteins, and now due to advances in protein chemistry, 11 routinely recommended vaccines contain fewer than 130 proteins in total [11].

The interpretation that "natural immunity" is superior to vaccine-induced immunity is often cited by vaccine-hesitant patients. Though this may be true for some diseases, the dangers of this approach far outweigh the relative benefits. For example, the risk of death in gaining immunity to measles through contracting the disease is one in five hundred. In contrast, the risk of a severe allergic reaction from a measles, mumps, and rubella (MMR) vaccine is less than one in one million [12]. These general misconceptions that vaccines are "unnatural," not effective, and may contain harmful elements, are often perpetuated by nonmedical sources and nontraditional media. There is no scientific evidence to support that low levels of formaldehyde, mercury, or aluminum found in vaccines can be harmful. The US Food and Drug Administration (FDA) and CDC state that formaldehyde produced by our own metabolic systems is found in higher levels in our bodies than the trace levels found in vaccines [12].

Misinformation regarding vaccines is often perpetuated by sources that do not subscribe to scientific principles and guidelines. The anti-vaccine lobby groups propagate misinformation and lies and manipulate research and data, which leads to public confusion. Their sources for information do not usually come from traditional media or scientific journals. Many parents commonly use the Internet and social media, as opposed to traditional media, as the source for their vaccine information. The negative influence of print, broadcast, internet, and social media sources on parents exacerbates the parental misperception of harm from vaccines [13]. People often perpetuate misinformation simply by repeating it or forwarding an email or Facebook post. Often social media and Internet depictions of vaccines include emotionally charged personal accounts of children, apparently harmed by vaccines, to which parents can easily relate. Celebrities who endorse false science can also have a great impact on the public. Jenny McCarthy, an American Playboy playmate turned actress and talk-show host, has widely promoted the false idea that vaccines cause autism, using her son's autism diagnosis as proof. Pro-vaccine advocates and websites find it difficult to counterbalance and repudiate such erroneous messages and fears in an understandable way by use of scientific facts. Put simply, it is more difficult to "take away the fear" once doubts have been raised than to instill fear around vaccines.

Framing the message of vaccines as a positive one, namely, that vaccines are safe and are the most effective means to protect children and adults from disease, needs to be the focus of future educational interventions. These interventions can utilize successful anti-vaccine strategies to stress the benefits of vaccination through personal storytelling with the focus on first person accounts of harmful effects of VPDs [14]. In this writer's opinion, CDC started an effective print and television campaign in 2016 to educate parents about the cancer-preventive benefits of the HPV vaccine through personal storytelling depicting children and young adults speaking to their parents about HPV-related cancers. However, more research is needed to know to what extent social media interactions with government agencies and professional organizations such as CDC, American Academy of Pediatrics (AAP), and AAFP can address parents' vaccine questions [15]. Education and communication around vaccines must be maintained with up-to-date, credible information online. Though there is not much data yet available, there appears to be great potential for improving vaccine uptake and vaccine coverage by implementing programs and interventions that apply new media, as defined by text messaging, smartphone applications, YouTube videos, Facebook, targeted websites and portals, software for physicians and health professionals, and email communication. Further research on these interventions and cost-effectiveness assessments is needed [16].

Proven Ways to Improve Community Demand   Activities and interventions that help improve community demand are identified in a large Cochrane database of systematic reviews performed in 2014. The implementation of the following activities/practices has shown statistically significant results to increase community demand for vaccination:

- Client reminder and recall systems – reminding members of a target population that vaccinations are due (reminders) or late (recall). These reminders may be delivered by various methods: telephone, letter, postcard, or other means such as text messages.

- Clinic-based patient education – face-to-face education or use of brochures, videotapes, posters, and vaccine information statements (VIS).

However, implementing these suggestions may be difficult to accomplish in many clinical practices as these vaccine improvement efforts take time, money, and personnel, often scarce resources for the average physician in practice. Community-wide immunization coalitions [17] may strive to increase demand for vaccines through a variety of nonclinical methods, including educational health fairs, billboards, and mass media. However, barriers to increasing community-wide immunization coalitions may be found at many levels: at the level of the primary care physician/practice, at a local government level, and at a national level. The lack of reimbursement for time spent on such community efforts creates a barrier to clinicians to attend the coalition meetings to coordinate these clinical and nonclinical efforts. City and state-funded events and educational campaigns also take time, money, and personnel and the support of local legislators. National campaigns to increase education on the importance of vaccines and disease prevention are often affected by political ideology or corporate self-interest. Reliable, unbiased sources of support for public health education about the importance, effectiveness, and safety of vaccines are difficult to find, and there exists much public mistrust of governmental declarations within the healthcare system.

Barrier Lack of Physician Knowledge

Physician knowledge deficits on vaccine science and immunization recommendations may also present a barrier to improved immunization rates of patients. Deficits in vaccine knowledge may be traced back to insufficient medical school education for some physicians and/or insufficient training during residency. There is no uniform required curriculum for teaching immunization and vaccine science across medical schools. The Liaison Committee on Medical Education (LCME), the accrediting body for programs leading to an MD degree in the US, does not specifically set educational vaccine science standards in its current published document: *Functions and Structure of a Medical School* (2016) for standards and elements effective July 1, 2017. In contrast, the Commission on Osteopathic College Accreditation (COCA) identifies the need for vaccine science education. COCA allows individual medical schools to set educational vaccine science and immunization standards in congruence with recommendations and best practices established by Centers for Disease and Prevention (CDC).

Furthermore, there is little uniform vaccine science curriculum required in graduate medical education for primary care residencies. The Accreditation Council for Graduate Medical Education (ACGME) is a private, 501(c)(3), not-for-profit organization that sets standards for US graduate medical education (residency and fellowship) programs and the institutions that sponsor them and renders accreditation decisions based on compliance with these standards. Those residencies associated with primary care include family medicine, pediatrics, internal medicine, and internal medicine-pediatrics. There are no specific ACGME vaccine science requirements for primary care residencies. Curriculum in vaccine science is left up to individual residency programs to create and impart.

A poll of obstetrics and gynecology (OB/GYN) residents (trained to deliver primary care for women) shows resident knowledge deficits regarding Advisory Committee on Immunization Practices (ACIP) guidelines. ACIP states pneumococcal vaccination is indicated for pregnant women with certain medical conditions. Many of the OB/GYN residents polled stated they do not recommend the vaccine when indicated, expressing uncertainty around the recommendations. They cited that uncertainty as one of the top reasons they do not vaccinate their pregnant patients against pneumococcus [18].

Post residency, practicing physicians may be undereducated in vaccine science and have knowledge deficits about current recommendations. Moreover, they may find it difficult to keep up with the ever-growing ACIP recommendations and changes in immunization guidelines. There are several proven, effective methods to address physician knowledge deficits. Educational programs that incorporate a didactic lecture, printed educational materials, and periodic email reminders are effective [19]. Brief, structured presentations can improve knowledge. Presentations given to several hundred healthcare workers including physicians, medical students, nurses, and other healthcare staff were shown to increase HPV knowledge significantly in that group [20].

It is helpful and necessary for physicians and other immunization providers to keep abreast of current guidelines through regular review of annual updates of ACIP recommendations. This may be accomplished by receipt of *Morbidity and Mortality Weekly Review (MMWR)*. A free electronic subscription may be obtained at http://www.cdc.gov/mmwr/index.html. The use of online resources and apps to help with decision-making for vaccine recommendations is helpful. *Shots Immunizations*, a free app for smartphones, is one such example of a useful app, produced by the Society of Teachers of Family Medicine (STFM) Group on Immunization Education (GIE). The Immunization Action Coalition (IAC), with financial support from CDC, offers one of the largest immunization resources for educational materials for health professionals and the public. IAC information is available at: http://www.immunize.org.

For those clinicians who have difficulty keeping up with immunization updates, the suggestion that more guideline advertisement may help them improve their patients' immunization rates seems reasonable. However, increasing awareness and familiarity with clinical practice guidelines *alone* has limited effect on physician behavior and improving patient outcomes. Other additional education techniques are needed. One suggestion to implement into physician practices is the addition of interactive techniques. These techniques include audit or feedback (e.g., the reporting of an individual clinician's vaccination rates compared with their partners' rates or desired, target rates), academic detailing or outreach, and reminders by way of electronic or other alerts. Audit or feedback takes advantage of many physicians' competitiveness to do better and is shown to be more effective than guidelines and didactic presentation alone to improve immunization rates [20, 21].

Barrier Lack of Regular Assessment of Vaccine Status and Missed Opportunities to Vaccinate

Patients' vaccine status and discussion around vaccines should ideally be a part of every clinical encounter in any primary care setting. Unfortunately, it is not. Most clinicians agree that health maintenance exams (annual physicals, well-child checks, etc.) are an appropriate patient care visit type to discuss vaccine status. However, patients see their physicians for many other types of office visits such as follow-up visits, visits for acute (urgent) care or chronic care, and for procedures. Consideration is to be given to update immunizations for all patients at all visit types. Clinic policies and physician preferences that limit vaccinating to only health maintenance visits increase missed opportunities to vaccinate and put up unnecessary barriers to improving immunization rates [21a]. Less than half of over one thousand family physicians and pediatricians polled reported discussing adolescent vaccines at sick visit types for 11- and 12-year-old patients with mild complaints. They reported that vaccination is better suited for a health maintenance, or "well" visit. The most commonly cited reasons for not vaccinating children at a sick visit were vaccination takes too long to discuss, and parents may blame the vaccine if the child's illness worsens [22]. It is clear physician preferences and clinic policies may need to change to improve vaccination rates [23–25].

In addition, concomitant (same-day or simultaneous vaccination) delivery of two or more vaccines is safe, effective, and efficient and may increase vaccination rates. Unfortunately, there are many missed opportunities to give needed vaccinations concomitantly to adolescents and adults. ACIP recommends that adolescents aged 11–12 years routinely receive three vaccines: tetanus toxoid, reduced diphtheria toxoid, and acellular pertussis vaccine (Tdap), quadrivalent meningococcal conjugate vaccine (MenACWY), and human papilloma virus (HPV) vaccine. Of surveyed adolescents who had initiated vaccination, two-thirds or less received two or more of the three adolescent vaccines during the same healthcare visit [26]. A 2014 CDC study estimated that routine concomitant vaccination among female adolescents could almost double the rates of HPV vaccine initiation and thus substantially reduce the risk of HPV-associated diseases [27].

In addition to the failure to give vaccines concomitantly when indicated, vaccine series are often initiated, but not completed. With younger children who generally come to the doctor's office more often than adolescents and young adults, there are more opportunities to give vaccinations outside of well visits and complete vaccine series already initiated. To increase completion rates of vaccination series for adolescents and young adult patients, appointments for immunizations should be made at time of checkout when the initial vaccine of the series is given. For example, schedule the second and third (if needed) HPV vaccine administration appointments when the patient leaves the office after the first HPV immunization administration [28].

Barrier Poor Patient Access to Vaccinations

Patients may have difficulty accessing vaccines. Patients that move frequently have limited access to transportation and work multiple jobs or nontraditional hours may have difficulties getting vaccinated. Per the US Bureau of Labor and Statistics,

15 million Americans work overnight hours, either on a regular or occasional basis. By contrast, most traditional primary care physician offices administer vaccinations during traditional clinic hours, 9:00 a.m. to 5:00 p.m., Monday through Friday [29]. Some workers may not have opportunity to take time away from their work to seek healthcare during traditional available clinic hours. Having vaccination services available during more nontraditional hours and days including early morning hours, lunchtime, evening hours, and Saturdays will help increase immunization rates.

Community pharmacies are uniquely positioned to increase immunization rates in the US by offering vaccination during nontraditional hours and days including holidays, Saturdays, and Sundays. One large study evaluated the more than six million vaccinations administered in more than 7500 pharmacies nationwide and found that almost 30% of the study population received one or more vaccinations during off-clinic hours. More than one million vaccinations took place during lunch hours (11:00 am to 1:00 pm), possibly demonstrating use of these hours by patients working traditional workday hours of 9:00 am to 5:00 pm. Almost 200,000 patients were vaccinated on a federal holiday, most often Columbus Day and Veterans Day. Furthermore, the more than 150,000 vaccinations that occurred during the overnight hours of 10:00 pm to 9:00 am demonstrate the value that 24-h community pharmacies may provide to nightshift workers [30].

There exist some challenges in more nontraditional delivery of vaccines, such as availability of treatment for adverse reactions [31]. Furthermore, the reality is that most pharmacies do not provide childhood vaccines or vaccines to the uninsured. While many pharmacies provide adult vaccines to insured patients, many pharmacies are reluctant to develop protocols to administer Vaccines for Children (VFC) vaccines to the uninsured or to children with Medicaid. In addition, adding an additional step requiring a patient to go to a local pharmacy or other healthcare site away from the patient medical home (PCMH) to obtain a vaccine may result in a missed opportunity to vaccinate. A patient may choose to not follow through on the referral given to vaccinate if an additional stop is needed at an outside pharmacy.

Barrier Complex Vaccination Schedules

The increasing complexity of medical decision-making required to properly implement ACIP recommendations makes it difficult for clinicians to stay abreast of immunization standards of care, for both children and adults [32]. The number of vaccines in the childhood and adolescent immunization schedule has more than doubled over the past 30 years. In 1985, ACIP recommendations called for only seven antigens in a maximum of two injections and one oral dose per clinic visit. By 2016, ACIP recommended coverage for 16 antigens (not including serotypes) in a maximum of six to eight injections and one oral dose at the 15-month well-child clinic visit (Table 6.1). For healthy children in the United States, from birth to age 6 years, ACIP recommends a cumulative total of 29–35 injections and four oral doses of routine vaccinations. The numerous vaccines, each with multiple doses, make completing the recommended schedule on time logistically challenging, even for families with significant motivation, social support, and economic resources. An analysis of data from the National Immunization Survey showed that only about

Table 6.1 Increasing numbers of ACIP-recommended childhood vaccines

1985	Diphtheria-tetanus-pertussis, polio, measles-mumps-rubella
1995	Diphtheria-tetanus-pertussis, polio, measles-mumps-rubella, hepatitis B, varicella, *Haemophilus influenzae* type b
2006	Diphtheria-tetanus-pertussis, polio, measles-mumps-rubella, hepatitis B, varicella, *Haemophilus influenzae* type b, hepatitis A, influenza, pneumococcus, rotavirus, meningococcus ACWY, human papilloma virus
2016	Diphtheria-tetanus-pertussis, polio, measles-mumps-rubella, hepatitis B, varicella, *Haemophilus influenzae* type b, hepatitis A, influenza (inactivated influenza vaccine IIV3 now also IIV4), pneumococcus (PCV7 now PCV13), rotavirus, meningococcus ACWY, meningococcus B, human papilloma virus (HPV2 and 4 now HPV9)

From Ref. [32a]

70% of children completed all doses of six recommended vaccines on time by 24 months of age [33]. The attempt to reduce the number of vaccines by the offer of multi-vaccine combinations may also create untoward barriers to vaccination. The pentavalent combination vaccines (DTaP-IPV-Hib, Pentacel® and DTaP-HepB-IPV, Pediarix®) lower the number of required injections but force clinics and health systems into choosing between two competing interlocking groups of vaccines (Table 6.2). Patients may move, change jobs, and/or change health insurance, and vaccine availability of interlocking groups of vaccines by office sites may also change, leading to an increase in the complexity of decision-making physicians and clinic staff face to properly vaccinate their patients.

Frequent ACIP changes in recommendations also add barriers to improved immunization rates. ACIP changes occur regularly and continually in response to emerging data as the 15 voting members of ACIP meet every fourth month. Patients and clinicians alike may be confused by the seemingly contradictory ACIP recommendations made over the past few years. For example, ACIP recommendations for live, attenuated influenza vaccine (LAIV) in young children changed three times in 3 years. Based on two studies [34, 35] showing better protection for young children, ACIP issued a *preferential recommendation* for LAIV over inactivated influenza vaccines (IIV) for children aged 8 years and younger for the 2014–15 influenza season [36]. This was the first time ACIP had preferentially recommended a specific presentation of one vaccine over another. For the 2015–2016 influenza season [37], citing observational studies [37a, 37b] showing intranasal LAIV was not superior to intramuscular IIV, the preference for LAIV over IIV was not renewed. The influenza recommendation reverted to the former recommendation of *either* LAIV or IIV without preference. Subsequently, in a third change in as many years, and only a few months before the start of the 2016–2017 influenza season, ACIP reversed its guidance by recommending *against* LAIV, thereby eliminating the potentially less painful intranasal option for influenza vaccination for persons aged 2–49 years.

Such a reversal in recommendations over such a short time span could decrease trust in ACIP's recommendation process especially in patients and clinicians who already have a tendency toward mistrust of authorities in government, healthcare, and scientific research. In response to the sentiments often expressed that CDC "got

Table 6.2 Interlocking combinations of immunizations

When using Pediarix®, DTaP-HepB-IPV			
Recommended childhood vaccines 2–15 months	2–15 months	2–15 months	4–6 years
combination vaccination covering 6 VPDs	Individual vaccines to complete recommendations	Individual vaccines to complete recommendations	Individual vaccines to complete recommendations
DTaP, HepB, IPV	+ *Haemophilus influenzae* (Hib)	Booster Tdap and IPV age 12–15 months (no need for HepB or HIB)	Booster Tdap and IPV age 4–6 years (no need for HepB or HIB)
Pediarix® (DTaP-HepB-IPV) 2, 4, 6 months	PedvaxHib® 2 and 12–15 months	Infanrix® (DTaP-IPV) 2, 4, 6 months	Kinrix® (DTaP-IPV) 4–6 years
Pediarix® 2, 4, 6 months	Hiberix® (Hib) (2, 4, 6, 15 months)	Infanrix® (DTaP-IPV) 2, 4, 6 months	Kinrix® (DTaP-IPV) 4–6 years
Pediarix® 2, 4, 6 months	ActHIB® (Hib) (2, 4, 6, 15 months)	Infanrix® (DTaP-IPV) 2, 4, 6 months	Kinrix® (DTaP-IPV) 4–6 years
When using Pentacel®, DTaP-IPV/Hib			
Combination vaccination covering 6 VPDs		Individual Vaccines to complete recommendations	Individual vaccines to complete recommendations
DTaP, IPV, Hib		+ HepB	Booster DTaP-IPV age 4–6 years
Pentacel® DTaP-IPV/Hib 2, 4, 6, and 15–18 months		RecombivaxHB® (0, 2, 6 months)	Quadracel® 4–6 years
Pentacel® 2, 4, 6, and 15–18 months		Engerix-B® (0, 2, 6 months)	Quadracel® 4–6 years

it wrong" about vaccine recommendations, clinicians ought to remind their patients and the public that ACIP recommendations change over time in response to currently available evidence, with the goal of ensuring safety and maximal effectiveness in preventing disease. In other words, changes in ACIP recommendations can be framed as *reassuring* given that the science behind vaccines is so carefully reviewed and reassessed with diligence.

Permissive (Category B) ACIP recommendations for vaccines may also provide confusion for clinicians and patients alike. Most clinicians are familiar with ACIP Category A recommendations, made for all persons in an age-based or risk factor-based format. Category A recommendations are clear and not left to interpretation. Category B recommendations, on the other hand, are made with the expectation that individual clinical decision-making is necessary when vaccines are offered and discussed with patients.

HPV vaccine recommendations exemplify changing ACIP category recommendations from Category B to Category A for males and the confusion that arose from different ACIP Category A and B HPV vaccination recommendations for different patient populations based on gender and age. HPV vaccination was originally published as a Category A recommendation in 2006 for females only, excluding males. Then in October 2009, ACIP issued a Category B recommendation for vaccinating *all males* ages 9–26 years against HPV. In 2011 ACIP again changed the HPV recommendation to Category A for *all males* ages 11–21 years and *males* ages 22–26 who have human immunodeficiency virus (HIV) that are immunocompromised or in special populations, including men who have sex with men (MSM). In addition, the Category B recommendation remained for all males 9 through 10 and 22 through 26 years without special conditions who wished to get the vaccine. These variations and differences in the recommendations within the male population as compared to the female population become confusing. Unfortunately, most family physicians and pediatricians did not consistently recommend HPV to males during ACIP's permissive (only) recommendation period between 2009 and 2011 [38], and the immunization rates for males lagged far behind females [39]. Only more recently do rates of HPV vaccination for males begin to approach those of females (Fig. 6.3).

The permissive recommendation for meningococcal B (MenB) vaccine for adolescents made in 2015 is another example of a situation where ACIP recommendations create confusion. The vaccine was licensed for use in the United States under an accelerated approval process in response to outbreaks on college campuses [40]. The full ACIP MenB recommendation is worded as follows:

A serogroup B meningococcal (MenB) vaccine series may be administered to adolescents and young adults 16 through 23 years of age to provide short term protection against most strains of serogroup B meningococcal disease. The preferred age for MenB vaccination is 16 through 18 years of age. [41]

Lack of available data is the reason ACIP made the decision to recommend MenB as a Category B rather than a Category A recommendation like the meningococcal quadrivalent (MenACWY) recommendation. The unavailable data included breadth of coverage of serogroup B strains circulating in the US, magnitude and duration of vaccine effectiveness, impact on carriage and herd immunity, and safety post-licensure [42]. Many physicians consider the vaccine's short duration of protection and the relative high-cost burden of vaccinating so many adolescents for a disease with a relatively low incidence rate in their decision to offer the vaccine. These reasonable and scientifically sound concerns may increase the indecision and confusion clinicians have in recommending MenB vaccination for adolescents.

In addition to confusion over permissive language, confusion over time-sensitive administration recommendations of vaccines may lead to poor vaccination rates. ACIP added pneumococcal *conjugate* vaccination (PCV13, Prevnar®) to the previously recommended pneumococcal *polysaccharide* vaccine (PPSV23, Pneumovax®) for all adults age 65 years and older [43]. Because studies show lower immune response when PPSV23 is given within the year before PCV13, ACIP preferentially recommends PCV13 be given before PPSV23 with established time intervals, depending on medical conditions present. ACIP recommendations in August 2014 included 6–12-month and 8-week intervals between the two vaccines if PCV13 was given first and PPSV23 given second, but a 12-month interval between the two if PPSV23 was given first and PCV13 given second [44]. These multiple time intervals are difficult to remember in busy clinical settings and very difficult to program into forecasting software used in medical records and immunization registries. In addition, Medicare rejects claims billing for two pneumococcal vaccinations of any type within 12 months' time. Given the medical equivalence and logistical superiority of a simplified regimen, ACIP in June 2015 changed the recommended interval to 12 months between pneumococcal vaccinations for all adults 65 years and older regardless of which type (PCV13 or PPSV23) is given first [45].

Other complex vaccination schedules are encountered for patients who are behind schedule, who have certain medical conditions (e.g., immunocompromised or chronically ill patients), who travel overseas, or have occupation exposures. Generally, *catch-up schedules* involve using minimum intervals. However, minimum intervals for some vaccines differ at different patient ages (e.g., Hib and PCV13). For *Haemophilus influenzae* type b (Hib) and PCV13 vaccines, the numbers of doses in catch-up schedules decrease as healthy children reach the age at which they are no longer at increased risk for those infections against which immunizations protect [46, 47]. These variable recommendations by age make the catch-up immunization schedules for Hib and PCV13 burdensome to interpret.

Some of the most complex ACIP recommendations involve *medical conditions* that put patients at risk for vaccine-preventable diseases. For example, persons with heart disease, asthma, or HIV require more vaccines than other otherwise healthy adults. Anticipation of iatrogenic risks for vaccine-preventable diseases, such as splenectomy, cochlear implant surgery, or chemotherapy, also trigger specific recommendations for vaccines against polysaccharide-encapsulated bacteria (meningococcus, Hib, and pneumococcus) [48, 49]. Within this high-risk category of patients, there exist additional distinctions and recommendations which may be confusing. For example, a patient with a nonfunctioning or missing spleen is recommended to receive two doses of PPSV23 before age 65. This represents one dose more than adults with asthma are recommended to receive before age 65. Moreover, healthy adults are not recommended to receive any PPSV23 vaccine *until* age 65.

Anticipation of *travel* to areas with ongoing transmission of vaccine-preventable diseases activates recommendations for catch-up and travel-related schedules for certain routinely recommended vaccines (e.g., MMR, hepatitis A [HepA], meningococcal) and for other travel-specific vaccines not routinely recommended to non-travelers (e.g., typhoid, yellow fever). Recommendations that involve anticipating future events present significant challenges to the forecasting algorithms of state immunization registries and the medical records used by health care systems.

Other new, novel recommendations have evolved out of a response to changes in epidemiology. For example, infant risk of death from pertussis is highest in the newborn period, before infants are eligible for vaccination. As the recommended doses of pertussis vaccine is given at 2, 4, and 6 months, infant death rates to pertussis infection taper off quickly (Fig. 6.2). In response to increases in pertussis cases in 2013, ACIP made a new Tdap recommendation for pregnant women, recommending every pregnant woman receive Tdap in her third trimester with every pregnancy. This recommendation affords transplacental immunity to newborns. However, the implementation of new immunization recommendations often takes years to be effected in clinical practice. Moreover, new recommendations may be especially difficult to implement in age groups with less frequent health maintenance visits than young children, namely, adolescents [50] (Fig. 6.3) and adults [25] (Fig. 6.4).

The use of online resources and apps to help with decision-making for vaccine recommendations for patients with certain medical conditions may be helpful. *Shots Immunizations*, mentioned earlier, produced by STFM GIE and CDC online sites and apps are helpful resources.

Barrier Systemic Processes

Protocols in health systems, practices, and governmental policies sometimes complicate vaccination practices unnecessarily. Sometimes it is the lack of certain protocols such as those stipulating the use of vaccine standing orders or the absence of a vaccine champion and practice care team that may create barriers to vaccination. The creation of system-based interventions can help improve immunization rates [51]. Moreover, governmental changes in supervision and accountability for the pneumococcal immunization rates of older adults add to poor immunization rates of adults.

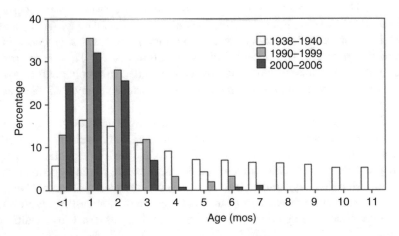

Fig. 6.2 Proportion of reported infant pertussis deaths, by age – US 1938–1940*, 1990–1999†, and 2000–2006§. *Source: Sako et al. [104]. $N = 7123$ reported infant pertussis deaths. †Source: Vitek et al. [105]. $N = 93$ reported infant pertussis deaths. §Source: CDC, unpublished data, 2007. $N = 145$ reported infant pertussis deaths

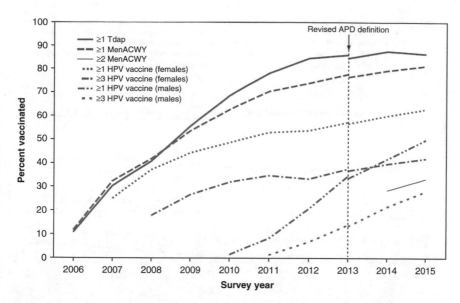

Fig. 6.3 Estimated vaccination coverage with selected vaccines and doses* among adolescents aged 13–17 years, by survey year – National Immunization Survey-Teen, United States, 2006–2015[†] [50]. Abbreviations: *ACIP* Advisory Committee on Immunization Practices, *APD* adequate provider data, *HPV* human papillomavirus, *MenACWY* quadrivalent meningococcal conjugate vaccine, *NIS-Teen* National Immunization Survey-Teen, *Tdap* tetanus toxoid, reduced diphtheria toxoid, and acellular pertussis vaccine. *Tdap: ≥1 dose Tdap at or after age 10 years; ≥1 MenACWY: ≥1 dose MenACWY or meningococcal-unknown-type vaccine; ≥2 doses MenACWY: ≥2 doses MenACWY or meningococcal-unknown-type vaccine, calculated only among adolescents aged 17 years at time of interview (does not include adolescents who received their first dose of MenACWY at or after 16 years of age); ≥1 HPV vaccine: ≥1 dose HPV vaccine, 9-valent (9vHPV), quadrivalent (4vHPV) or bivalent (2vHPV); ACIP recommends 9vHPV, 4vHPV, or 2vHPV for females and 9vHPV or 4vHPV for males (the routine ACIP recommendation was made for females in 2006 and for males in 2011); ≥3 HPV vaccine: ≥3 doses HPV vaccine. † NIS-Teen implemented a revised APD definition in 2014 and retrospectively applied the revised APD definition to 2013 data. Estimates using different APD definitions may not be directly comparable

Confusing changes in pneumococcal recommendations for adults age 65 years for PCV13 and PPSV23 coincided in 2014 with the removal of pneumococcal vaccination rates from national inpatient quality measures:

> Effective 1/1/2014 due to variances in guidelines and vaccine administration recommendations, … collection [of pneumococcal immunization rates] was suspended for The Joint Commission and is voluntary for CMS [Centers for Medicare & Medicaid Services]. [52]

Thus, some hospitals discontinued previously enforced standing orders for pneumococcal vaccination on discharge. Perhaps the time and effort to develop new complicated protocols and train nursing staff to implement them correctly were felt to be cumbersome. Perhaps hospital systems were concerned over an increased likelihood of medical errors. Perhaps the concern was over reimbursement. Whatever the reason, shifting the burden for pneumococcal vaccination from inpatient towards

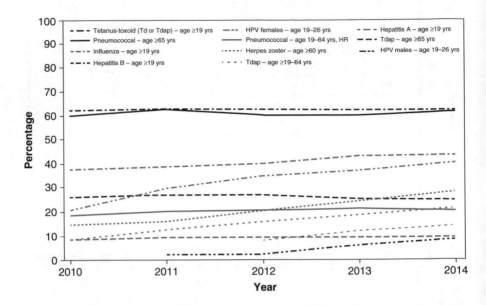

Fig. 6.4 Estimated proportion of adults aged ≥19 years who received selected vaccinations, by age group and high-risk status – National Health Interview Survey, United States, 2010–2014 [25]

outpatient settings did not reduce the complexity of the medical decision-making process and added to missed opportunities to vaccinate.

To improve vaccine rates, many health systems and practices have a *practice care team* and a *vaccine champion* to oversee quality improvement and work to generate support and cooperation from co-workers. Those practices without a practice care team and a vaccine champion may have lower immunization rates than those with them [53]. Traditionally, vaccine recommendations have been solely the responsibility of the physicians within a practice. The practice team, based on the PCMH model, includes physicians, nurse practitioners and/or physician assistants, nurses, medical assistants, pharmacists, social workers, and other staff. The PCMH team model can facilitate a shift of vaccine-ordering responsibilities from physicians to other team members. Nurses, medical assistants, and other PCMH team members can take responsibility in recommending vaccines [53, 54]. Vaccine champions may be any member of the PCMH. They should keep abreast of new vaccine recommendations and relay that information to the practice through regular staff meetings, announcements, and office postings. Pre-visit planning for immunizations can also be supervised by the vaccine champion [54, 55].

Another system-based practice that has been shown to improve vaccination rates is the use of standing orders. Standing orders to vaccinate allow nurses and other appropriately trained health care personnel to assess immunization status and administer vaccinations according to protocol without a physician's exam [56, 57]. Standing orders have been shown to increase vaccination rates in adults in a variety of inpatient and outpatient settings, including long-term-care facilities, managed-care organizations, assisted living facilities, correctional facilities, pharmacies, adult workplaces, and home healthcare agencies. Without standing orders, opportunities to give immunizations may be missed during a busy clinic day. ACIP recommends standing orders under supervision of a medical director as a national health priority for influenza and pneumococcal vaccinations in adults in all long-term, inpatient, and outpatient facilities [58].

Barrier Financial Incentives/Disincentives

Financial incentives for physicians that give rewards for various health metrics outside of improved vaccination rates can interfere with obtaining higher vaccination rates. For example, financial incentives that reward physicians to see more patients and incentives that reward high patient satisfaction scores may negatively impact vaccination rates. On the other hand, incentives that specifically reward higher vaccination rates may positively impact overall vaccination rates for some but may raise the risk of patient discrimination for others.

Financial incentives that encourage physicians to see more numbers of patients per month (fee for service) create time constraints on physicians with each patient encounter. Physicians may feel they do not have enough time to educate patients about vaccination, especially vaccine-hesitant patients who may require time-consuming conversations to address their concerns and questions. Physicians may feel the more time spent with one patient discussing vaccines or determining appropriate recommendations for those with chronic disease or special circumstances may mean less time left to see other patients and generate more revenue. In addition they worry that income-generating activities such as in-office procedures and acute care visit overbooks may be sacrificed to the time needed to make complex vaccination decisions for patients [59, 60].

The Affordable Care Act (ACA) signed into law by President Obama in March 2010 increased the number of insured patients and reduced patient out-of-pocket expenses for preventive services [64]. However, the resulting increased patient panel sizes seen in many primary care practices added to time constraints physicians felt in the office. As shown by increased use of emergency departments since the ACA initiation, physician availability for routine care was reduced, and urgent care takes priority over preventive services, including vaccinations [61].

Another financial incentive creating a barrier to improved vaccination rates is imposed by health insurance plans and healthcare systems that tie high patient satisfaction measures to physician reimbursement. Physicians fear that addressing vaccine hesitancy will upset patients and lead to decreased patient satisfaction scores. Unfortunately, these fears are substantiated. An inverse relationship between vaccine acceptance and visit experience is shown in a study of clinicians in a pediatric practice. Those clinicians who used more assertive, presumptive communication formats (assuming vaccination) showed increased vaccine rates and parental acceptance of vaccines over those clinicians who used participatory formats (collaborative discussions). Sadly, those same clinicians using presumptive communication formats inversely saw their patient-visit satisfaction rates go down, and they scored lower than their partners, whose patients had a happier experience, but left without their children immunized [62]. A similar realization is shown in the context of other health outcomes: patient satisfaction is shown to be inversely related to health outcomes, health care utilization, and expenditure [63]. Further supporting this frustrating phenomenon is the correlation that increased physician adherence to clinical preventive services recommended by USPSTF is associated with lower patient satisfaction scores [64].

Unfortunately, the ACA also indirectly led to decreased delivery of vaccinations by local health departments. Since 1962, the United States Congress has authorized funds for vaccinations through the Section 317 of the Public Health Service Act. These funds are to be used at local health departments for immunizing priority populations [65]. Prior to October 1, 2012, CDC did not require local health departments to strictly exclude insured patients from their immunization services: both insured and uninsured patients were able to get vaccinated at local health departments. As the ACA has been implemented, however, the patient population in local health departments has narrowed to a priority population of strictly underinsured children not eligible for Vaccines for Children (VFC) and uninsured adults [66]. As of October 1, 2012, only adults with no insurance coverage for vaccines (eligible for Section 317 coverage) and children 18 years and younger on Medicaid, with no insurance, or who are Native American (eligible for the VFC program) may receive vaccinations at local health departments.

Furthermore, because vaccines had been accessible through local health departments to all patients, with and without insurance, prior to October 2012, many small independent health clinics and practices did not provide vaccines. They instead chose to refer all their patients to health departments, thereby avoiding all the financial risk incurred with vaccines including the purchase, maintenance and storage of expensive vaccines, and reimbursement uncertainties. In addition, clinical staff expenses required to properly maintain vaccine stock in stringently monitored temperatures in designated refrigerators was averted. In some rural and inner city areas, the local health departments, with nursing staff well versed in storing and handling relatively large amounts of vaccines for patients, became a centralized source for vaccinations.

In addition, for those practices that already offer vaccines, the storage of both VFC and privately purchased vaccines is made complicated because of federal government rules requiring strict physical separation of VFC and private vaccines in separate refrigerators. These rules are mandated in the contracts the federal government negotiates when purchasing VFC vaccines from manufacturers at deep discounts as compared to private stock [67]. Therefore, many small, independent clinics who do not carry vaccines today are unlikely to start carrying vaccines in the future or add VFC vaccines to their inventory due to the many costs associated.

More health insurance plan-directed physician financial incentives to vaccinate, on the other hand, may improve vaccination rates. Currently, high immunization rates represent about four of several dozen measures that health insurance plans use to motivate healthcare systems to improve health outcomes of the populations they serve [68]. Evidence weakly supports financial incentives for individual clinicians to push harder to immunize patients [69]. One worries, though, that if insurance plans were to more strongly tie targeted immunization rates to financial incentives, that action may create financial imbalances within physician groups and create patient discrimination. Increased financial incentives to immunize might perversely incentivize physicians and healthcare systems to discharge or refuse to accept vaccine-hesitant patients. This practice is currently observed in Ann Arbor, Michigan, where a large healthcare system reportedly does not accept patients who are anti-vaccine into its pediatric practices. Several pediatrics practices in California are also dismissing patients from their practices if they do not vaccinate [70]. These actions thereby disproportionately overload those nearby practices with vaccine-hesitant patients, helping to raise the rewards of financial incentives to the discriminating practices and lowering the rewards of financial incentives to the rest.

Barrier Limited Use of Electronic Records, Tools, and Immunization Registries

Immunization information systems (IISs), also known as immunization registries, are defined by CDC as confidential, population-based, computerized databases that record all immunization doses administered by participating providers to persons residing within a given geopolitical area. Per CDC, IISs provide aggregate data at the population level on vaccinations for use in surveillance and program operations. IISs guide public health action with the goals of improving vaccination rates and reducing vaccine-preventable disease [71]. CDC further stipulates that at the point of clinical care, an IIS can provide consolidated immunization histories for use by a vaccination provider in determining appropriate client vaccinations. Electronic alerts, represent *best practice* recommendations, are "pop-up" notices in the electronic medical record intended to help physicians in prescribing and in clinical decision support for patient care. These are often implemented to remind physicians when vaccines are due. Limited or lack of IIS use and electronic alerts may present barriers to improved immunization rates.

Even with an IIS, determining recommendations for current and future immunizations for patients is time-consuming and may present another barrier to improved vaccination rates. The *look-up* function of electronic medical records and/or immunization registries refers to the identification of which vaccines a patient received previously. The *forecasting* function refers to patient vaccination needs at the time of their clinic visit. If one's medical record system is not electronically linked to the state registry, entering vaccination histories (on which the look-up and forecasting functions are based) into both an immunization registry and a medical record system may involve labor-intensive manual double entry. Some systems rely on automated data dumps of billing information into immunization registries to update patient and state records. This process may introduce inaccuracies and delays in data entry if the data dumps are scheduled weekly or monthly rather than daily [72, 73].

Electronic alerts in an electronic health record may help improve immunization rates but may also present some difficulties in doing so. These alerts advance the basic *look-up* and *forecasting* functions by one step but may require real-time data exchange between registries maintained by state health departments and medical records maintained by health systems. Moreover, Internet firewalls and requirements for data-sharing agreements often make achieving interoperability between medical records and immunization registries challenging [74]. Clinicians with office-based patient electronic health records that do not "talk" to their state registry may receive inaccurate alerts. If the forecast from the registry conflicts with the interpretation of ACIP recommendations by clinicians or the clinical alerts programmed into the electronic medical record, then confidence in registry falls and confusion about vaccination recommendations increase. "Clicking out" of the electronic health record and into the registry to resolve such conflicts adds to the burdens of practice in both time and energy that frustrate clinicians. This inconvenience in finding accurate, clinically relevant information may lead to missed opportunities to vaccinate.

IISs can generate reports that identify patients who are behind on vaccinations, and vaccination rates may be calculated through use of IISs within the populations they serve. Clinicians and healthcare systems may use this surveillance data to target educational efforts and clinical policies and deliver patient reminders for vaccinations. However, patient vaccination lists generated internally from a physician office or health system may show many discrepancies when compared to IIS lists. The identification of patients' primary care physicians and PCMHs is sometimes difficult to recognize and more complex than the definition of who is a resident under a health department's jurisdiction. Patients change physician practices and change home addresses. The immunization registry lists are not always up to date and may contain patients who are no longer active patients at the offices and clinics where they previously received vaccines. Inaccuracies in patient lists are exacerbated by patients moving between states. Currently, no national immunization registry exists and the prospect of one is unlikely. Some states are negotiating legal agreements and getting divergent information systems to communicate with each other, but so far this represents a piecemeal effort [75, 75a].

Though in general, use of IISs helps improve vaccination rates, some IIS features may cause additional barriers. Take, for example, some IIS requirements that include inventory control functions [76]. Some states require that clinics order stock from VFC programs via the advanced functions of the state registry [76a]. Advanced functions of registries require clinical staff to receive extensive training and practice to use these functions efficiently and effectively to prevent potential financial losses accrued through the vaccine stock expiration. Furthermore, the incompatibility of inventory and lot number record-keeping processes between registry and clinical processes might result in on site vaccine shortages [32].

Barrier Patient Hesitancy and Vaccine Refusal

Despite the small vocal minority of patients and parents that actively refuse and/or speak against vaccination, the social norm in America is for patients and parents to trust the advice of their physicians that vaccines are safe and effective. There are patients who accept all vaccines without reservations. There are also other patients who are hesitant to accept vaccines. Vaccine hesitancy among patients includes varying degrees of indecision and acceptance. To a degree, hesitancy is understandable to those uninformed. Vaccine-preventable diseases are rare. Vaccine doses are numerous and painful. Complacency about vaccines results paradoxically from the success of vaccines at making once common life-threatening infections exceptionally rare.

Patients (and clinicians) with no vaccine-preventable diseases experience tend to undervalue the importance of vaccines given the rarity of the diseases that they prevent. Public health messages focusing on the dangers of vaccine-preventable diseases unfortunately may increase vaccine hesitancy since the messages delivered do not fit the frame of reference of most patients [77]. These messages may be perceived as condescending to vaccine-hesitant parents as they perceive the value of their concerns about the safety of their children being questioned.

Many variables factor into patient acceptance of vaccination. Patient confidence about and ultimate acceptance of vaccines revolves around trust of physicians, health systems, vaccine manufactures, researchers, and government officials and agencies. Many parents have concerns regarding the safety of vaccines. These concerns range from what ingredients go into vaccines, how vaccines are tested, and when to give vaccines. In a survey of 376 parents of children aged 6 years or less, 26% believed that ingredients in vaccines are unsafe, and 17% felt that vaccines are not tested enough for safety. Only 23% had no concerns about childhood vaccines. Many parents were unaware it is safe to vaccinate children when the child has a mild illness [15]. These beliefs suggest that many people are unaware of the stringent regulatory quality and safety processes involved in vaccine development. These processes monitor and respond to safety signals that may appear during vaccine use in large populations not only during vaccine research but also during development, manufacturing, and post-licensure [78]. Clearly, more education regarding safety measures surrounding vaccine production and testing is needed.

In addition to vaccine safety, patients also worry about how officials and experts make policies and recommendations about vaccines: how scientists conduct research, and how manufacturers might influence research processes to raise profits. Patients' unfamiliarity with the scientific method and their tendency to suspect the motives of officials based on personal experience or historical events may also influence their likelihood to accept vaccinations. Their world view, as framed by religion and/or politics, is often an influence.

Modern-day parental refusal of childhood vaccines is a growing public health concern. Some parents accept only select vaccines while delaying or refusing others for their children. A small group of patients refuse all vaccines for their children (Table 6.3). Those who are opposed to all vaccines are known as anti-vaxxers. Vaccine hesitancy and refusals may lower vaccination rates enough to result in the failure to achieve or sustain herd immunity [79], allowing for outbreaks of infectious diseases. In looking at parent groups about their inclination to accept vaccination for their children, parents can be divided into five broad groups: unquestioning acceptors, cautious acceptors, hesitators, selective acceptors, and refusers. Unquestioning acceptors of vaccination form the largest group at 30–40%. They see the importance and safety of vaccination even though they tend to have less detailed knowledge about vaccines. They trust that medical professionals put their children's best interests first and foremost. The next largest group of parents, at 25–35%, cautiously accepts vaccination. They recognize that vaccines carry rare but serious side effects and hope that their children are not affected. A significant minority of parents (20–30%) hesitate but still mainly vaccinate their children despite significant concerns.

Table 6.3 Spectrum of vaccine hesitancy: five parental groups

Unquestioning acceptor	30–40%
Cautious acceptor	25–35%
Hesitant acceptor – "fence sitters" who require discussions, mostly comply with vaccination	20–30%
Later or selective acceptor – choose to delay or refuse some vaccines	2–27%
Refuser of all vaccines	<2%

Source: Leask et al. BMC Pediatrics 2012, 12:154. www.biomedcentral.com/1471-2431/12/154

These "fence sitters" generally desire discussions with knowledgeable health professionals who can answer their questions with relevant information. Some parents (2–27%) doubt the safety and necessity of vaccines and choose to delay or refuse one or more vaccines. Such late, or selective, vaccinators know more about vaccines than other groups, perhaps because they ask many questions. However, they struggle with whom to trust, and worry about the safety on some vaccines. The very small number (<2%) of parents who refuse all vaccines for their children cite medical mistrust or philosophical/religious beliefs. They seek alternative health professionals who accept their decisions about vaccinations and tend to cluster in communities who share their beliefs. They have less accurate knowledge about vaccination than all other groups except the "acceptor" group of parents [80].

Laws requiring vaccination help improve vaccination rates. In the US, the federal government makes vaccine recommendations and individual states mandate laws that require vaccination for children entering schools and daycare. Currently, all states require children to be vaccinated against certain communicable diseases as a condition for school attendance. In most instances, state vaccination laws apply not only to children attending public schools but also to those attending private schools and daycare facilities. In addition to vaccination requirements for school children, state laws establish the process for obtaining exemptions from those requirements and the implications of an exemption in the event of an outbreak. Few states allow no exemptions to immunizations aside from medically indicated ones. Most states allow nonmedical exemptions from vaccines for one or more of the following reasons: philosophical, religious, and personal reasons. California is the first state to bar all religious and personal vaccine exemptions for schoolchildren when Governor Jerry Brown signed legislation in law effective July 1, 2016 [81]. There exist nine different variations on state school vaccination exemption laws with variations of different combinations of medical, religious, and philosophical exemptions allowed in each state. [http://www.cdc.gov/phlp/docs/school-vaccinations.pdf].

In those states that allow personal or philosophical exemptions from vaccines required for school, the states that have an easier process by which to obtain the exemptions encourage parents to act on their vaccine hesitancy. In some states, claiming a personal exemption is as easy as downloading a form from the internet, filling it out, and submitting it to a child's school. The state of Michigan was one such state for several years. In 2014, state vaccination rates for Michigan children were fourth worst in the nation. Then, the Michigan Joint Committee on

Administrative Rules approved a new educational requirement for parents wishing to waive their children from getting vaccinated before entering school. Effective January 1, 2015, any parent or guardian in Michigan who wants to claim a nonmedical waiver must receive education regarding the benefits of vaccination and the risks of disease from a county health department official. Only after that requirement is met can the parent obtain a certified nonmedical waiver from the health department. After the first year of this legislative change, the Michigan Department of Health and Human Services documented 9377 fewer waiver requests, a 35.4% overall reduction in exemptions.

In addition to lenient exemption laws, patient hesitancy may be unwittingly facilitated through physician and staff misconceptions of patient beliefs. For example, incorrect perceived parental beliefs that the HPV vaccine will promote sexual activity may lead physicians to present the need for HPV vaccination differently than other medically recommended vaccines and inadvertently facilitate vaccine hesitancy. Clinicians and staff in two Los Angeles, California, clinics serving a predominant Hispanic population [82] mistakenly overvalued the parental belief that receipt of the HPV vaccine promotes sexual activity. Clinicians mistakenly thought that parents were more concerned with the idea that the HPV vaccine may cause increase promiscuity than they actually were [83]. This same misperception of parental concerns was demonstrated again when nearly half of pediatricians and family physicians surveyed in another study incorrectly reported that many parents of adolescent patients are concerned that vaccination against HPV may encourage earlier or riskier sexual behavior. The reality is that only 8% of Latino mothers surveyed reported those concerns [84]. Similar findings substantiating lower parental concerns were also found in population-based studies with only 0.5–7.6% of parents citing concerns about the effect on their daughter's sexual behavior as reasons not to vaccinate [85, 86].

Barrier Poor Physician Communication Regarding Vaccine Recommendations

Health literacy deficits affect half the American patient population and are linked to poor health, ineffective disease management, and high rates of hospitalization. Effective physician oral literacy, with clear communication between clinicians and patients, is required to improve patient health literacy and optimize healthcare outcomes, including immunization rates [87, 88]. It is not only important *what* clinicians say to patients regarding vaccine recommendations but also *how* clinicians communicate with a focus on the *style of communication*. Poor clinician communication contributes to rejection of vaccines and increases missed opportunities to vaccinate. Effective interactions and communication can address the concerns of vaccine supportive parents and motivate a vaccine-hesitant parent or patient toward vaccine acceptance [80]. Subtle modifications of the wording of questions and inquiries can affect response outcomes.

For example, the implementation of the word *some* in language when used to elicit patient concerns was more effective than the use of the word *any* in the same situation.

Do you have **any** concerns over this immunization?

is considered negatively polarized and is not as effective in eliciting patient concerns as

Do you have **some** questions or concerns regarding this immunization? [89]

Furthermore, in addition to the words used, clinicians need to be aware of their physical presence when recommending vaccines as well as their oral and visual presentation of their recommendations. When concentrating, people tend to look away. They inhibit eye contact and shift eye gaze as a way to sharpen their attention and enhance information retrieval [90]. If clinicians look away when recommending vaccination, the resulting lack of eye contact and wayward eye gaze may be interpreted by patients that the clinician may be detached or not speaking personally and intentionally to them. Patients may feel that perhaps they are being lectured to and they are not engaging in a two-way discussion [91].

Effective physician communication is especially important because it is well documented that physicians are highly influential in determining a patient's decision to vaccinate. A *strong* recommendation to vaccinate made by a healthcare provider influences a patient's decision to vaccinate [92–94]. In comparing teen girls who were unvaccinated against HPV to girls who were fully vaccinated, researchers found that the most important independent predictor associated with being fully vaccinated against HPV was having a clinician who is a positive influence on parents' decision to vaccinate their daughter against HPV. Clinicians influence decisions by talking to parents about the HPV vaccine, giving parents enough time to discuss the HPV vaccine, and by making a strong recommendation for administration of the HPV vaccine [28]. Further support of the assertion that a strong recommendation improves vaccination rates is illustrated in a study on pregnant women. Regardless of their perceptions of vaccination safety or effectiveness, pregnant women offered influenza vaccination by their healthcare provider are more likely to be vaccinated than those not offered vaccination. They are more likely to have positive attitudes about the effectiveness of influenza vaccination and the safety of influenza vaccination for themselves and for their infants [95]. In an anonymous questionnaire, most of over 1400 pregnant women surveyed report willingness to receive the influenza vaccine during pregnancy if their healthcare provider recommended it [96]. Moreover, women with a negative attitude toward vaccination who received a clinician's offer of vaccination are more likely to be vaccinated than women who have a positive attitude toward vaccination, but did not receive a clinician's offer [95]. It is therefore imperative that physicians and other vaccine providers communicate well with a *strong recommendation* when recommending vaccines.

Communication Styles There are several models of communication and communication styles within the doctor/patient relationship. Different styles of communication result in different health outcomes and levels of patient satisfaction. Three communication models are particularly pertinent to conversation around vaccinations: (1) traditional paternalism, (2) pure informed decision-making, and (3) shared decision-making.

There has been a historical trend in standard clinical practice to move from the traditional paternalistic model of communication toward informed and shared decision-making. In the paternalistic model, "the doctor knows best." Patient involvement in decision-making is limited to giving consent to the treatment advised and advocated by a physician without discussion. This model assumes primacy for the clinician's technical knowledge and makes no concessions to the patients' values or preferences. It is considered "old style" and dates back hundreds of years when patients were not expected to ask many questions and physicians did not offer many explanations to their prescriptions and advice. Physicians commonly withheld diagnostic information from patients. This type of communication style is no longer favored in most instances of physician/patient communication in the USA. An example of this communication style is exemplified in a medical school graduation speech given by Oliver Wendell Holmes in 1871:

> Your patient has no more right to all the truth you know than he has to all the medicine in your saddlebags. He should get only just so much as is good for him. Some shrewd old physicians have a few phrases always on hand for patients who insist on knowing the pathology of their complaints without the slightest capacity of understanding the scientific explanation. I have known the term 'spinal irritation' to serve well on such occasions. [97]

Another type of communication style and decision-making involves the pure informed model, where the patient (and perhaps the patient's family/friends in consultation with the patient) makes decisions about their healthcare after a physician provides information. With this model, it is assumed a patient is given all necessary information so that he/she can decide on their own healthcare. Patients' preferences are most highly valued in this model and a physician's role is reduced to that of only providing technical information to support a patient's decision [98].

A third type of decision-making is *shared* decision-making. In this method both the process of decision-making and the ultimate decision-making is a shared venture between a physician and patient, with agreement on the decision reached in the end. Recently, there has been a shift toward this model of doctor/patient communication within the concept of "patient-centered care" where a patient's viewpoint is taken into consideration more than ever before. The shared decision-making model as described by Charles et al. [99] stipulates that both the physician and patient participate in the process of treatment decision-making with a prerequisite of information sharing. A treatment decision is made with both parties in agreement. The clinician acknowledges the legitimacy of the patient's preferences, and the patient accepts shared responsibility for the treatment decision.

As mentioned earlier, communication styles can also be described as participatory or presumptive. Participatory communication implies more of informed consent decision-making; vaccine decisions are left up to parents. However, some parents may be vaccine-hesitant and subscribe to misinformation. In this instance, the physician unspokenly acknowledges the possibility of controversy and vaccine hesitancy. Alternatively, the use of the presumptive format, whereby the physician assumes that vaccination is the norm, without acknowledgment of controversy, takes a more traditional, paternalistic approach. The physician supposes that vaccines are not a medically debatable issue. When recommending childhood vaccines to parents of children due for vaccines, these two different types of communication formats were tested. There was a difference in vaccination uptake between the patients of the clinicians who used each style. When clinicians used participatory formats to initiate vaccine discussion with parents of children needing vaccinations such as

Well, what do you want to do about Teddy's shots today?

parents were more likely to voice initial resistance to vaccines than when clinicians used presumptive formats that assumed vaccination:

Well, we have to give Teddy some shots today.

Ultimately, those parents who experienced the participatory communication were less likely to vaccinate their children than those who experienced the presumptive communication style. Of note, when patients voiced resistance to vaccination, no matter which style was initially used, the clinicians' *pursuit* of their original vaccine recommendations such as

Teddy really needs these shots!

changed nearly half of parents' vaccine decision.

Unfortunately, as mentioned earlier, this study also showed an inverse relationship between parental acceptance of vaccines and visit experience. Those parents who left the office with their children vaccinated rated their healthcare experience lower than those parents who left with their children unvaccinated. The use of the presumptive format that assumes vaccination increased acceptance of immunizations but decreased the visit experience, whereas the use of the participatory format that provided parents more decision-making latitude appeared to do the opposite. This makes the two desirable outcomes (increased vaccine acceptance and increased patient satisfaction) mutually exclusive in the context of a single visit [100]. Nonetheless, what may be more important than either the presumptive or the participatory initial approach to a parent of a child needing vaccines is the commitment to pursuing parental resistance. Perhaps a combination of styles is in order. Following the use of participatory initiation format (which aligns with better patient satisfaction) with a firm recommendation, followed by persistence in recommendation to those who are hesitant (which increases vaccination rates), may therefore represent a communication strategy that attains the best possible vaccine acceptance and parent/patient satisfaction [100].

I recommend Teddy get his shots today. I realize you may have some questions.

Recommendation Emphasis   Not only is the communication style used in recommending vaccines important, but so is the emphasis placed on vaccine promotion. Vaccines are best recommended as *routine*, *standard*, and *customary*. All vaccines should be presented in a similar manner with equal importance. No vaccine should be presented with preference or presented differently than others [101]. This is especially true in the case of the HPV vaccine, which is considered controversial by a subset of parents and clinicians. Attention should be paid specifically to the *order* of the listing of recommended vaccines. For adolescents who are due for several immunizations during one office visit, clinicians ought to list the HPV vaccine as *routine* and not prioritize other vaccines. HPV vaccination should not be described with special circumstances attached and/or left for last in a list of immunizations presented. Disappointingly, a large national survey of over 1000 family physicians and pediatricians showed that when recommending vaccines to parents of adolescents, 64% of physicians did preferentially recommend certain adolescent vaccines. These physicians reported that for patients ages 11–12, they usually discussed the vaccines in a particular order and with varying degrees of endorsement. They indicated they endorsed HPV vaccination less strongly than Tdap or meningococcal vaccines. Tdap was discussed first by 73% of the physicians and 70% of them discussed HPV last. Parents may perceive more moderate endorsement of the HPV vaccine as indicative of physicians' ambivalence or concern of importance [22, 102].

On the flip side, too much unsolicited detail with an unnecessarily long explanation of HPV to try to justify its importance may reduce patient acceptance of vaccine recommendations. It is preferable to say:

> Christina is due for her meningitis, HPV, and her Tdap vaccines today.
>
> Vs.
>
> Christina is due for her meningitis and her Tdap vaccine. She can also get the HPV vaccine today – this is to protect her from the HPV virus which causes cervical cancer in patients that harbor the virus for a long time – usually ten years or more – and it is a sexually transmitted virus.

In the second example, the choice of the word "can": "Christina *can* get the vaccine" (as opposed to: "Christina *should* get her vaccine" or "Christina *is due for* her vaccine") does not make a strong endorsement for vaccination and allows parents to choose NOT to vaccinate [103]. Furthermore, the listing of the HPV vaccine last may imply less endorsement. Better to list the tetanus vaccine last, as there is far greater public acceptance to this vaccine. The long explanation/justification about the reasons for recommendation also indicates a less strong endorsement for the vaccine. The explanation goes overboard to "legitimize" the vaccine's value that is out of proportion to explanations given about other vaccines. The sexual reference gives parents the option of declining the vaccine, especially if parents do not believe their child is yet sexually active. A small minority of parents may erroneously think their child does not need the vaccine prior to sexual debut or believe the vaccine will increase sexual promiscuity. Recent ACIP changes to decrease the HPV vaccine series from a three-dose to a two-dose series for those younger than 15 years of age, because of better immune response seen in younger adolescents, may help convince parents on the fence about vaccinating their "virgin" children. Physicians need not discuss teenage sex and sexual activity when providing HPV vaccine recommendations, just as they need not routinely discuss future sexual activity as a justification for giving the hepatitis B vaccine at birth. Both vaccines prevent cancer. Morality and concerns about when sexual debut may occur is not an issue requiring discussion.

Conclusion

There are many barriers to improved vaccination rates in children and adults. These include a lack of community demand for vaccination, poor patient access to vaccinations, and patient misinformation about vaccinations leading to vaccine hesitancy. Lack of physician knowledge of vaccine recommendations, complex vaccination schedules, arbitrary state laws, and limited use of electronic records and tools also create barriers to improved immunization rates. Additionally, the lack of regular assessment of vaccine status, poor healthcare system and financial incentives to vaccinate, and missed opportunities for vaccination lead to less than optimal vaccination rates. Perhaps one of the biggest barriers to improved vaccination rates is poor clinician communication, especially with vaccine-hesitant patients. Poor communication regarding *what* to say when recommending vaccines and *how* to recommend vaccines reduces immunization rates. Without effective communication, even those clinicians with excellent knowledge, support systems, tools, and incentives will have difficulty improving immunization rates. The use of the *presumptive* style of communication in recommending vaccines, presented as *routine,* with use of good eye contact and with a *strong endorsement*, increase vaccination rates. The *persistence* in recommendation with those who are vaccine-hesitant is also effective to increase vaccination rates. Ongoing clinician education combined with the use of vaccine standing orders and coordination of a practice team with a vaccine champion also helps increase vaccination rates. As healthcare systems further develop coordination between electronic health records and state registries, vaccination rates may improve in the years ahead.

References

1 Centers for Disease Control and Prevention (CDC). Impact of vaccines universally recommended for children – United States, 1990–1998. MMWR Morb Mortal Wkly Rep [Internet]. 1999;48(12):243–8. [cited 2016 Sep 1]. Available from: http://www.ncbi.nlm.nih.gov/pubmed/10220251

2 Centers for Disease Control and Prevention (CDC). Ten Great Public Health Achievements – United States, 2001-2010. MMWR Morb Mortal Wkly Rep [Internet]. 2011;60(19):619–23. Available from: http://www.cdc.gov/mmwr/preview/mmwrhtml/mm6019a5.htm

2a. Centers for Disease Control and Prevention (CDC). Vaccine-specific coverage among children 19–35 months, National Immunization Survey, 1994–2014. www.cdc.gov/vaccines/imz-managers/coverage/nis/child/figures/2014-map.html

3. McIntosh AM, McMahon J, Dibbens LM, Iona X, Mulley JC, Scheffer IE, et al. Effects of vaccination on onset and outcome of Dravet syndrome: a retrospective study. Lancet Neurol [Internet]. 2010;9(6):592–8. [cited 2016 Sep 1]. Available from: http://www.ncbi.nlm.nih.gov/pubmed/20447868

4. Clemmons NS, Gastanaduy PA, Fiebelkorn AP, Redd SB, Wallace GS, Centers for Disease Control and Prevention (CDC). Measles – United States, January 4–April 2, 2015. MMWR Morb Mortal Wkly Rep [Internet]. 2015;64(14):373–6. [cited 2016 Sep 1]. Available from: http://www.ncbi.nlm.nih.gov/pubmed/25879894

5. Office of Disease Prevention and Health Promotion, US Department of Health and Human Services. Immunization and Infectious Diseases in Healthy People 2020. [Internet]. [cited

2017 Jan 4]. Available from: https://www.healthypeople.gov/2020/topicsobjectives/topic/immunizationand-infectious-diseases/objectives

6. Johnson DR, Nichol KL, Lipczynski K. Barriers to adult immunization. Am J Med [Internet]. 2008;121(7 Suppl 2):S28–35. [cited 2016 Sep 1]. www.amjmed.com/article/S0002-9343(08)00468-3/pdf

6a. Ventola CL. Immunization in the United States: recommendations, barriers, and measures to improve compliance. P T. 2016;41(7):426–36 and (8):492–506. www.ncbi.nlm.nih.gov/pmc/articles/PMC4927017

7. Williams WW, Lu P-J, O'Halloran A, Kim DK, Grohskopf LA, Pilishvili T, et al. Surveillance of vaccination coverage among adult populations – United States, 2014. MMWR Surveill Summ [Internet]. 2016;65(1):1–36. [cited 2017 Jan 3]. Available from: http://www.cdc.gov/mmwr/volumes/65/ss/ss6501a1.htm

8. Ehresmann KR, Ramesh A, Como-Sabetti K, Peterson DC, Whitney CG, Moore KA. Factors associated with self-reported pneumococcal immunization among adults 65 years of age or older in the Minneapolis-St. Paul metropolitan area. Prev Med (Baltim) [Internet]. 2001;32(5):409–15. [cited 2016 Sep 2]. Available from: http://www.ncbi.nlm.nih.gov/pubmed/11330990

9. Schneeberg A, Bettinger JA, McNeil S, Ward BJ, Dionne M, Cooper C, et al. Knowledge, attitudes, beliefs and behaviours of older adults about pneumococcal immunization, a Public Health Agency of Canada/Canadian Institutes of Health Research Influenza Research Network (PCIRN) investigation. BMC Public Health [Internet]. 2014;14:442. [cited 2016 Aug 20]. Available from: http://www.ncbi.nlm.nih.gov/pubmed/24884433

10. Qutaiba B, Al-lela O, Bahari MB, Al-Qazaz HK, Salih MRM, Jamshed SQ, Elkalmi RM. Are parents' knowledge and practice regarding immunization related to pediatrics' immunization compliance? a mixed method study. BMC Pediatr [Internet]. 2014;14:20. [cited 2016 Aug 27]. Available from: http://www.ncbi.nlm.nih.gov/pubmed/24460878

11. Offit PA, Quarles J, Gerber MA, Hackett CJ, Marcuse EK, Kollman TR, et al. Addressing parents' concerns: do multiple vaccines overwhelm or weaken the infant's immune system? Pediatrics. 2002;109(1), 124–129.

12. Vaccine Myths Debunked | PublicHealth.org [Internet]. [cited 2017 Jan 4]. Available from: http://www.publichealth.org/public-awareness/understanding-vaccines/vaccine-myths-debunked/

13. Brunson EK. The impact of social networks on parents' vaccination decisions. Pediatrics [Internet]. 2013;131(5):e1397–404. [cited 2016 Sep 3]. Available from: http://www.ncbi.nlm.nih.gov/pubmed/23589813

14. Healy CM. Commentary on "Parental vaccine-hesitancy: Understanding the problem and searching for a resolution". Hum Vaccin Immunother [Internet]. 2014;10(9):2597–9. [cited 2016 Aug 27]. Available from: http://www.ncbi.nlm.nih.gov/pubmed/25483476

15. Kennedy A, Lavail K, Nowak G, Basket M, Landry S. Confidence about vaccines in the United States: understanding parents' perceptions. Health Aff (Millwood) [Internet]. 2011;30(6):1151–9. [cited 2016 Sep 2]. Available from: http://www.ncbi.nlm.nih.gov/pubmed/21653969

16. Odone A, Ferrari A, Spagnoli F, Visciarelli S, Shefer A, Pasquarella C, et al. Effectiveness of interventions that apply new media to improve vaccine uptake and vaccine coverage. Hum Vaccin Immunother [Internet]. 2015;11(1):72–82. [cited 2016 Aug 27]. Available from: http://www.ncbi.nlm.nih.gov/pubmed/25483518

17. About Immunization Coalitions – Immunization Coalitions Network [Internet]. Available from: http://www.immunizationcoalitions.org/about-coalitions/

18. Fay EE, Hoppe KK, Schulkin J, Eckert LO. Survey of obstetrics and gynecology residents regarding pneumococcal vaccination in pregnancy: education, knowledge, and barriers to vaccination. Infect Dis Obstet Gynecol [Internet]. 2016;2016:1752379. [cited 2016 Aug 27]. Available from: http://www.ncbi.nlm.nih.gov/pubmed/26949324

19. Ngamruengphong S, Horsley-Silva JL, Hines SL, Pungpapong S, Patel TC, Keaveny AP. Educational intervention in primary care residents' knowledge and performance of hepa-

titis B vaccination in patients with diabetes mellitus. South Med J [Internet]. 2015;108(9):–510, 5. [cited 2016 Aug 24]. Available from: http://www.ncbi.nlm.nih.gov/pubmed/26332473

20. Berenson AB, Rahman M, Hirth JM, Rupp RE, Sarpong KO. A brief educational intervention increases providers' human papillomavirus vaccine knowledge. Hum Vaccin Immunother [Internet]. 2015;11(6):1331–6. [cited 2016 Aug 24]. Available from: http://www.ncbi.nlm. nih.gov/pubmed/25945895

21. Bloom BS. Effects of continuing medical education on improving physician clinical care and patient health: a review of systematic reviews. Int J Technol Assess Health Care [Internet]. 2005;21(3):380–5. [cited 2016 Aug 24]. Available from: http://www.ncbi.nlm.nih.gov/pubmed/16110718

21a. Standards for pediatric immunization practices. Recommended by the National Vaccine Advisory Committee. MMWR Recomm Rep. 1993;23;42(RR-5):1–10. CDC. http://www.cdc.gov/mmwr/preview/mmwrhtml/00020935.htm

22. Gilkey MB, Moss JL, Coyne-Beasley T, Hall ME, Shah PD, Brewer NT. Physician communication about adolescent vaccination: how is human papillomavirus vaccine different? Prev Med (Baltim). 2015;77:181–5.

23. Nichol KL. Ten-year durability and success of an organized program to increase influenza and pneumococcal vaccination rates among high-risk adults. Am J Med [Internet]. 1998;105(5):385–92. [cited 2016 Aug 20]. Available from: http://www.ncbi.nlm.nih.gov/pubmed/9831422

24. Nowalk MP, Zimmerman RK, Feghali J. Missed opportunities for adult immunization in diverse primary care office settings. Vaccine [Internet]. 2004;22(25–26):–3457, 63. [cited 2016 Aug 27]. Available from: http://www.ncbi.nlm.nih.gov/pubmed/15308372

25. Williams WW, Lu P-J, O'Halloran A, Kim DK, Grohskopf LA, Pilishvili T, et al. Surveillance of vaccination coverage among adult populations – United States, 2014. MMWR Surveill Summ [Internet]. 2016;65(1):1–36. [cited 2016 Aug 27]. www.cdc.gov/mmwr/volumes/65/ss/ss6501a1.htm

26. Moss JL, Reiter PL, Brewer NT. Concomitant adolescent vaccination in the U.S., 2007–2012. Am J Prev Med [Internet]. 2016.; [cited 2016 Aug 27]Available from: http://www.ncbi.nlm.nih.gov/pubmed/27374208

27. Stokley S, Jeyarajah J, Yankey D, Cano M, Gee J, Roark J, et al. Human papillomavirus vaccination coverage among adolescents, 2007–2013, and postlicensure vaccine safety monitoring, 2006–2014 – United States. MMWR Morb Mortal Wkly Rep [Internet]. 2014;63(29):620–4. [cited 2016 Aug 27]. Available from: http://www.ncbi.nlm.nih.gov/pubmed/25055185

28. Smith PJ, Stokley S, Bednarczyk RA, Orenstein WA, Omer SB. HPV vaccination coverage of teen girls: the influence of health care providers. Vaccine [Internet]. 2016;34(13):1604–10. [cited 2016 Aug 24]. Available from: http://www.ncbi.nlm.nih.gov/pubmed/26854907

29. Schoen C, Osborn R, Huynh PT, Doty M, Peugh J, Zapert K, et al. Health Aff (Millwood) [Internet]. 25(6):w555–71. [cited 2016 Aug 27]. Available from: http://www.ncbi.nlm.nih.gov/pubmed/17102164

30. Goad JA, Taitel MS, Fensterheim LE, Cannon AE. Vaccinations administered during off-clinic hours at a national community pharmacy: implications for increasing patient access and convenience. Ann Fam Med [Internet]. 2013;11(5):429–36. [cited 2016 Aug 27]. Available from: http://www.ncbi.nlm.nih.gov/pubmed/24019274

31. Postema AS, Breiman RF, National Vaccine Advisory Committee. Adult immunization programs in nontraditional settings: quality standards and guidance for program evaluation. MMWR Recomm Rep [Internet]. 2000;49(RR-1):1–13. [cited 2016 Sep 1]. Available from: www.cdc.gov/mmwr/preview/mmwrhtml/rr4901a1.htm

32. Institute of Medicine, Committee on Immunization Finance Policies and Practices. National Academies Press, Washington, DC. 2000. Calling the shots: immunization finance policies and practices. [Internet]. Available from: http://www.ncbi.nlm.nih.gov/pubmed/25077270

32a. Centers Disease for Control and Prevention (CDC). Past immunization schedules. www.cdc.gov/vaccines/schedules/past.html

33. Kurosky SK, Davis KL, Krishnarajah G. Completion and compliance of childhood vaccinations in the United States. Vaccine [Internet]. 2016;34(3):387–94. [cited 2016 Sep 1].
Available from: http://www.sciencedirect.com/science/article/pii/S0264410X15016163
34. Belshe RB, Edwards KM, Vesikari T, Black SV, Walker RE, Hultquist M, et al. Live attenuated versus inactivated influenza vaccine in infants and young children. N Engl J Med
[Internet]. 2007;356(7):685–96. [cited 2016 Sep 1]. Available from: http://www.ncbi.nlm.
nih.gov/pubmed/17301299
35. Ashkenazi S, Vertruyen A, Arístegui J, Esposito S, McKeith DD, Klemola T, et al. Superior
relative efficacy of live attenuated influenza vaccine compared with inactivated influenza
vaccine in young children with recurrent respiratory tract infections. Pediatr Infect Dis
J [Internet]. 2006;25(10):870–9. [cited 2016 Sep 1]. Available from: http://www.ncbi.nlm.
nih.gov/pubmed/17006279
36. Grohskopf LA, Olsen SJ, Sokolow LZ, Bresee JS, Cox NJ, Broder KR, et al. Prevention and
control of seasonal influenza with vaccines: recommendations of the Advisory Committee on
Immunization Practices (ACIP) – United States, 2014–15 influenza season. MMWR Morb
Mortal Wkly Rep [Internet]. 2014;63(32):691–7. [cited 2016 Sep 1]. Available from: www.
cdc.gov/mmwr/preview/mmwrhtml/mm6332a3.htm
37. Grohskopf LA, Sokolow LZ, Olsen SJ, Bresee JS, Broder KR, Karron RA. Prevention
and control of influenza with vaccines: recommendations of the Advisory Committee on
Immunization Practices, United States, 2015–16 influenza season. Am J Transplant [Internet].
2015;15(10):2767–75. [cited 2016 Sep 1]
37a. Advisory Committee on Immunization Practices (ACIP). Summary report: October 29–30,
2014 (Meeting minutes). Washington, DC: US Department of Health and Human Services,
CDC; 2014. Available at www.cdc.gov/vaccines/acip/meetings/downloads/min-archive/min-
2014-10.pdf
37b. Advisory Committee on Immunization Practices (ACIP). Summary Report: February 26,
2015 (Meeting minutes). Washington, DC: US Department of Health and Human Services,
CDC; 2015. Available at www.cdc.gov/vaccines/acip/meetings/downloads/min-archive/min-
2015-02.pdf
38. Malo TL, Giuliano AR, Kahn JA, Zimet GD, Lee J-H, Zhao X, et al. Physicians' human
papillomavirus vaccine recommendations in the context of permissive guidelines for male
patients: a national study. Cancer Epidemiol Biomarkers Prev [Internet]. 2014;23(10):–2126,
35. [cited 2016 Aug 20]. Available from: http://cebp.aacrjournals.org/cgi/doi/10.1158/1055-
9965.EPI-14-0344
39. Rahman M, Islam M, Berenson AB. Differences in HPV immunization levels among young
adults in various regions of the United States. J Community Health [Internet]. 2015;40(3):404–
8. [cited 2016 Aug 22]. Available from: http://www.ncbi.nlm.nih.gov/pubmed/25669443
40. National Meningitis Association. Serogroup B meningococcal disease outbreaks
on U.S. College Campuses [Internet]. Available from: http://www.nmaus.org/
disease-prevention-information/serogroup-b-meningococcal-disease/outbreaks/
41. CDC. Use of serogroup B meningococcal vaccines in adolescents and young adults: recommendations of the Advisory Committee on Immunization Practices, 2015 [Internet].
Available from: http://www.cdc.gov/mmwr/preview/mmwrhtml/mm6441a3.htm
42. Advisory Committee on Immunization Practices (ACIP). Summary Report: June 24, 2015
(Meeting minutes). Washington, DC: US Department of Health and Human Services, CDC;
2015. Available at: www.cdc.gov/vaccines/acip/meetings/downloads/min-archive/min-2015-
06.pdf
43. Isturiz R, Webber C. Prevention of adult pneumococcal pneumonia with the 13-valent pneumococcal conjugate vaccine: CAPiTA, the community-acquired pneumonia immunization
trial in adults. Hum Vaccin Immunother [Internet]. 2015;11(7):1825–7. [cited 2016 Sep 10].
Available from: http://www.ncbi.nlm.nih.gov/pubmed/26076136
44. Tomczyk S, Bennett NM, Stoecker C, Gierke R, Moore MR, Whitney CG, et al. Use of
13-valent pneumococcal conjugate vaccine and 23-valent pneumococcal polysaccha-

ride vaccine among adults aged ≥65 years: recommendations of the Advisory Committee on Immunization Practices (ACIP). MMWR Morb Mortal Wkly Rep [Internet]. 2014;63(37):822–5. [cited 2016 Sep 10]. Available from: www.cdc.gov/mmwr/preview/mmwrhtml/mm6337a4.htm

45. Kobayashi M, Bennett NM, Gierke R, Almendares O, Moore MR, Whitney CG, Pilishvili T. Intervals between PCV13 and PPSV23 vaccines: recommendations of the Advisory Committee on Immunization Practices (ACIP). MMWR Morb Mortal Wkly Rep. 2015;64(34):944–7. [cited 2017 June 12]. www.cdc.gov/mmwr/preview/mmwrhtml/mm6434a4.htm. [Internet]

46. Nuorti JP, Whitney CG, Centers for Disease Control and Prevention (CDC). Prevention of pneumococcal disease among infants and children – use of 13-valent pneumococcal conjugate vaccine and 23-valent pneumococcal polysaccharide vaccine – recommendations of the Advisory Committee on Immunization Practices (ACIP). MMWR Recomm Rep [Internet]. 2010;59(RR-11):1–18. [cited 2016 Sep 10]. www.cdc.gov/mmwr/preview/mmwrhtml/rr5911a1.htm#Tab8. Available from: http://www.ncbi.nlm.nih.gov/pubmed/21150868

47. Briere EC, Rubin L, Moro PL, Cohn A, Clark T, Messonnier N, Division of Bacterial Diseases, National Center for Immunization and Respiratory Diseases, CDC. Prevention and control of haemophilus influenzae type b disease: recommendations of the Advisory Committee on Immunization Practices (ACIP). MMWR Recomm Rep [Internet]. 2014;63(RR-01):1–14. www.cdc.gov/mmwr/preview/mmwrhtml/rr6301a1.htm

48. Robinson CL, Romero JR, Kempe A, Pellegrini C, et al. Advisory Committee on Immunization Practices Recommended Immunization Schedule for Children and Adolescents Aged 18 Years or Younger – United States, 2017. MMWR Morb Mortal Wkly Rep [Internet]. 2017;66(5):134–5. [cited 2017 June 12]. www.cdc.gov/mmwr/volumes/66/wr/mm6605e1.htm

49. Kim DK, Riley LE, Harriman KH, Hunter P, Bridges CB. Advisory Committee on Immunization practices recommended immunization schedule for adults aged 19 years or older – United States, 2017. MMWR Morb Mortal Wkly Rep [Internet]. 2017;66(5):136–8. [cited 2017 June 12]. Available from: http://www.cdc.gov/mmwr/volumes/66/wr/mm6605e2.htm

50. Reagan-Steiner S, Yankey D, Jeyarajah J, Elam-Evans LD, Curtis CR, MacNeil J, et al. National, regional, state, and selected local area vaccination coverage among adolescents aged 13–17 years – United States, 2015. MMWR Morb Mortal Wkly Rep [Internet]. 2016;65(33):850–8. [cited 2016 Sep 1]. www.cdc.gov/mmwr/volumes/65/wr/mm6533a4.htm#F1_down

51. Rockwell PG. What you can do to improve adult immunization rates. J Fam Pract [Internet]. 2015;64(10):625–33. [cited 2016 Sep 11]. Available from: http://www.ncbi.nlm.nih.gov/pubmed/26551470

52. Immunization. The Joint Commission. [Internet]. [cited 2017 June 12]. Available from: https://www.jointcommission.org/immunization/

53. Gannon M, Qaseem A, Snooks Q, Snow V. Improving adult immunization practices using a team approach in the primary care setting. Am J Public Health [Internet]. 2012;102(7):e46–52. [cited 2016 Aug 20]. Available from: http://www.ncbi.nlm.nih.gov/pubmed/22594743

54. Bottino CJ, Cox JE, Kahlon PS, Samuels RC. Improving immunization rates in a hospital-based primary care practice. Pediatrics [Internet]. 2014;133(4):e1047–54. [cited 2016 Aug 20]. Available from: http://www.ncbi.nlm.nih.gov/pubmed/24664096

55. Hainer BL. Vaccine administration: making the process more efficient in your practice. Fam Pract Manag [Internet]. 2007;14(3):48–53. [cited 2016 Aug 20]. Available from: http://www.ncbi.nlm.nih.gov/pubmed/17408132

56. Recommendations regarding interventions to improve vaccination coverage in children, adolescents, and adults. Task Force on Community Preventive Services. Am J Prev Med [Internet]. 2000;18(1 Suppl):92–6. [cited 2016 Aug 20]. Available from: http://www.ncbi.nlm.nih.gov/pubmed/10806981

57. Zimmerman RK, Albert SM, Nowalk MP, Yonas MA, Ahmed F. Use of standing orders for adult influenza vaccination a national survey of primary care physicians. Am J Prev Med

[Internet]. 2011;40(2):144–8. [cited 2016 Aug 27]. Available from: http://www.ncbi.nlm.nih. gov/pubmed/21238862

58. Use of standing orders programs to increase adult vaccination rates, Recommendations of the Advisory Committee on Immunization Practices. Centers for Disease Control and Prevention (CDC), et al. MMWR Morb Mortal Wkly Rep [Internet]. 2000;49(RR01):15–26. Available from: http://www.cdc.gov/mmwr/preview/mmwrhtml/rr4901a2.htm

59. Freed GL, Cowan AE, Clark SJ. Primary care physician perspectives on reimbursement for childhood immunizations. Pediatrics [Internet]. 2009;124:S466–71. [cited 2016 Sep 10]. Available from: http://www.ncbi.nlm.nih.gov/pubmed/19948578

60. Hurley LP, Bridges CB, Harpaz R, Allison MA, O'Leary ST, Crane LA, et al. U.S. physicians' perspective of adult vaccine delivery. Ann Intern Med [Internet]. 2014;160(3):161. [cited 2016 Sep 10]. Available from: http://www.ncbi.nlm.nih.gov/pubmed/24658693

61. Dresden SM, Powell ES, Kang R, McHugh M, Cooper AJ, Feinglass J. Increased emergency department use in Illinois after implementation of the patient protection and Affordable Care Act. Ann Emerg Med [Internet]. 2016.; [cited 2016 Sep 11]; Available from: http://www.ncbi. nlm.nih.gov/pubmed/27569108

62. Opel DJ, Mangione-Smith R, Robinson JD, Heritage J, DeVere V, Salas HS, et al. The influence of provider communication behaviors on parental vaccine acceptance and visit experience. Am J Public Health [Internet]. 2015;105(10):1998–2004. [cited 2016 Aug 27]. Available from: http://www.ncbi.nlm.nih.gov/pubmed/25790386

63. Fenton JJ, Jerant AF, Bertakis KD, Franks P. The cost of satisfaction: a national study of patient satisfaction, health care utilization, expenditures, and mortality. Arch Intern Med [Internet]. 2012;172(5):405–11. [cited 2016 Aug 21]. Available from: http://www.ncbi.nlm. nih.gov/pubmed/22331982

64. Weyer SM, Bobiak S, Stange KC. Possible unintended consequences of a focus on performance: insights over time from the research association of practices network. Qual Manag Health Care [Internet]. 2008;17(1):47–52. [cited 2016 Sep 10]. Available from: http://www. ncbi.nlm.nih.gov/pubmed/18204377

65. Hinman AR, Orenstein WA, Rodewald L. Financing immunizations in the United States. Clin Infect Dis [Internet]. 2004;38(10):1440–6. [cited 2016 Sep 11]. Available from: http://www. ncbi.nlm.nih.gov/pubmed/15156483

66. Questions answered on vaccines purchased with 317 funds. National Center for Immunization and Respiratory Diseases, CDC. [Internet]. [cited on 2017 June 12]. Available from: http:// www.cdc.gov/vaccines/imz-managers/guides-pubs/qa-317-funds.html

67. Knowing Cost (of Immunizations). American Academy of Pediatrics. [Internet]. [cited on 2017 June 12]. Available from: https://www.aap.org/en-us/advocacy-and-policy/aap-health-initiatives/immunization/Pages/knowing-cost.aspx

68. FACT SHEET measuring performance in Accountable Care Organizations.

69. Fairbrother G, Hanson KL, Friedman S, Butts GC. The impact of physician bonuses, enhanced fees, and feedback on childhood immunization coverage rates. Am J Public Health [Internet]. 1999;89(2):171–5. [cited 2016 Sep 11]. Available from: http://www.ncbi.nlm.nih. gov/pubmed/9949744

70. Doctors turning away unvaccinated children – LA Times [Internet]. [cited 2017 Jan 4]. Available from: http://www.latimes.com/science/la-me-vaccination-policy-20150210-story. html

71. IIS | About | Immunization Information System | CDC [Internet]. Available from: http://www. cdc.gov/vaccines/programs/iis/about.html

72. Immunization Information System (IIS) Functional Standards. National Center for Immunization and Respiratory Diseases, CDC. [Internet]. [cited 2017 June 12]. Available from: http://www.cdc.gov/vaccines/programs/iis/func-stds.html

73. Urquhart GA. Immunization Information Systems Current Status. National Vaccine Advisory Committee. Slides dated September 11, 2012. Available at: https://www.hhs.gov/sites/ default/files/nvpo/nvac/meetings/pastmeetings/2012/immunization_registries.pdf

74. Dombkowski KJ, Clark SJ. Redefining meaningful use: achieving interoperability with immunization registries. Am J Prev Med [Internet]. 2012;42(4):e33–5. [cited 2016 Sep 1]. Available from: http://www.ncbi.nlm.nih.gov/pubmed/22424260

75. Martin K. Overview and findings from Association of State and Territorial Health Officials' (ASTHO's) IIS interstate data sharing meeting. Slides dated April 22, 2015. Available at: http://www.immregistries.org/resources/iis-meetings/Wednesday_Closing_Plenary-_ASTHO.pdf Discussion Guide.

75a. Petit A, Muscoplat M. Immunization data exchange between Minnesota and Wisconsin. Slides presented at American Immunization Registry Association (AIRA) National Meeting on April 6, 2016. http://www.immregistries.org/resources/iis-meetings/Evaluation_of_Interstate_Immunization_Data_Exchange_between_Minnesota_and_Wisconsin.pdf

76. Recommendations of the American Immunization Registry Association (AIRA), Modeling of Immunization Registry Operations Work Group (MIROW) decrementing inventory via electronic data exchange. 2016 [cited 2016 Sep 4]; Available from: http://www.immregistries.org/resources/aira-mirow

76a. Vaccine Management Business Improvement Project (VMBIP), Vaccine Tracking System (VTrckS), Page accessed: August 8, 2016. Page last updated: December 22, 2015. Content source: National Center for Immunization and Respiratory Diseases, Centers Disease for Control and Prevention, Atlanta, GA. Available at http://www.cdc.gov/vaccines/programs/vtrcks/vmbip.html

77. Nyhan B, Reifler J, Richey S, Freed GL. Effective messages in vaccine promotion: a randomized trial. Pediatrics [Internet]. 2014;133(4):e835–42. [cited 2016 Sep 1]. http://pediatrics.aappublications.org/content/pediatrics/early/2014/02/25/peds.2013-2365.full.pdf

78. Hardt K, Schmidt-Ott R, Glismann S, Adegbola RA, Meurice FP. Sustaining vaccine confidence in the 21st century. Vaccines [Internet]. 2013;1(3):204–24. [cited 2016 Aug 27]. Available from: http://www.ncbi.nlm.nih.gov/pubmed/26344109

79. Jacobson RM, St Sauver JL, Finney Rutten LJ. Vaccine hesitancy. Mayo Clin Proc [Internet]. 2015;90(11):1562–8. [cited 2016 Aug 21]. Available from: http://www.ncbi.nlm.nih.gov/pubmed/26541249

80. Leask J, Kinnersley P, Jackson C, Cheater F, Bedford H, Rowles G. Communicating with parents about vaccination: a framework for health professionals. BMC Pediatr. 2012;12:154.

81. California Governor Signs School Vaccination Law. The two-way: NPR [Internet]. [cited 2017 Jan 3]. Available from: http://www.npr.org/sections/thetwo-way/2015/06/30/418908804/california-governor-signs-school-vaccination-law

82. Javanbakht M, Stahlman S, Walker S, Gottlieb S, Markowitz L, Liddon N, et al. Provider perceptions of barriers and facilitators of HPV vaccination in a high-risk community. Vaccine [Internet]. 2012;30(30):–4511, 6. [cited 2016 Aug 20]. Available from: http://www.ncbi.nlm.nih.gov/pubmed/22561142

83. Yeganeh N, Curtis D, Kuo A. Factors influencing HPV vaccination status in a Latino population; and parental attitudes towards vaccine mandates. Vaccine [Internet]. 2010;28(25):4186–91. [cited 2016 Aug 25]. Available from: http://www.ncbi.nlm.nih.gov/pubmed/20417261

84. Daley MF, Crane LA, Markowitz LE, Black SR, Beaty BL, Barrow J, et al. Human papillomavirus vaccination practices: a survey of US physicians 18 months after licensure. Pediatrics [Internet]. 2010;126(3):425–33. [cited 2016 Aug 20]. Available from: http://www.ncbi.nlm.nih.gov/pubmed/20679306

85. Constantine NA, Jerman P. Acceptance of human papillomavirus vaccination among Californian parents of daughters: a representative statewide analysis. J Adolesc Health. 2007;40(2):108–15.

86. Bair RM, Mays RM, Sturm LA, Zimet GD. Acceptability of the human papillomavirus vaccine among Latina mothers. J Pediatr Adolesc Gynecol. 21:329–34.

87. Dempsey AF, Pyrzanowski J, Lockhart S, Campagna E, Barnard J, O'Leary ST. Parents' perceptions of provider communication regarding adolescent vaccines. Hum Vaccin Immunother [Internet]. 2016;12(6):1469–75. [cited 2016 Aug 27]. Available from: http://www.ncbi.nlm.nih.gov/pubmed/27078515

88. Rosenthal SL, Weiss TW, Zimet GD, Ma L, Good MB, Vichnin MD. Predictors of HPV vaccine uptake among women aged 19–26: importance of a physician's recommendation. Vaccine [Internet]. 2011;29(5):890–5. [cited 2016 Aug 21]. Available from: http://www.ncbi.nlm.nih.gov/pubmed/20056186

89. Heritage J, Robinson JD, Elliott MN, Beckett M, Wilkes M, et al. J Gen Intern Med [Internet]. 2007;22(10):1429–33. [cited 2016 Aug 21]. Available from: http://www.ncbi.nlm.nih.gov/pubmed/17674111

90. Galluscio EH, Paradzinski P. Task-specific conjugate lateral eye movements. Percept Mot Skills [Internet]. 1995;81(3 Pt 1):755–62. [cited 2016 Aug 24]. Available from: http://www.ncbi.nlm.nih.gov/pubmed/8668432

91. Roter DL, Erby LH, Larson S, Ellington L. Assessing oral literacy demand in genetic counseling dialogue: preliminary test of a conceptual framework. Soc Sci Med [Internet]. 2007;65(7):1442–57. [cited 2016 Aug 24]. Available from: http://www.ncbi.nlm.nih.gov/pubmed/17614177

92. Rosenthal SL, Weiss TW, Zimet GD, Ma L, Good MB, Vichnin MD. Predictors of HPV vaccine uptake among women aged 19–26: importance of a physician's recommendation. Vaccine [Internet]. 2011;29(5):890–5. [cited 2016 Aug 22]. Available from: http://www.ncbi.nlm.nih.gov/pubmed/20056186

93. Zimmerman RK, Santibanez TA, Janosky JE, Fine MJ, Raymund M, Wilson SA, et al. What affects influenza vaccination rates among older patients? An analysis from inner-city, suburban, rural, and Veterans Affairs practices. Am J Med [Internet]. 2003;114(1):31–8. [cited 2016 Aug 22]. Available from: http://www.ncbi.nlm.nih.gov/pubmed/12543287

94. Smith PJ, Kennedy AM, Wooten K, Gust DA, Pickering LK. Association between health care providers' influence on parents who have concerns about vaccine safety and vaccination coverage. Pediatrics [Internet]. 2006;118(5):–e1287, 92. [cited 2016 Aug 24]. Available from: http://www.ncbi.nlm.nih.gov/pubmed/17079529

95. Centers for Disease Control and Prevention (CDC), et al. MMWR Morb Mortal Wkly Rep [Internet]. 2011;60(32):1078–82. [cited 2016 Aug 27]. Available from: http://www.ncbi.nlm.nih.gov/pubmed/21849964

96. Moniz MH, Vitek WS, Akers A, Meyn LA, Beigi RH. Perceptions and acceptance of immunization during pregnancy. J Reprod Med [Internet]. 2013;58(9–10):383–8. [cited 2016 Aug 27]. Available from: http://www.ncbi.nlm.nih.gov/pubmed/24050026

97. Laine C, Davidoff F. Patient-centered medicine. A professional evolution. JAMA [Internet]. 1996;275(2):152–6. [cited 2016 Aug 21]. Available from: http://www.ncbi.nlm.nih.gov/pubmed/8531314

98. Coulter A. Partnerships with patients: the pros and cons of shared clinical decision-making. J Health Serv Res Policy [Internet]. 1997;2(2):112 21. [cited 2016 Aug 20]. Available from: http://www.ncbi.nlm.nih.gov/pubmed/10180362

99. Charles C, Gafni A, Whelan T. Shared decision-making in the medical encounter: what does it mean? (or it takes at least two to tango). Soc Sci Med [Internet]. 1997;44(5):681–92. [cited 2016 Aug 21]. Available from: http://www.ncbi.nlm.nih.gov/pubmed/9032835

100. Opel DJ, Mangione-Smith R, Robinson JD, Heritage J, DeVere V, Salas HS, et al. The influence of provider communication behaviors on parental vaccine acceptance and visit experience. Am J Public Health [Internet]. 2015;105(10):1998–2004. [cited 2016 Aug 5]. Available from: http://www.ncbi.nlm.nih.gov/pubmed/25790386

101. Hunter P. Tell Parents Immunizations Key to Children's Health, Well-being [Internet]. Available from: http://www.aafp.org/news/opinion/20150331ge-vaccines.html

102. Gilkey MB, Moss JL, Coyne-Beasley T, Hall ME, Shah PD, Brewer NT. Physician communication about adolescent vaccination: How is human papillomavirus vaccine different? Prev Med. 2015;77:181–5.

103. Hughes CC, Jones AL, Feemster KA, Fiks AG, et al. BMC Pediatr [Internet]. 2011;11:–74. [cited 2016 Aug 24]. Available from: http://www.ncbi.nlm.nih.gov/pubmed/21878128

104. Sako W, Treuting WL, Witt DB, Nichamin SJ. Early immunization against pertussis with alum precipitated vaccine. JAMA. 1945;127:379–84.

105. Vitek CR, Pascual FB, Baughman AL, Murphy TV. Increase in deaths from pertussis among young infants in the United State in the 1990s. Pediatr Infect Dis J. 2003;22:628–34.
106. Community Preventive Services Task Force. Vaccination Programs: Community-Based Interventions Implemented in Combination. [Internet] [cited 2017 June 17] https://www.thecommunityguide.org/findings/vaccination-programs-community-based-interventions-implemented-combination
107. National Vaccine Program Office. National Adult Immunization Plan, Goal 3. [Internet] [cited 2017 June 17] https://www.hhs.gov/nvpo/nationaladult-immunization-plan/goal-3/index.html

Chapter 7
Models of Health Behavior and Systems and Overcoming Barriers to Improved Immunization Rates

Jonathan M. Raviotta and Richard K. Zimmerman

Introduction

Despite major advances in immunization science with the licensure of effective vaccines, they are often underused. To a clinician, the patient sitting in the exam room suffering from a particular disease seems far more compelling than all of the unseen, averted cases prevented by excellent care. Perhaps it is part of a healer's nature to focus on disease rather than on health. Health seems nebulous and precarious, while disease is concrete and measurable. Yet, one of the top ten achievements of modern medicine is immunization [1].

Immunization is an exemplar of successful public health programming. In one of the greatest cooperative achievements of humankind, smallpox was declared globally eradicated a mere 200 years after the initial discovery of variation. Given that this was accomplished during the infancy of modern epidemiologic surveillance techniques and vaccine manufacturing processes and before the age of rapid international travel, our modern challenges to routine vaccination seem trivial compared with those faced by early vaccination pioneers [2]. By learning from experience and systematically building on success, the eradication of smallpox was just the beginning of mass prevention of infectious diseases. With the eradication of polio in sight, our global community has demonstrated that even the most obstinate barriers to immunization can be overcome [3].

J.M. Raviotta, MPH (✉)
Department of Family Medicine and Clinical Epidemiology,
University of Pittsburgh School of Medicine, Pittsburgh, PA, USA
e-mail: raviottaj@upmc.edu

R.K. Zimmerman, MD, MPH
University of Pittsburgh School of Medicine,
4420 Bayard Street, Suite 520, Pittsburgh, PA 15260, USA
e-mail: zimmer@pitt.edu

© Springer International Publishing AG 2017
P.G. Rockwell (ed.), *Vaccine Science and Immunization Guideline*,
DOI 10.1007/978-3-319-60471-8_7

While global eradication of a virulent pathogen is a noble objective, the routine control of the cadre of less spectacular illnesses has an even greater ability to extend life. Between 1900 and 1997, average life expectance in the United States was extended by 29.2 years, largely due to the reduction of mortality from infectious diseases in children under 5 years of age [4]. Even mediocre success in controlling influenza (the most devious of vaccine preventable diseases) has resulted in the estimated prevention of up to 6.6 million cases and 79,000 hospitalizations *per year* in the United States between 2005 and 2013 [5]. Despite these obvious public health triumphs, the US vaccination program is still far from perfect.

Vaccination opportunities still exist and with varying degrees of severity. In Healthy People 2020 [6], the CDC reports vaccination coverage rates are below target for ≥4 doses of diphtheria, tetanus, and acellular pertussis vaccine (DTaP), the full series of *Haemophilus influenzae* type b (Hib) vaccine, hepatitis B (HepB) birth dose, ≥4 doses pneumococcal conjugate vaccine (PCV), ≥2 doses of hepatitis A, the full series of rotavirus vaccine, and the combined vaccine series; [7] human papillomavirus (HPV) vaccine in adolescents; [8] and seasonal influenza vaccination [5, 9]. However, a more troubling observation than subpar vaccine-specific rates is the systematically low rates of vaccination among entire demographics, particularly adults [10] and the underprivileged and vulnerable [7].

Improving universal vaccination coverage in the United States will certainly take resources, determination, and effort. However, let the example of global smallpox eradication, led by D.A. Henderson, reveal the true scale of the obstacles to improving vaccination rates [11]. By adopting the same unwavering conviction and steadfast tenacity, we can, and will, overcome the barriers to immunization.

In the first part of this chapter, we examine the public health dynamics of the US immunization program to learn why many common theoretical models of health behavior are insufficient to fully capture all of the components of immunization practice and explore an alternative framework with greater utility. Part II of this chapter will expose the reader to the operational constructs in the field of implementation science and equip the reader to plan an immunization improvement intervention. We conclude this chapter with a review of the most effective evidence-based interventions designed to improve immunization coverage and present a taxonomy of critical leverage points that will guide the selection of quality improvement strategies.

Part I: Theoretical Models Relevant to the US Immunization System

Social Context of Immunization Behavior

The behavior of vaccination is simple, in comparison to other health behaviors. For some vaccine preventable diseases (VPD), even a single inoculation is sufficient to provide lifelong protection. As compared to weight loss, smoking cessation, or the maintenance of healthy levels of physical activity, the binary decision associated with vaccination should be less difficult than avoiding the onslaught of temptations that threaten the daily confirmation of healthy lifestyle decisions. Therefore, it seems logical to focus considerable effort at the individual level to have patients say, "yes" to vaccination at the point of care. However, the application of individual-level theories, while important, is unlikely to drive results at a population level.

As is discussed in Part III, manipulation of individual-level constructs like knowledge, attitudes, and beliefs about immunization is necessary but insufficient to substantially improve vaccination rates. The models that seem applicable in a patient-provider visit, such as the health belief model [12], protection motivation theory [13], and the theory of planned behavior [14], can still be useful in developing decision aids or in framing educational messages [15, 16]: however, they are inadequate as a guiding framework to improve population outcomes at either the practice or regional levels. These limitations become more apparent by examining the societal context of the immunization system.

Immunization Services at a Societal Level

The social ecological model [17], as depicted in Fig. 7.1, defines a nested hierarchy of social-psychological influences that account for variances in behavior. For example, in an analysis of the uptake of the 2009 H1N1 influenza vaccine among US adults, Kumar et al. [18] found that each social ecological level was a significant predictor of both intention and uptake. The variances in vaccine uptake were the individual level (53%), the interpersonal level (47%), the organizational level (34%), the community level (8%), and the public policy level (8%). In combination, all levels explained 65% of the variance in uptake which suggests that a systemic approach could achieve more than interventions targeting any single level.

Leveraging the multiplicative effects that come from multi-system interventions is critical to maximizing the effectiveness of vaccination interventions. Though the prior statistics may sound optimistic, the difference between *percentage of explained variance* and *percentage uptake* can be confusing. The results presented above quantify the influence of each of the levels of the social ecological model. While 65% sounds like a high number, it actually means that the model can account for most of the reasons why participants did, or did not, receive the vaccine. What it does not report, however, is how many people actually did receive the vaccine. That figure is much less encouraging. The US Centers for Disease Control and Prevention (CDC) estimated that only 20.1% of US adults were vaccinated with the 2009 H1N1 influenza vaccine [19]. The 2009 H1N1 influenza pandemic is a frightening example of how far our public health system needs to advance to truly protect the population. If the 2009 pandemic had been as virulent as the 1918 Spanish flu pandemic, a meager 20.1% coverage rate would leave millions of adults susceptible to a potentially deadly infection.

Fig. 7.1 Socio-ecological
model. Reprinted with
permission [79]

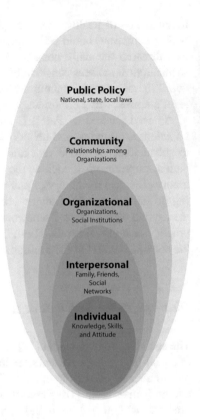

If the social ecological model can account for most of the variance in immunization behavior, then why are coverage levels lower than desired? First, the application of multilevel models, like the example above, is an avant-garde approach to
conceptualizing health outcomes. As evidenced by the corpus of immunization
publication, a great deal of scientific effort has focused on the individual predictors
of health behavior with decreasingly less rigorous scrutiny applied to the ascending intermediate social levels. The analysis from Kumar et al. [18] presented above
mirrors this supposition. While it is possible that the ascending social strata are less
predictive of individual behavior, it is also possible that the current extra-personal
interventions are too feeble to produce a substantial effect. For example, our
national plan includes some specific interventions in public policy, including
publicly subsidized vaccinations and compulsory vaccination programs, but those
policies have been inconsistently applied to the population by largely excluding
adults. Additionally, immunization interventions at the interpersonal level (like
social marketing [20]), the organizational level (like employer-mandated vaccination [21]), and at the community level (like pharmacist administration of vaccine

[22]) are all fairly new efforts. For these reasons, future analyses of health behavior may find that the broader levels of the social ecological hierarchy will contribute an increasing greater proportion of influence.

In addition to the novelty of the simultaneous application of multilevel interventions, the second reason for suboptimal outcomes is that the interdependencies among levels are not well understood. Acknowledging that immunization interventions need to target multiple levels of the social ecological hierarchy is good; intervening at multiple levels simultaneously is better but still difficult. To coordinate maximum impact on immunization rates, the entire US society (and, arguably, the global society) must be viewed as a complex dynamic system. The simplistic diagram of social ecological levels discretely nested like Russian dolls one inside another ignores the tangled network of interdependencies woven within, between, and among all of the levels of social organization [23].

Immunization Services as a Complex Adaptive System

Like many other public health initiatives, the US immunization program functions as a complex adaptive system. A complex adaptive system is a collection of entities that produce an outcome through dynamic, interrelated processes. Complexity occurs when the variability in the relationships among the elements in the system becomes important. Note that being complex is different from being complicated. A system can be complicated without being complex. Complicated systems are characterized by long chains of if-then operations. This logic can even branch out into many alternate pathways, but the final outcome can always be anticipated by a logical flow of predictable intermediate outcomes. A complex system also has predictable processes, but the outcome is dependent on how these processes interact with one another. In a complex system, causal pathways circle back to prior processes to create feedback loops.

For example, vaccine manufacturers want to produce as much vaccine as is necessary to immunize the population without creating a surplus that expires. A complicated version of the system would proceed linearly. Epidemiologists would estimate the required monthly inventory, and the manufacturer would produce some fraction of that inventory with every production run. Then clinicians would administer doses. In this system, oversupply or shortage is inevitable since the supply chain has no awareness of the demand. Adding a feedback loop to the system makes it adaptable to fluctuations in demand. Such a feedback loop might be a weekly inventory monitoring system where some number of doses is established as a reserve. If the reserve is full, production is halted. If the reserve is not full, production continues. If the reserve is ever emptied, production accelerates, and the reserve number is increased. If doses in the reserve ever expire, the reserve number is decreased. Now the system is taking feedback from one process and turning that into an input for another process, thus making the system adaptable. Because of this ability to modify one process in response to another, the system maintains stability even under inconsistent conditions [24].

The broader immunization system functions in a similar way, albeit with many more processes occurring at a larger scale. Consider the introduction of the HPV vaccine. Initially, demand for the vaccine and uptake were nil because a vaccine was not available. Once the vaccine was approved for use in the population, demand and uptake rose; however, the vaccine was only licensed and recommended for females. Because the primary aim of the program was vaccinee protection from HPV-related cancers, marketing, education, and clinician training centered on the vaccination of preteen and teenage girls. When the Advisory Committee on Immunization Practices (ACIP) recommended the routine immunization of 11- and 12-year-old girls against HPV, CDC added the licensed vaccine to the Vaccines for Children (VFC) Program which guarantees that low-income and impoverished children have access to all recommended vaccines. This system *should have* demonstrated increasing levels of coverage among girls and decreasing prevalence of cervical cancers later in life. However, several important relationships in the system created unintended feedback loops that inhibited the rapid adoption that was initially predicted.

First, cost and convenience of the vaccine were a substantial barrier. Not all vaccine providers accept VFC and thus some could not access VFC vaccine. Some vaccine providers did not stock HPV vaccine. Furthermore, the three-dose series over 6 months is recommended at an age when children typically make only annual visits. Second, the selective recommendation fueled a public debate about the perceived risks of the possible sexual disinhibition of vaccinated children, and concerns about vaccine safety arose [25]. In a complex adaptive system, stability can be a benefit if the observed outcome is desirable; however, in this case, the observed outcome (low rates) was undesirable. Because the feedback loops in the system (high cost, a three-dose series, and perceived risks of vaccination) were stronger than the effects of clinician counseling, widespread uptake was limited [26]. Changing the outcome in a system like this will not happen without modifying the underlying system dynamics. No amount of clinician education would prove sufficient to overcome the existing feedback loops [27].

Fortunately, policy makers, clinicians, and scientists recognized the problems and altered the assumptions of the original population models. By including boys and young men in the vaccination effort, women would experience greater protection from HPV-related cancers. Vaccination became "routinized" and large education efforts to prevent cancer occurred in the lay and provider communities. Also, in the face of low rates, the economic benefits of the reduction of other HPV-related diseases, like genital warts and head and neck, anal, and penile cancers, further argued for an expansion of the ACIP HPV recommendations [28]. Subsequently the vaccine was licensed for boys and recommended by the ACIP for all adolescents. This expanded the VFC formulary to include males, and coverage under the Affordable Care Act occurred. Also, the universal recommendation has likely diminished the strength of the effect of parental refusal. Though risk perception is still cited as a barrier, the shift in public policy may have softened objections enough that clinicians are now able to overcome parental hesitancy. The result of increased access, enhanced publicity, and routinized vaccine provider recommendations is increasing levels of coverage [29, 30].

As this example illustrates, an individual's health is determined by factors well beyond that person's locus of control. While it is tempting to believe that every person can autonomously choose his or her own state of health through rational decision-making, the truth is that all people are subject to unexpected tangential influences that serve to limit the breadth of options available at the individual level.

The Social Determinants of Health as a Framework for Immunization Services

The Commission on Social Determinants of Health was established in 2005 by the World Health Organization (WHO). This commission was charged with building a model of the social inputs to individual health. The resulting conceptual framework, the social determinants of health (SDH) [31], pictured in Fig. 7.2, overcomes the limitations of the social ecological model by describing health as the result of a multilevel social structure that acts as a complex adaptive system. [A complete discourse on the Social Determinants of Health is beyond the scope of this chapter. For more information, the curious reader is directed to the excellent resources available through WHO at http://www.who.int/social_determinants/en/.]

This framework is useful in planning and evaluating intervention strategies as potential leverage points can be examined within the system dynamics. This contextualization allows for the identification of unintended consequences resulting from nonobvious interactions among system variables.

Similar to the social ecological model, the SDH places the individual within a mosaic of social institutions. Unlike the social ecological model, the SDH provides relationships among all of the components of the social hierarchy through explicit causal pathways. According to this framework, individual health is the product of the structural determinants of the society which produce intermediary determinants that feed back to the structural level in a cycle. The structural determinants are (1) the socioeconomic and political context, including laws and policies, and cultural and societal values and (2) the individual's socioeconomic position, which is the product of social class factors including education, occupation, and income. This structural context defines the boundaries of the health environment available to member of the society. An individual's health state is further constrained by the additional influence of the intermediary determinants: material circumstances, behaviors and biological factors, psychosocial factors, and the health system as moderated by social cohesion and social capital. Finally, the resultant health states

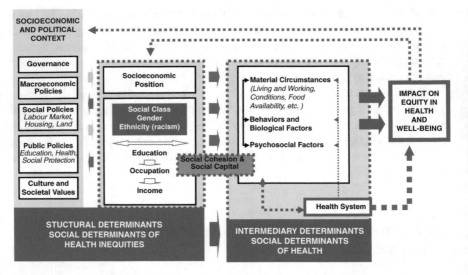

Fig. 7.2 Conceptual framework of the social determinants of health (Reprinted with permission [31])

of the members of the population influence the structural determinants for all of the society [31]. To clarify the operation of this framework, consider US seasonal influenza policy.

At the structural level, influenza policy is established by valuing the potential economic and social costs of various policy alternatives, weighed against the potential economic and social benefits of those alternatives. An extreme example might be the comparison between the policies of optional seasonal influenza vaccination vs. compulsory vaccination for everyone in the population. An analysis of these alternatives might find that compulsory vaccination could prevent the most cases of disease but that the cost of policing universal coverage and the restrictions on individual liberty outweigh the expected health benefits. If, however, the political context was colored by a recent pandemic resulting in mass casualties, the expected benefits might supersede the costs of enforcement and the reduction in civil liberties. In addition to explicit policy directives, the socioeconomic context includes other seemingly unrelated factors. Structural elements such as urban design, availability of mass transportation, funding for local health departments, school class sizes, and more can all play a role in the epidemiology of seasonal outbreaks. Thus, the decisions made at a societal level can exert additional influences on population health. This effect is translated to individuals through socioeconomic position.

Those with advantageous socioeconomic positions receive greater benefit, or suffer less, from coincidental structural influences. Suppose that a policy of compulsory vaccination for children and optional vaccination for adults were to be adopted. An individual's likelihood of being vaccinated would be a function of their socioeconomic position. An unintended consequence of this policy manifesting in socioeconomic position might be the allocation of the available vaccine stock to the more profitable insured market resulting in a disruption in supply to the VFC program. This would leave some of the most vulnerable children unprotected. In the adult population, a large proportion of the more educated and higher-earning citizens might opt out of vaccination due to misinformation and pseudoscientific deception.

Resolving an individual's health state during a pandemic would occur by first solving for the structural effects given the individual's socioeconomic position, then subtracting the effects of the intermediary determinants, adjusting for moderating effects from social capital, and then adding effects from the health system. An unvaccinated impoverished child would fare poorly. In addition to contracting the virus, his/her health might be further compromised by caustic environmental conditions more common in low-income housing, delayed or neglected medical care from overworked or absent parents, and compounded by the endemic levels of psychological stress associated with poverty. Contrariwise, a middle-class vaccine abstainer might experience less severe outcomes as his/her illness may not be compounded by additional environmental and psychological stressors.

Social capital and the health system provide feedback loops from the intermediary determinants to the structural determinants. Social capital moderates the effects of socioeconomic position, while the health system mediates effects in individual health. For the low-income child, a lack of social capital would offer no counterbalance to the negative socioeconomic effects, while the more affluent adult might be able to further reduce illness intensity by taking advantage of available social supports such as using a family member to help with childcare and cooking for the family.

A final opportunity to adjust health occurs when the individual interfaces with the health system. As a result of these individual's socioeconomic positions, it is likely that the child may never receive medical care or that it may be deferred until the symptoms become so severe that they become an additional household stressor, while the middle-class adult might access care early enough to benefit from antivirals which prevent additional disruption to daily activities.

At the end of this chain of events, the resulting health states of the impoverished child and the middle-class vaccine objector will feed back to the socioeconomic context for each individual and may establish a new socioeconomic position prior to the next medical crisis. The child who could not be vaccinated suffered a more intense illness as a result of socioeconomic position, the lack of social capital, and minimal mitigation by the health system; this child did not improve in socioeconomic standing and may have even fallen below the starting position. The flu-stricken adult experienced a reduction in the potential severity of the illness resulting from the absence of poverty-related stressors, available social capital, and early access to the health system. While this individual probably did not improve in socioeconomic standing during the illness, the reduced severity likely prevented a drop in standing if, for example, he/she were to have lost a job due to illness.

The final dynamic in this system occurs when the aggregate experiences of all members of society inform policy, programming, and cultural values. If the impoverished child scenario becomes too common or is widely publicized, it may lead to changes in structural-level interventions for the disadvantaged. Likewise, the minimized consequences of illness for the vaccine abstainer might lead others to believe that vaccination is unnecessary. If that erroneous belief were translated into structural inputs (e.g., abolishing compulsory childhood vaccinations), the entire society would suffer as more people contract VPD.

Part II: Implementation Science

By definition, overcoming barriers necessarily requires change. While some barriers are outside of the sphere of influence of primary care providers, others can be surmounted by modifications at the practice level. Before presenting those opportunities, we need to add one more layer of theory to understand the process of change. The following section discusses the process of integrating evidence-based innovations into clinical practice.

Those who have tried to maintain a New Year's resolution for an entire year are aware that change is hard. Resolutions like quitting smoking, or incorporating exercise into most days, often end only a few short weeks or possibly months later but certainly before the first blossoms of spring appear. Why are people successful at some resolutions and not others? There are probably dozens of factors that influence each success and each failure. The same is true of organizations that try to make changes. Some changes stick, while others are forgotten almost immediately.

The field of implementation science addresses the process of translating research into practice through change. Change occurs during implementation or the institutionalization of the set of conditions and behaviors required to successfully execute an evidence-based practice. Implementation science is not a replacement for health behavior theory nor a substitute for effective health interventions, rather it is a unifying framework that describes the relationships among factors in the external environment, the characteristics of the organization, the characteristics of the innovation, and the process of deploying the innovation [32]. This systematic study of change reveals solutions and problems outside of the innovation's clinical effectiveness that also contribute to an intervention's success or failure.

Surprisingly, this is a new field of research evolving from the methodical development of evidence-based practices and programs. Though researchers have become better at manipulating health outcomes in small samples of the health system, they have struggled to complete the next logical step which is to consistently replicate and scale these programs in the larger population. Thus, implementation science was born to bridge this chasm between research and practice [33]. As the study of translation progresses, clinicians adopting new innovations will begin to achieve closer results to those predicted in clinical trials.

While implementation science can benefit the deployment of even simple innovations, it is most useful when the innovation targets a complex system with a complex intervention. As presented in the prior section, the scope of immunization covers every level of the social ecological hierarchy and has inputs and outputs in all levels of the social determinants of health. Moreover, most single-component interventions will fail to produce a significant change in immunization rates. Achieving measurable improvement requires multicomponent interventions for which the emerging field of implementation science offers guidance to minimize the risk of program rejection and to maximize the effectiveness of a successful system change.

Box 7.1 Implementation Reflection 1

Consider how a primary care office might use the current best practices from implementation science to inform a new immunization initiative. The National Implementation Research Network (NIRN) has generated and continued to refine an excellent model of the implementation process. Interested readers will benefit from a more thorough study of the resources cited in this section especially [34]. Imagine that you are a managing clinician in a midsize family medicine practice. Your practice is part of a larger healthcare system, so while you have clinical autonomy, your practice is accountable to the management and operational processes of your business unit. Your practice is staffed with several physicians, a nurse practitioner, a few RNs, and several medical assistants. This clinical team is supported by a practice manager, a social worker, and a cadre of clerical staff.

You have volunteered to lead a task force charged with improving the immunization rates in all family medicine practices in your business unit. To support the effort, your company is willing to invest a reasonable amount of capital and to provide administrative support for the project. Take a moment to digest that assignment. Can you recall any similar situations from your experience? Perhaps you have walked out a meeting having "volunteered" for a project with a similarly audacious mandate. Before reading on, take some notes on that project or think about how you might tackle your new assignment. Answer the questions below to capture your thoughts:

1. What was/is the desired outcome?
2. How did/will you know the project succeeded?
3. How did/will you decide what to do to reach the outcome?
4. What were/are the challenges you had (will have to) to overcome at the beginning of the project?
5. What new challenges occurred/will occur after some time had passed?
6. What kind of leadership was/is required for the project?
7. How did/will personnel learn what to do?
8. What support was provided (or is needed) from your organization?

Stages of Evidence-Based Program Implementation

The successful implementation of a complex evidence-based program is a process that will pass through the four stages pictured in Fig. 7.3: (1) exploration, (2) installation, (3) initial implementation, and (4) full implementation. Note that this timeline is lengthy. For ambitious projects, such as a new immunization improvement program (IIP), full implementation may take months or longer to achieve. Also note that the process may continue indefinitely. This is certainly true of immunization. New vaccines will be released, recommendations will change, and staff will turn over. These time-related characteristics should shape expectations of the new project. The first step is to come to understand the implementation environment. This happens in the exploration stage.

Exploration

As the name implies, exploration involves setting aside one's own opinions and seeking to understand the implementation environment from the perspective of other stakeholders. Everybody wants to offer the best patient care and probably agrees that immunization should be a priority. If that is true, then why are rates as low as they are? In truth, there are reasons beyond individual effort that multiplicatively contribute to suboptimal results. The first task during the exploration stage is to understand what these issues are and why they occur (assess needs). The second task is to review available interventions that have demonstrated improvement to the target outcome in other similar environments (examine intervention components) [Bertram et al. [34] categorize intervention components with further refinement as

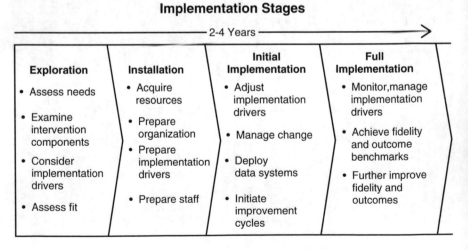

Fig. 7.3 The stages of implementation (Reprinted with permission [34])

Box 7.2 Key Questions During the Exploration Stage
1. Assess needs – What factors contribute to current results?
2. Examine intervention components – What evidence-based interventions have demonstrated effectiveness with these factors? Or what are the components of the assigned intervention and how do they work?
3. Consider implementation drivers – What resources are necessary and available within the organization to support the intervention?
4. Assess fit – Given this assessment of the implementation environment, what intervention/components are likely to achieve the most success?

(a) model definition, (b) theory bases supporting those elements and activities, (c) the model's theory of change, (d) target population characteristics, and (e) alternative models. We have omitted discussion of these intervention components in favor of presenting primary care physicians with a more accessible approach to implementation of an existing evidence-based immunization intervention]. And the third task is to evaluate the capacity of the organization to support the necessary strategies (consider implementation drivers). With that information at hand, one will be able to select the right intervention or components from an assigned intervention (assess fit). That is, will the proposed strategy solve the identified problems within the constraints of the organizational capacity?

These tasks remain the same for implementations of any size. The present example assumes an intervention on multiple practices, but the tasks of exploration are the same even when deploying strategies to a single small practice. However, the methodology used to arrive at an assessment of fit may need to be scaled up or down accordingly. In a small practice, it may be practical to interview members of the staff informally over the course of a few workdays, while in a multi-site healthcare system, you may need to collect data through questionnaires, interviews, participant observation sessions, and focus groups or even hire trained personnel to assist with assessment. Regardless of the scale of the program, the questions in Box 7.2 should be addressed before moving to the next stage, installation.

Installation

During the installation stage, the implementation team should prepare all of the individuals and resources necessary to perform the intervention. This step is frequently overlooked in one's eagerness to take action. In general, people don't like to be surprised with sweeping changes. When business processes are suddenly changed, people are rarely immediately supportive and need some time to "come around" to the idea. Advanced warning helps to smooth acceptance of the changes. Installation is as much about achieving the social-psychological milestone of buy-in, as it is about logistics. If this stage is skipped, the success of the implementation will be jeopardized, or at least delayed, to remediate the oversight and to attempt to hastily acquire necessary resources and/or overcome nagging resentments from staff.

Before the involvement of any non-project personnel, secure the needed resources. This may be training materials, an expense account, protected staff time, software, hardware, custom programming, or other reserves dictated by the selected intervention. Procuring resources is often subject to delays, so insuring that all materials are available prior to mobilization is critical. Next the organization should be alerted of the project and informed of the rationale and goals of the initiative. It may be helpful if this notice is proffered by stakeholders from each of the domains of the organization that will be affected by the implementation. For example, the division medical director, human resources representative, accounts manager, information technology liaison, and implementation team members may all prepare a memorandum and newsletter article including frequently asked questions and the contact information of team members. Though it may seem unnecessary to reiterate the message over numerous communication channels, overcommunication is preferable to surprise. Create a plan that keeps the appropriate members of the organization apprised of the program and begin to publish periodic updates within the communication avenues of your organization for as long as the implementation is active. This exposure will also aid in the next objective which is to prepare implementation drivers.

The ultimate change in outcomes is dependent on the three interrelated and compensatory implementation drivers of competency, organizational systems and culture, and leadership, which will be more fully discussed in the following section. During the exploration stage, the implementation team reviewed the requirements of the program and the available skills and resources in the organization. Now in installation, each of the three drivers will be bolstered by initiating training, installing systems, and empowering leadership. Once the appropriate staff have been prepared for execution of the program activities, the project is ready to move into initial implementation.

Initial Implementation

After months, or even years, of planning and development, a new immunization improvement program is ready to be deployed. The organization and staff have been prepared with frequent communication, appropriate trainers have been empowered, the organization has provisioned all the resources that are required by the project, and the project leadership team is ready to launch. Initial implementation is the time to turn excitement and anticipation into action. While it is theoretically possible that all of the preparation will result in a unilaterally adopted and flawlessly executed intervention, the more likely scenario is that it will encounter unanticipated problems, unexpected obstacles, and unpredictable behavior. The primary objectives during the initial implementation stage are resolving these problems, overcoming these obstacles, and managing these behaviors.

Successful navigation of this tumultuous stage will be least stressful by adopting the philosophy of kaizen, or continuous improvement [35]. [While a full discourse of modern process improvement ideology is outside of the scope of this narrative, any individual who finds him-/herself routinely involved in project management or quality improvement will benefit from a dedicated study of business practices evolving from Sakichi Toyoda's and Taiichi Ohno's substantial contributions to the product development cycles used throughout the world today. See also the Toyota Production System and Lean manufacturing [35, 36].

In this paradigm, perfection is unattainable and problems are unavoidable, but *improvement* is well within reach. Adopting an attitude of continuous improvement positions the implementation team for success without compromising quality even in uncertain conditions. Though simple and powerful, this philosophy is counter to the way many people tackle implementation. Fully adopting kaizen requires that one abandon the search for "the correct" way to achieve a goal, opting instead, for the discovery of incrementally "better ways." In practice, this means that during the initial implementation stage, the organization will conduct an experiment, measure the results, recalibrate the approach, and then try again. With each successive iteration, the team will learn what implementation drivers need to be adjusted and see what unanticipated issues arise.

The characteristics of the intervention being implemented will define the scope of each "experiment." It may make sense to consider a single iteration as the deployment of a single process like the addition of a clinical decision aid within the EHR. Perhaps it might make more sense to deploy the total intervention to a pilot group of practices or maybe to stage the intervention by job role. The key is to take small steps through the initial implementation process to afford the implantation team, as well as the organization, the opportunity to learn from experience and to adapt implementation drivers accordingly. Full implementation begins when the program activities occur as a matter of course and the new processes start to become routine.

Full Implementation

Some interventions may never achieve full implementation, while others may become institutionalized rapidly. The speed and degree of adoption are related to the complexity of the change and the fit between the program activities and the skills and resources available to support the implementation drivers. When an organization can meet a program's requirements for staff competency, systems and resources, and leadership dynamics, full implementation will occur with greater fidelity to the prescribed activities than when there is a mismatch between requirements and skills [37]. The initial implementation stage is the time to adjust one or both of these parameters until program fidelity can be achieved.

Once the organization is reliably performing the specified activities, focus will shift to maintenance of the new processes and evaluation of outcomes. All of the hard work prior to full implementation has occurred with the educated assumption that outcomes will improve as a result of the installation of new processes and behaviors. Now is the time to evaluate that hypothesis at scale. If there is a large discrepancy between the expected and observed outcomes, one can employ the kaizen philosophy to achieve better program fidelity through the implementation drivers or begin a new exploration phase to choose an intervention with a better fit. Otherwise, the improved outcomes should be monitored for consistency through time. We will explore the relationships among the implementation drivers and program outcomes next.

> **Box 7.3 Implementation Reflection 2**
> Review your answers to the questions in **Box 7.1**. Questions 6–8 address each of the implementation drivers of leadership, competency, and organizational resources. Do you see relationships between your project's outcomes and your responses to items 6–8? What changes in outcomes might you expect if you were to modify one or more of the answers to those questions?

Implementation Drivers

Implementation drivers are the most important determinants of implementation success. The three components of competency, leadership, and organizational environment presented in Fig. 7.4 all contribute equally to the intervention's potential effectiveness. Competency drivers are largely influenced by human resources and staff performance management. Organization drivers reflect the translation of changes in external policies and conditions to internal business practices or treatment protocols. Lastly, leadership drivers include the availability and characteristics of project leadership [34]. All of these drivers are addressed throughout all of the stages of implementation. In the exploration stage, the implementation team compares what is required by the intervention with what is available within the organization. In the installation stage, the systems and processes that support the program are deployed. During initial implementation, the program is tested and the implementation drivers are adjusted. Finally, in full implementation, the organization executes the intervention activities with fidelity and continues to build on successes.

The overarching goal in aligning implementation drivers is to achieve program fidelity [33]. While there is considerable flexibility in how the program is installed and in what components are selected as an appropriate fit for the environment, the actual execution of the prescribed activities should remain as close to those that have demonstrated population-level effectiveness as possible. For example, an organization conducting an immunization improvement intervention may choose to assess vaccination status for every patient prior to their appointment as a program strategy. Depending on the organizational supports available, they might choose to either assign a staff person to look up each patient at the start of the day and list

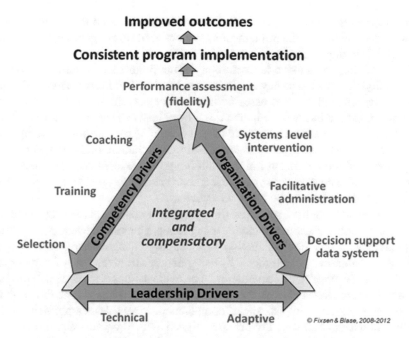

Fig. 7.4 Implementation drivers (Reprinted with permission [34]; © Fixsen & Blase, 2008–2012)

needed vaccines on the schedule or to activate an EHR module that automatically reports this information.

Even this simple example implies parameters for all three drivers. The availability of automatic vaccination assessment through the EHR is an organizational driver that will determine the level of training and supervision necessary to insure competency, which affects the type of leadership required to install either comprehensive training in vaccination assessment or the activation of a new technical feature in the EHR. Notice that the drivers are integrated and compensatory which implies that deficits in one area can be mitigated by adjusted effort in other areas. Imagine the following extension of the scenario. The organizations decide to try manual vaccination assessment at the start of each day performed by a nurse but find that despite thorough training and coaching, staff are having a difficult time accurately identifying vaccination status. The project lead has been focused on the technical challenge of installing sufficient training, which seems to be falling short, so a change in tactics to a more adaptive leadership style is required. Through troubleshooting, observation, and staff interviews, the team lead discovers that nurses know how to assess vaccination status but that the patient's vaccination history cannot be trusted. From this, the team deduces that the activities in the competency driver are working and the problem truly lies in the organizational domain. Upon investigation of possible solutions with the EHR vendor, the organization finds that connecting the EHR with state vaccine registries would cost more than the organization is willing to spend. Under these conditions, the implementation team needs to compensate for the identified deficit in organizational drivers.

Still utilizing an adaptive leadership style, the project lead returns to the clinicians to find that most gaps in vaccination can be identified from the medical record and that the remainder can be assessed through contact with the patient's insurance provider or patient interview. Finally, the project lead can switch back to technical leadership to manage the deployment of a new training module about finding accurate vaccination status for patients with missing information. In the end, nurses will have to expend more effort in training and in vaccine assessment activities to supplement the missing data system, but the compromise is acceptable to project stakeholders in order to realize the financial savings.

In this section, we have reviewed the operational constructs relevant to the process of translating research to practice using implementation science. A fundamental challenge in any implementation is managing change. Disruption from the process of change can be minimized by using findings from the field of implementation science. Successful implementation of an evidence-based practice will progress through the four stages of exploration, installation, initial implementation, and full implementation. During each stage, competency drivers, leadership drivers, and organizational environment drivers are aligned with program requirements and organizational capacity to insure implementation fidelity. Execution of the program components with fidelity to the evidence-based model will result in a change in practice outcomes. Next we will turn our attention to the currently recommended programs to overcome the barriers to immunization.

Part III: Strategies to Overcome Barriers to Immunization

The Community Guide

In this section, we review the Community Guide, its strengths, and possible limitations. The Community Preventive Services Task Force (Task Force) is charged with systematically reviewing and synthesizing the results of peer-reviewed intervention studies across a spectrum of population health conditions. The Community Guide, available at http://www.thecommunityguide.org, contains the findings and recommendations reported by the Task Force and includes an extensive section on increasing appropriate immunization. Because the Task Force conducts rigorous evaluations that are peer-reviewed by stakeholders from research, policy, practice, and government agencies, including the Centers for Disease Control and Prevention, the Community Guide is a trustworthy and comprehensive resource [38].

In the evaluation of interventions to increase universally recommended vaccinations, the Community Guide presents the findings from 22 recent systematic reviews and recommends 15 of the evaluated strategies. The Task Force suggests that additional research is necessary to issue an opinion on the remaining seven strategies and did not "recommend against" any of the reviewed strategies [38]. The review's logic model groups interventions into the five categories: (1) interventions enhancing access to immunization services, (2) interventions to increase community demand for immunizations, (3) provider-based interventions, (4) interventions to promote seasonal influenza vaccinations among healthcare workers, and (5) interventions to promote seasonal influenza vaccinations among non-healthcare workers [39, 40].

One strength of the Community Guide is its "stock and flow" perspective which assumes that increasing demand for immunization and/or increasing access to immunization will increase the number of patients seeking vaccination. When those patients engage with the healthcare system, provider-based interventions will increase the proportion of vaccinated individuals. This framework is logical from a population-based disease transmission perspective as it mirrors the common susceptible, infected, recovered (SIR) model that is very familiar to epidemiologists [41].

Another strength is that on-the-ground immunization champions would likely agree with common themes in the recommendations of the Community Guide. First, simply increasing access to immunization is effective in multiple settings and across diverse populations. Reducing financial burdens, reducing opportunity costs, and offering more convenient locations for vaccination all contribute to increased uptake. Second, many people seem willing to be vaccinated when they are reminded, it is routine or required, or influential social factors are leveraged to encourage vaccination intention. However, knowledge of vaccine status and vaccine education are necessary but insufficient to elicit vaccination intention. Third, practitioner-based interventions are sensitive to increased system efficiency and automation and achieve maximal effectiveness when implemented in combination with other strategies. Finally, clinicians respond to motivation.

Limitations exist; a review of Table 7.1 illustrates that this framework has limited use from a patient panel, clinician-centered perspective, since the organizational scheme used in the Community Guide blends the intention of the intervention (enhancing access and increasing demand) with the locus of intervention (provider, system, or workplace). Additionally, many of the strategies involve socioecological levels outside of a clinician's sphere of influence. Thus, practitioners who want to overcome barriers to immunization need a more action-oriented framework to conceptualize possible intervention strategies.

The 4 Pillars™

Zimmerman et al. present the following themes to primary care practitioners as the 4 Pillars™, which are (1) convenience and access, (2) patient communication, (3) enhanced vaccination systems, and (4) motivation. The 4 Pillars™ Practice Transformation Program operationalizes these principles by assisting primary care

Table 7.1 Task Force recommendations and findings to increase appropriate vaccination [38]

	Recommended	Insufficient evidence	Recommend against
Enhancing access to vaccination services			
Home visits to increase vaccination rates	X		
Reducing client out-of-pocket costs	X		
Vaccination programs in schools and organized childcare centers	X		
Vaccination programs in WIC settings	X		
Increasing community demand for vaccinations			
Client or family incentive rewards	X		
Client reminder and recall systems	X		
Community-based interventions implemented in combination	X		
Vaccination requirements for childcare, school, and college attendance	X		
Client-held paper immunization records		X	
Clinic-based education when used alone		X	
Community-wide education when used alone		X	
Monetary sanction policies		X	
Provider or system-based interventions			
Healthcare system-based interventions implemented in combination	X		
Immunization information systems	X		
Provider assessment and feedback	X		
Provider reminders	X		
Standing orders	X		
Provider education when used alone		X	
Interventions to promote seasonal influenza vaccinations among healthcare workers			
Interventions with on-site, free, actively promoted vaccinations	X		
Interventions with actively promoted, off-site vaccinations		X	
Interventions to promote seasonal influenza vaccinations among non-healthcare workers			
Interventions with on-site, reduced cost, actively promoted vaccinations	X		
Interventions with actively promoted, off-site vaccinations		X	

clinicians and office staff to adopt and implement evidence-based strategies [42–44]. Clinical trials of the 4 Pillars™ Practice Transformation Program have shown increased uptake of seasonal influenza vaccine in children [45–48] and seasonal influenza, pneumococcal, and pertussis vaccines in adults [42, 49]. Also, evaluation of the clinical implementation supports the Community Guide recommendations for multifaceted healthcare system-based interventions [38, 50].

Pillar 1: Convenience and Access

Access to care is a strikingly complex barrier to immunization. Truly providing complete access to all patients is elusive and can be frustrating as barriers are removed only to reveal new hidden obstacles [51]. Similarly, some practitioners may overlook opportunities to increase access to immunization by focusing on the societal-level impediments rather than the myriad small ways they can make vaccines more widely available to their patients. A useful way to overcome these challenges is to consider the five As of access to care described below.

Penchansky and Thomas [52] suggest that access to care has five dimensions that describe a patient's "degree of fit" with the health system. Primary care providers can extend this taxonomy to describe a given patient's degree of fit with their practice, their vaccination services, and even a particular vaccine:

- *Availability* is the value of the relationship between supply and demand. A primary care provider is available when a community has enough clinicians to offer services to the population. Influenza vaccine is available when a provider has enough stock to immunize all the patients who are eligible to receive it during the flu season.
- *Accessibility* is a measure of the perceived distance between the location of the patient and service. A clinic is accessible if it is within a reasonable commute from a patient given the available transportation. A vaccine is accessible if it is administered at the patient's home or workplace.
- *Accommodation* describes the patient's perception of feasibility to receive care. A school teacher may perceive a clinic as accommodating if s/he can schedule an appointment after school hours or on the weekend. A provider who offers no-wait, walk-in flu shots is showing accommodation for flu vaccination.
- *Affordability* measures the patient's ability to pay for the services provided as well as their perceived value of the services and knowledge of payment options. A primary care provider is affordable if the patient can pay for routine and unexpected care without extraordinary financial burden. A vaccine administration is affordable if a patient is willing to sacrifice the time, money, and effort necessary to receive the vaccine as well as any research and paperwork necessary to receive reimbursement for out-of-pocket costs.
- *Acceptability* relates an individual's knowledge, attitudes, and beliefs about a resource to the actual characteristics of that resource. A PCP is more likely to be acceptable to a patient if the patient perceives the clinician as willing to listen. A vaccine is more likely to be acceptable to a patient if the clinician presents the benefits, common side effects, and the uncommon risks.

The preceding examples of access to primary care and access to immunization are only a start to the methods a practitioner might employ to increase access to vaccination services. Box 7.4 lists strategies from the 4 Pillars™ Practice Transformation Program that you might use to increase the convenience to and access of your vaccination services. If you are developing new strategies, consider the principles and questions in Fig. 7.5 to elicit creative solutions.

Box 7.4 Pillar 1: Convenience and Access Strategies
- Use every patient visit type as an opportunity to vaccinate, including nursing; acute, chronic care; and follow-up visits for visits for another vaccination.
- Offer open access/walk-in vaccination during office hours.
- Promote simultaneous vaccination (e.g., offer other vaccines at the time of influenza vaccination).
- Hold express vaccination clinics outside normal office hours where only vaccines are offered, with streamlined flow systems for check-in, screening, and record keeping.
- Create a dedicated vaccination station.
- Extend the influenza vaccination season by vaccinating as soon as supplies arrive and continuing to vaccinate as long as flu is circulating in the community.

©, 2012, University of Pittsburgh. All Rights Reserved.

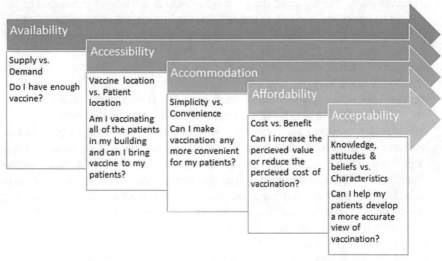

Fig. 7.5 Fundamental components of access to vaccination services (Copyright, © 2012, University of Pittsburgh. All Rights Reserved; Copyright, © 2016, University of Pittsburgh. Reprinted with permission)

Offering accessible vaccination services is key to reducing social and healthcare inequities [53]. Providing equal access means solving problems that are subtler than a simple determination of insurance coverage. While expanding the population of insured individuals may be out of the scope of an individual physician, that physician can certainly manipulate many elements of availability, accessibility, accommodation, affordability, or acceptability to increase access to vaccination services.

Pillar 2: Patient Communication

Patient refusal is one of the most obvious barriers to vaccination and is undoubtedly the most frequently blamed "reason" for suboptimal vaccination rates. Refusal is a problem but occurs much less frequently than one might imagine. Leask and Kinnersley [54] estimate that less than 2% of parents in a sample of western countries are absolute refusers with the remaining 98% ranging from late or selective to unquestioning acceptor. While one should consider how to communicate with vaccine refusers, one should also refrain from allowing the vocal minority to become overly distracting. In actuality, the most important instances of patient communication occur well before the point of asking for consent to vaccinate.

The "Communicate to vaccinate" project developed a taxonomy of communication objectives identified in published immunization interventions [55]. The range of potential audiences and communication strategies resulting from the project underscores the importance of examining every patient engagement for opportunities to optimize communication. Though all of the communication purposes presented in Fig. 7.6 are potentially useful, primary care providers will likely use the

Taxonomy Purposes

Inform or Educate
Interventions to enable consumers to understand the meaning and relevance of vaccination to their health and the health of their family or community. Interventions are sometimes tailored to address low literacy levels and can also serve to address misinformation.

Remind or Recall
Interventions to remind consumers of required vaccinations and to recall those who are overdue.

Teach Skills
Interventions to provide individuals with the ability to operationalise knowledge through the adoption of practicable skills.

Provide Support
Interventions to provide assistance or advice for consumers outside the traditional consultation environment.

Facilitate Decision Making
Interventions to help parents understand the personal benefits or harms of vaccination and to assist parents to actively participate in decision making.

Enable Communication
Interventions to make communication possible.

Enhance Community Ownership
Interventions to increase community participation and promote interaction between the community and health services. Interventions may build trust among consumers and generate awareness and understanding of vaccination. Interventions of this nature embrace collective decision making and community involvement in planning, program delivery, research, advocacy or governance.

Fig. 7.6 COMMVAC taxonomy purposes and definitions (Reprinted with permission [55])

objectives related to reminder and recall and patient education the most frequently. Of those two aims, reminder and recall interventions are more effective in increasing uptake if no other strategies are enlisted, while patient education requires the support of additional leverage points to achieve a noticeable increase in vaccine uptake [38, 39].

To many practitioners, patient education can become the default intervention strategy for every quality improvement program. This makes sense as clinicians are passionate about patients as individuals and want to achieve the most healthful outcome for every patient at every visit. While this is important, effective patient communication efforts must include strategies that act well outside of the exam room. Ideally, effective patient communication eliminates the need for intensive education because the patient walks into a visit asking for a vaccine. Additionally, focusing communication efforts on short, routine interactions can reach the largest number of patients with the least amount of effort.

Consider the time prior to a patient's appointment in the context of the transtheoretical model [56] as illustrated in Fig. 7.7. Prior to any external cues, all of the eligible and unvaccinated patients will exist in the precontemplation stage. Some proportion of these people may spontaneously schedule appointments for vaccination

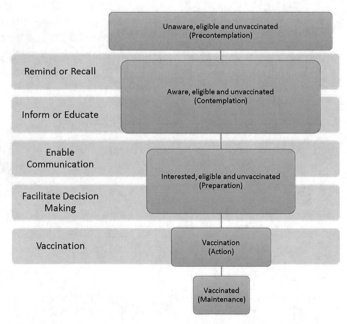

Fig. 7.7 Patient communication opportunities prior to and during appointment (Copyright, © 2012, University of Pittsburgh. All Rights Reserved; Copyright, © 2016, University of Pittsburgh. Reprinted with permission)

in response to school or workplace requirements and some others in response to media or other mass communication initiatives. The remainder (especially adults) will need to be shepherded onto the schedule with a *remind or recall* program. This initial contact is a moment to create awareness of vaccination and to move patients from a precontemplation stage into a contemplation stage. Every subsequent encounter prior to the visit offers another opportunity to *inform or educate* patients with positive messages or reminders about vaccination. Once in the office, posters, fliers, and decision aids can help patients work through the preparation stage or bring any precontemplators who ignored prior cues into the process. Rooming the patient and taking vital signs are opportune times to *enable communication* and to *facilitate decision-making* by checking vaccination status and exposing patients to more posters, fliers, and decision aids. If the practice has implemented standing order protocols for vaccination (see Pillar 3), all vaccines could be administered by the rooming medical assistant or nurse prior to the first contact with the clinician. Finally, during the clinician's consultation, any remaining objections to vaccination can be addressed. By the end of the communication cycle, all patients will have been given every possible opportunity to overcome any personal reluctance to immunization and to take action by accepting all overdue vaccines.

Communication with patients about immunization, however, is much more than carefully delivered monologues in the exam room. While skillfully responding to the concerns of vaccine-hesitant patients is important, a much larger audience exists outside of the office walls. Using every engagement with patients as an opportunity to enable communication and to provide a small dose of education or information will deliver a sustained and consistent message that cannot be duplicated in a single appointment. See Box 7.5 for a list of recommended patient communication strategies from the 4 Pillars™ Practice Transformation Program.

Box 7.5 Pillar 2: Patient Communication Strategies
- Enroll patients in electronic health portal.
- Provide information about vaccine preventable diseases at the beginning of every visit.
- Train staff to discuss vaccines during routine processes such as vital signs.
- Discuss the serious nature of vaccine preventable diseases.
- Promote 100% vaccination rates among staff to set a good example.
- Use on-hold messages, poster, fliers, electronic message board, website posting, and social media to promote vaccination.
- Reach out by email, phone, text, mail, health portal, etc. to recommend vaccines that are due and about arrival of influenza vaccine supplies.

©, 2012, University of Pittsburgh. All Rights Reserved

Pillar 3: Enhanced Vaccination Systems

For decades, epidemiologists, clinicians, policy makers, and manufacturers have continued to extend an increasingly robust immunization infrastructure closer and closer to each member of the population. As always, the familiar dyad of the physician and patient is left at the end of that complex chain to overcome any barriers. As a public health program, immunization is both blessed and cursed by a dependence on standardization and automation. Immunizing the entire human race can only be achieved through standardization, routinization, and complex systems support. This is a benefit to the program of immunization because ambiguity in any part of the process is systematically replaced with well-documented policies and procedures. This corpus of prescriptive information can then be transformed into algorithms, programs, and industrial processes that eliminate a great deal of human intervention. Unfortunately, this dependence on automation and standardization can introduce new problems. Errors can impact enormous numbers of people, and, conversely, improvements can take substantial time to deploy. This section will discuss opportunities to use automation and protocols to improve immunization coverage.

There are three major systems that have demonstrated positive influences on vaccination outcomes: (1) immunization information systems, (2) provider reminders, and (3) standing orders for vaccination. Additionally, clinicians should also consider how their unique office systems can be enhanced to support vaccination services. We will discuss each of these systems in this section.

Immunization Information Systems

An immunization information system (IIS) is a centralized repository of personally identifiable vaccination information for individual members of the served population. Nearly all US states now operate an active IIS; however, the features and functionality of each system are variable. During this period of transition to centralized vaccination registries, the Immunization Information Systems Support Branch, CDC – National Center for Immunization and Respiratory Diseases (NCIRD), directs expectations through an incrementally more complex set of functional standards for IIS. These standards were introduced in 2001, incremented in 2013, and will be evaluated again in 2017 [57]. The technical standards support the programmatic goals of CDC-funded immunization programs and state vaccine registries listed in Box 7.6: Programmatic Goals of CDC-Funded Immunization Programs.

In practice, this registry system will overcome the frustrating and all too common barrier of accurate assessment of vaccination status. When fully implemented, an IIS will programmatically record detailed information for all vaccine administrations and report relevant data to authorized requestors on demand. This simple concept will enable automated information sharing among vaccine service providers, public health services, consumers, and possibly other participants in the national immunization program [58]. Despite the obvious benefits to be gained from a fully implemented IIS and conceptual simplicity, national deployment has been slow.

> **Box 7.6 Programmatic Goals of CDC-Funded Immunization Programs [57]**
> 1. Support the delivery of clinical immunization services at the point of immunization administration, regardless of setting.
> 2. Support the activities and requirements for publicly purchased vaccine, including the Vaccines for Children (VFC) and state purchase programs.
> 3. Maintain data quality (accurate, complete, timely data) on all immunization and demographic information in the IIS.
> 4. Preserve the integrity, security, availability, and privacy of all personally identifiable health and demographic data in the IIS.
> 5. Provide immunization information to all authorized stakeholders.
> 6. Promote vaccine safety in public and private provider settings.

Offering access to sensitive health information to such a breadth of stakeholders has a monumental list of challenges and threats and has necessitated a strategy of slow and deliberate incremental advancement.

Unlike some other system enhancements, clinicians will likely have minimal involvement in the continued institutionalization of IIS but will reap ever-increasing rewards from background improvements to the infrastructure. The most important action item for providers is cooperation with any manual processes required to interface with the system, especially when accuracy can be compromised. Manually entering vaccination data into multiple databases, for example, may seem burdensome, but activities like this help every other stakeholders in the system to offer better services to patients. Ultimately, these chores will be replaced by the robust automation of the transfer of data between the EMR and the IIS. See Box 7.7 for some common strategies to maximally leverage IIS.

Provider Reminder Systems

Provider reminder systems notify clinicians that a vaccine should be administered to a particular patient at the point of care. The mechanism of this notification is less important than its existence and can take whatever form fits within the patient workflow. This strategy is effective for any vaccine and for any age patient and in nearly all clinical settings [38]. Reminders can be informally implemented as a note on a chart or formally implemented as programmatic notifications in the electronic medical record (aka, best practice alerts) [59, 60]. The most important considerations are that the provider responsible for vaccination takes notice of the reminder during the patient encounter and that the reminder is accurate.

The mechanism of action for provider notifications has not been well studied [61]. However, there are numerous reports in the medical informatics literature of implementation details in EHR systems that may have an impact on outcomes.' Additionally, there are some unintended consequences of the success of clinical decision supports like provider reminder systems. "Alert fatigue" and cognitive overload are certainly familiar concepts to clinicians who work with an EHR [62]. In planning a provider reminder strategy, one should consider the following:

- *What* is displayed in the content of the reminder.
- *How* the reminder is presented to the clinician. This may include the use of consistent colors, visual cues, and terminology as well as the required level of interruption to the patient care workflow.
- *Where* the reminder is presented in the salience hierarchy. For example, as a dialog box alert that appears immediately upon opening a patient record or as a footnote that is visible only after navigating deeply into the record.
- *When* the reminder is presented in the patient care workflow [63].

Because of the variability in office systems, primary care practices will need to implement provider reminders in whatever form makes the most sense within the business operational structure and patient care workflow. Some organizations will be able to simply turn on functionality provided by an EHR vendor, and some will need to define and enable custom prompts, while others will need to rely on the creativity of staff to create manual prompts outside of the EHR. Every implementation will have unique shortcomings, but reminders of nearly any description are better than missing an opportunity to vaccinate.

Standing Orders for Vaccination

Standing order protocols for vaccination (SOP) allow authorized healthcare staff to assess vaccination status and administer vaccines without an examination or specific order from a physician at the time of the administration. Standing orders are established by clearly defining a protocol for vaccine status assessment and vaccine administration. The SOP can range from broad, including many vaccines and many patent sets, to narrow including a single vaccine and a single patient set. This protocol is then approved by the appropriate personnel responsible for patient care and disseminated through training to all relevant clinical staff.

Standing orders for vaccination can be one of the more difficult to implement provider-based immunization interventions. However, the rewards in efficiency, increased vaccinations, and prevented cases of disease are well worth the effort, especially in the adult population [64, 65]. Both the Task Force on Community Preventive Services [66] and the Advisory Committee on Immunization Practices (ACIP) recommend the use of SOPs in many contexts [67]. In fact, the positive impact of SOPs can hardly be understated. Among a sample of elderly inpatient hospital stays, the use of SOPs increased the identification of pneumococcal vaccination opportunities from 8.6% to 59.1% [68]. In a randomized trial of 3777 hospitalized patients comparing SOPs to physician reminders, SOPs resulted in a 42% influenza vaccination rate vs. 30% from provider reminders and a 51% pneumococcal vaccination rate vs. 31% from provider reminders [69]. In a university-based practice, a retrospective analysis of patient visits over 4 years showed that the physicians who used SOPs achieved an influenza vaccination rate of nearly double of those who did not use SOPs (63% vs. 38%) [70]. Similarly, an implementation in an urban family medicine center resulted in a 1.4-fold increase in influenza vaccinations [71]. Clearly, all primary care clinicians should strongly consider adopting standing orders for vaccination.

Standing orders are regulated by state law [72]. Since standing orders can be used in many healthcare settings such as hospitals, clinics, medical offices, and long-term care facilities and can cover many provider roles such as nurses, pharmacists, and medical assistants, describing specific regulatory details is outside of the scope of this text. Hence, one should check state law and medical regulations in the covered locality prior to implementing SOPs. Despite the inherent regulatory complexity, standing orders are a well-known healthcare process with clear guidelines and prolific documentation [67]. Therefore, development and implementation of SOPs need not be stymied by excessive legal caution. [The George Washington University Center for Health Services Research and Policy and School of Public Health and Health Services provides a wealth of information regarding the governance of immunizations. Interested readers can access materials at http://publichealth.gwu.edu/departments/healthpolicy/immunization/.]

Unquestionably, implementing standing orders can be a challenge in some environments, but the healthcare benefits far outweigh the organizational effort. There are many excellent resources available from the CDC and other reputable partner organizations to help healthcare organizations and primary care providers plan and establish SOPs. A particularly useful library is maintained by the Immunization Action Coalition (IAC) at http://www.immunize.org/standing-orders.

Primary care providers must assess the office environment holistically to maximize the effectiveness of immunization systems, provider reminder systems, and standing orders for vaccination. See Box 7.7 for some common ways to enhance

---

Box 7.7 Pillar 3: Enhanced Vaccination System Strategies
- Ensure sufficient vaccine inventory to handle increased immunizations.
- Assess vaccination eligibility for every patient encounter by a systematic mechanism: (1) review of EMR prompts, (2) vaccination as a vital sign, and/or (3) create huddle report at the beginning of session of unvaccinated patients.
- Review accurate EMR vaccination record keeping.
- Update EMR with vaccinations as they are administered.
- Update EMR with vaccinations given elsewhere.
- Assess immunizations as part of vital signs.
- Establish standing order protocols for nursing and other patient care staff to vaccinate without an individual physician order.
- Develop systematic process for vaccinating every person with a vaccination need, such as standing orders or pending/queuing an order in the electronic health record.

primary care office systems for immunization. Every practice will have unique strengths and limitations in enhancing office systems for immunization. The key is to select strategies that make sense in the environment and to fully adopt these practices as part of the normal course of patient care and business operations. These deep-level alterations in routines, habits, and procedures will ultimately take less effort and result in much larger effects than from any campaign-oriented initiative.

Pillar 4: Motivation

The fourth pillar of the 4 Pillars™ Practice Transformation Program is motivation of the clinical team. Making changes to established workflows and to office systems is not easy. In our experience, the most common objection to any quality improvement program is almost always some variation on a lack of time and resources. From this perspective of resource scarcity, the very thought of conducting a deep, multi-system, multicomponent intervention is almost farcical. Yet if change in outcomes is expected, then some change must occur. Faced with this reality, many clinicians fall to the default intervention, education. The assumption is natural. One assumes that if he or she knows more or can teach patients more, then positive results will follow. Unfortunately, in the domain of immunization, education is necessary but not sufficient to achieve measurable changes in vaccination rates. The kinds of changes that are required stress leverage points at every level of the healthcare organization and beyond. Immunization interventions are complex and multifaceted and involve many stakeholders. All seasoned clinicians will likely admit to having participated in at least one spectacular failure of a complex intervention during his/her career; one that never got off the ground or if it did take flight, crashed into a wall of obstinate habits, stoic willfulness, or entrenched bureaucracy. Assuredly, those that have not, will. Motivation is the only fuel that can propel the albatross of quality improvement programs around obstacles, over barriers, and through storms.

An observant reader may have already noted that the majority of strategies to overcome immunization barriers are really designed, though automation and habituation, to overcome our shortcomings as human beings. It is laughably ironic that engineering around human fallibility is, itself, subject to yet another level of human interference. Even the most carefully orchestrated and flawlessly planned quality improvement program can be hamstrung at the human/plan interface. But, there is more to this story than fatalistic pessimism. How does one achieve change if it is so hard to do? How is it that some of the most haphazard and impromptu programs can succeed? Why do some practices consistently immunize the majority of their patients under the same organizational constraints? The answer, of course, is motivation [73, 74].

The Community Guide recommends assessing vaccine providers' performance and offering feedback [38]. Though there is considerable evidence that feedback on past vaccination performance tends to increase future performance, the active mechanisms are relatively unexplored. The exact nature of an "audit" and of "feedback" is highly variable. For example, in the literature reviewed by the Community Preventive Task Force, an audit may be conducted as infrequently as every 5 years or as often as weekly. Similarly, feedback may be a list of unvaccinated patients, provider education, or even financial incentives tied to vaccination rates. Also, few studies examine audit and feedback in isolation. Many reports include co-occurring interventions or are confounded by secular trends. More research will be necessary to isolate and test different methodologies and causal pathways [75].

Organizational motivation is a potential mediator in the effectiveness of audit and feedback strategies. Immunization interventions are complex and often involve individuals and business units who do not have close working relationships. Special care should be taken to engage all stakeholders in appropriate planning and preparation to secure institutional buy-in of the program. Failure to do so may result in insufficient institutional motivation or even overt sabotage that will derail the project [76]. To guard against these risks, consider the planning, deployment, and implementation of the program as carefully as each of the program activities.

Immunization programs are dependent on team participation. If clinicians improve individual performance with audits and feedback, it stands to reason that teams will improve group performance with the same. The 4 Pillars™ Practice Transformation Program recommends the nomination of an immunization champion (IC) to serve as a team motivator [49]. This individual should be respected by the staff as a leader and be able to guide staff through system changes [50]. The IC should also have strong interpersonal skills and enjoy frequent communication. The ideal IC finds win-win solutions to conflicts and demonstrates tenacity in overcoming roadblocks. Finally, the IC should be committed to the quality improvement goal and be nominated as the IC through purposeful consideration and not simply by default.

Box 7.8 lists strategies that the IC can employ to provide feedback to the team. A note of caution: in generating motivation, the quality of the audit is less important than the quality of the feedback. Obviously, audit results must be truthful, but abso-

---

Box 7.8 Pillar 4: Motivation Strategies
- Create a chart to track progress. Set an improvement goal and regularly track progress (e.g., daily or weekly). Post the graph of your progress in a prominent location and update it regularly.
- Provide ongoing feedback to staff on vaccination progress at staff meetings or through other forms of communication.
- Create a competitive challenge for the most vaccinations given among your staff.
- Provide rewards for successful results to create a fun-spirited environment.

Box 7.9 Implementation Reflection 3

Primary care providers should examine their own practices through the eyes of an unimmunized patient to uncover the unintentional barriers to vaccination institutionalized in habits, staff behavior, and office systems. Once identified, those points can be optimized to facilitate vaccination. As you enter your office as an unvaccinated patient, do you know that you need a vaccine? How do you know? Did you receive a reminder through the mail, text, internet, or phone? How do you feel about vaccination? Have you encountered any information from your provider in support of vaccination? On arrival for a visit, do you notice any decision aids or notices encouraging vaccination? During the capture of your vital signs, does the nurse or medical assistant also check immunization status? Does that individual offer to administer the missing vaccines? Is that staff person able to overcome objections with a tailored response? Are multiple vaccines administered whenever possible? Does your clinician make a strong recommendation for immunization? Can your physician tell you what vaccines you have had? What co-pay did you have to make? Were you referred to a pharmacy for a vaccination? How do you feel about that? Are you likely to follow through with vaccination? Does your pharmacy report to an IIS? All of these questions and more will help you to find the easiest places to start implementing change.

lute precision is unnecessary. ICs should use the data at hand to develop the best possible description of the practice's baseline vaccination rates, generate reasonable but challenging targets, and then start implementing strategies to try to improve rates. Someday all practices using an EHR will be able to summon an accurate population-based report of real-time vaccination rates. Until that day arrives, use the readily available reports and measure success as a changeover baseline. If no reports are available, simply tracking the number of doses administered per period or manually auditing some small sample of charts is preferable to implementing a quality improvement program with no measures of effectiveness.

Practice managers and organizational leadership can also provide a special kind of motivation. Operational policies like standing orders can be used to describe required job performance standards. By extension, employees can be compelled to fulfill these standards as a condition of employment. Though tempting, the formalization of best practices into job requirements may lead to more employee dissatisfaction than productivity [77].

In this section we have reviewed some important considerations in motivating a team at the practice level. Mobilizing and harnessing motivation are key drivers in implementation success. Though it may be tempting to dismiss the social-psychological needs of a team engaging in change, doing so can jeopardize the effectiveness of the entire intervention.

Conclusion

Immunization is one of the most effective medical interventions ever devised. Increasing rates of vaccination have extended the human lifespan, reduced childhood mortality, and significantly reduced, and even eliminated, the incidence of several infectious diseases. As a primary care clinician, insuring that all eligible patients are vaccinated is one of the best measures of preventative care that can be administered. By taking advantage of every opportunity to vaccinate and overcoming the barriers to immunization, PCPs are providing a service every bit as valuable as the police force and fire brigade. Immunization protects not only the vaccinee but also their friends, family, and community [78]. Vaccinating every patient extends protection to immunocompromised elderly parents. Vaccinating every patient extends protection to the children of misinformed vaccine-hesitant parents. Vaccinating every patient extends protection to infant grandchildren. Vaccinating every patient extends protection to society.

Every illness incurs both financial and psychological costs to the infirmed. Many VPD are so devastating that infection of the patient or a family member may mean a downward shift in socioeconomic position. By preventing unnecessary illness, vaccination avoids this potential consequence and offers patients and their families the best possible quality of life. This is especially important in the underprivileged and at-risk communities where vaccination rates are, unfortunately, the lowest. These individuals need every benefit available to escape from the cycle of poverty. Even though vaccine administration is far from glamorous, the unseen effects can be even more dramatic than the most complex surgical procedure.

While vaccine administration is simple, the public health program of immunization is both complicated and complex. With multiple points of failure, adopting a system-oriented perspective is crucial to the improvement of population coverage. Even physicians and office staff need to consider the system dynamics of their immunization services to make changes in their patient panel. The Social Determinants of Health model suggests that all citizens can help to improve the US immunization program. At the structural level, all clinicians can participate in policy-level activities such as contributing to the scientific literature, participating in immunization-related committees, development of vaccination standards by professional medical organizations, and political activism. At the intermediary level, clinician managers can support the effectiveness of the healthcare system by maintaining fair and equitable employment policies and work environments; deploy system changes that moderate the effects of vaccination services on patients' material circumstances, biologic factors, and psychosocial factors; and implement system change interventions with fidelity. Within the health system, all clinicians should commit to overcome barriers to immunization and to vaccinate every eligible patient and build social cohesion and social capital by championing vaccination within the health system.

References

1. Centers for Disease Control and Prevention. Ten great public health achievements in the 20th century online2013 [updated April 26, 2013. Available from: http://www.cdc.gov/about/history/tengpha.htm
2. Fenner F. Smallpox and its eradication. Geneva: World Health Organization; 1988. xvi, 1460 pp.
3. The Global Polio Eradication Initiative. Polio this week 2016. Available from: http://www.polioeradication.org/Dataandmonitoring/Poliothisweek.aspx
4. Centers for Disease Control and Prevention. Control of infectious diseases. MMWR Morb Mortal Wkly Rep. 1999;48(29):621–9.
5. Reed C, Kim IK, Singleton JA, Chaves SS, Flannery B, Finelli L, et al. Estimated influenza illnesses and hospitalizations averted by vaccination--United States, 2013-14 influenza season. MMWR Morb Mortal Wkly Rep. 2014;63(49):1151–4.
6. Healthy People 2020. Immunization and infectious diseases national snapshots. Washington, DC: U.S. Department of Health and Human Services, Office of Disease Prevention and Health Promotion; 2016. Updated 07/27/16. Available from: https://www.healthypeople.gov/2020/topics-objectives/topic/immunization-and-infectious-diseases/national-snapshot
7. Hill HA, Elam-Evans LD, Yankey D, Singleton JA, Kolasa M. National, state, and selected local area vaccination coverage among children aged 19-35 months – United States, 2014. MMWR Morb Mortal Wkly Rep. 2015;64(33):889–96.
8. Reagan-Steiner S, Yankey D, Jeyarajah J, Elam-Evans LD, Singleton JA, Curtis CR, et al. National, regional, state, and selected local area vaccination coverage among adolescents aged 13–17 years--United States, 2014. MMWR Morb Mortal Wkly Rep. 2015;64(29):784–92.
9. Appiah GD, Blanton L, D'Mello T, Kniss K, Smith S, Mustaquim D, et al. Influenza activity – United States, 2014-15 season and composition of the 2015-16 influenza vaccine. MMWR Morb Mortal Wkly Rep. 2015;64(21):583–90.
10. Williams WW, Lu PJ, O'Halloran A, Kim DK, Grohskopf LA, Pilishvili T, et al. Surveillance of vaccination coverage among adult populations – United States, 2014. Morb Mortal Wkly Rep Surveill Summ (Washington, DC: 2002). 2016;65(1):1–36.
11. Belongia EA, Naleway AL. Smallpox vaccine: the good, the bad, and the ugly. Clin Med Res. 2003;1(2):87–92.
12. Rosenstock IM. The health belief model: explaining health behavior through expectancies. In: Glanz K, Lewis FM, Rimer BK, editors. Health behavior and health education: theory, research, and practice. San Francisco: Jossey-Bass; 1990. p. 39–62.
13. Maddux JE, Rogers RW. Protection motivation and self-efficacy: a revised theory of fear appeals and attitude change. J Exp Soc Psychol. 1983;19(5):469–79.
14. Ajzen I. Theories of cognitive self-regulation: The theory of planned behavior. Organ Behav Hum Decis Process. 1991;50(2):179–211.
15. Gerend MA, Shepherd JE. Predicting human papillomavirus vaccine uptake in young adult women: comparing the health belief model and theory of planned behavior. Ann Behav Med. 2012;44(2):171–80.
16. Montano DE. Predicting and understanding influenza vaccination behavior. Alternatives to the health belief model. Med Care. 1986;24(5):438–53.
17. McLeroy KR, Bibeau D, Steckler A, Glanz K. An ecological perspective on health promotion programs. Health Educ Q. 1988;15(4):351–77.
18. Kumar S, Quinn SC, Kim KH, Musa D, Hilyard KM, Freimuth VS. The social ecological model as a framework for determinants of 2009 H1N1 influenza vaccine uptake in the United States. Health Educ Behav. 2012;39(2):229–43.
19. Centers for Disease Control and Prevention. Interim results: state-specific influenza A (H1N1) 2009 monovalent vaccination coverage – United States, October 2009–January 2010. MMWR Morb Mortal Wkly Rep. 2010;59(12):363–8.

20. Andreasen AR. Marketing social marketing in the social change marketplace. J Public Policy Market. 2002;21(1):3–13.
21. Backer H. Counterpoint: in favor of mandatory influenza vaccine for all health care workers. Clin Infect Dis. 2006;42(8):1144–7.
22. Hogue MD, Grabenstein JD, Foster SL, Rothholz MC. Pharmacist involvement with immunizations: a decade of professional advancement. J Am Pharm Assoc. 2006;46(2):168–82.
23. Diez Roux AV. Complex systems thinking and current impasses in health disparities research. Am J Public Health. 2011;101(9):1627–34.
24. Miller JH, Page SE. Complex adaptive systems: an introduction to computational models of social life. Princeton: Princeton University Press; 2007. xix, 263 pp.
25. Brewer NT, Fazekas KI. Predictors of HPV vaccine acceptability: a theory-informed, systematic review. Prev Med. 2007;45(2–3):107–14.
26. Charo RA. Politics, parents, and prophylaxis--mandating HPV vaccination in the United States. N Engl J Med. 2007;356(19):1905–8.
27. Centers for Disease Control and Prevention. Human papillomavirus vaccination coverage among adolescent girls, 2007–2012, and postlicensure vaccine safety monitoring, 2006–2013-United States. MMWR Morb Mortal Wkly Rep. 2013;62(29):591.
28. Elbasha EH, Dasbach EJ. Impact of vaccinating boys and men against HPV in the United States. Vaccine. 2010;28(42):6858–67.
29. Holman DM, Benard V, Roland KB, Watson M, Liddon N, Stokley S. Barriers to human papillomavirus vaccination among US adolescents: a systematic review of the literature. JAMA Pediatr. 2014;168(1):76–82.
30. Stokley S, Jeyarajah J, Yankey D, Cano M, Gee J, Roark J, et al. Human papillomavirus vaccination coverage among adolescents, 2007-2013, and postlicensure vaccine safety monitoring, 2006-2014--United States. MMWR Morb Mortal Wkly Rep. 2014;63(29):620–4.
31. Commission on Social Determinants of Health. Closing the gap in a generation: health equity through action on the social determinants of health: final report of the commission on social determinants of health. WHO 2008.
32. Fisher ES, Shortell SM, Savitz LA. Implementation science: a potential catalyst for delivery system reform. JAMA. 2016;315(4):339–40.
33. Fixsen DL, Naoom SF, Blase KA, Friedman RM, Wallace F. Implementation research: A synthesis of the literature. Tampa, FL: University of South Florida, Institute LdlPFMH; 2005. FMHI Publication #231
34. Bertram RM, Blase KA, Fixsen DL. Improving programs and outcomes: implementation frameworks and organization change. Res Soc Work Pract. 2014;25(4):477–87.
35. Sutherland JV. Scrum: the art of doing twice the work in half the time. 1st ed. New York: Crown Business; 2014. viii, 248 pp.
36. Tno T. Toyota production system: beyond large-scale production. Cambridge, MA: Productivity Press; 1988. xix, 143 pp.
37. Fixsen DL, Blase KA, Naoom SF, Wallace F. Core Implementation Components. Res Soc Work Pract. 2009;19(5):531–40.
38. Task Force on Community Preventive Services. Guide to community preventive services – increasing appropriate vaccination. Online updated April 26, 2016. Available from: www.thecommunityguide.org/vaccines/index.html
39. Task Force on Community Preventive Services. Vaccine-preventable diseases: improving vaccination coverage in children, adolescents, and adults. A report on recommendations from the Task Force on Community Preventive Services. MMWR Recommendations and reports: Morbidity and mortality weekly report Recommendations and reports / Centers for Disease Control. 1999;48(RR-8):1–15.
40. Task Force on Community Preventive Services, Zaza S, Briss P, Harris KW. Vaccine preventable diseases. The guide to community preventive services: what works to promote health? Atlanta: Oxford University Press; 2005. p. 223–303.

41. Allen LJS. Some discrete-time SI, SIR, and SIS epidemic models. Math Biosci. 1994; 124(1):83–105.
42. Nowalk MP, Nolan BA, Nutini J, Ahmed F, Albert SM, Susick M, et al. Success of the 4 pillars toolkit for influenza and pneumococcal vaccination in adults. J Healthc Q Off Publ Natl Assoc Healthc Q. 2014;36(6):5–15.
43. Zimmerman RK, Nowalk MP. Implementing the 4 pillars immunization toolkit in adolescent populations: randomized controlled trial. 2014.
44. Zimmerman RK, Nowalk MP. The 4 Pillars™ Practice Transformation Program. Available from: http://www.4pillarstoolkit.pitt.edu/
45. Nowalk MP, Zimmerman RK, Lin CJ, Reis EC, Huang HH, Moehling KK, et al. Maintenance of increased childhood influenza vaccination rates 1 year after an intervention in primary care practices. Acad Pediatr. 2016;16(1):57–63.
46. Lin CJ, Nowalk MP, Zimmerman RK, Moehling KK, Conti T, Allred NJ, et al. Reducing racial disparities in influenza vaccination among children with asthma. J Pediatr Health Care Off Publ Natl Assoc Pediat Nurse Assoc Pract. 2016;30(3):208–15.
47. Zimmerman RK, Nowalk MP, Lin CJ, Hannibal K, Moehling KK, Huang HH, et al. Cluster randomized trial of a toolkit and early vaccine delivery to improve childhood influenza vaccination rates in primary care. Vaccine. 2014;32(29):3656–63.
48. Nowalk MP, Lin CJ, Hannibal K, Reis EC, Gallik G, Moehling KK, et al. Increasing childhood influenza vaccination: a cluster randomized trial. Am J Prev Med. 2014;47(4):435–43.
49. Nowalk MP. Using the 4 pillars™ practice transformation program to increase adult Tdap immunization in a randomized controlled cluster trial. J Am Geriatr Soc 2016.
50. Hawk M. Using a mixed methods approach to examine practice characteristics associated with implementation of an adult immunization intervention using the 4 pillars™ immunization toolkit. J Healthc Q Off Publ Natl Assoc Healthc Q. 2016;39(3):153–67.
51. McLaughlin CG, Wyszewianski L. Access to care: remembering old lessons. Health Serv Res. 2002;37(6):1441–3.
52. Penchansky R, Thomas JW. The concept of access: definition and relationship to consumer satisfaction. Med Care. 1981;19(2):127–40.
53. Downs LS Jr, Scarinci I, Einstein MH, Collins Y, Flowers L. Overcoming the barriers to HPV vaccination in high-risk populations in the US. Gynecol Oncol. 2010;117(3):486–90.
54. Leask J, Kinnersley P, Jackson C, Cheater F, Bedford H, Rowles G. Communicating with parents about vaccination: a framework for health professionals. BMC Pediatr. 2012;12(1):154.
55. Willis N, Hill S, Kaufman J, Lewin S, Kis-Rigo J, Freire SBDC, et al. "Communicate to vaccinate": the development of a taxonomy of communication interventions to improve routine childhood vaccination. BMC international health and human rights. 2013;13(1):1.
56. Prochaska JO, Velicer WF. The transtheoretical model of health behavior change. Am J Health Promot AJHP. 1997;12(1):38–48.
57. Centers for Disease Control and Prevention. Immunization Information System (IIS) Functional Standards Online updated December 18, 2012. Available from: https://www.cdc.gov/vaccines/programs/iis/func-stds.html
58. National Center for Immunization and Respiratory Diseases. Summary of IIS Strategic Plan v1.3. Online: Centers for Disease Control and Prevention, 2013 11/30/2013. Report No.
59. Patwardhan A, Kelleher K, Cunningham D, Spencer C. Improving the influenza vaccination rate in patients visiting pediatric rheumatology clinics using automatic best practice alert in electronic patient records. Pediatr Rheumatol. 2012;10(1):1–2.
60. Burns IT, Zimmerman RK, Santibanez TA. Effectiveness of chart prompt about immunizations in an urban health center. J Fam Pract. 2002;51(12):1018.
61. Baron JM, Lewandrowski KB, Kamis IK, Singh B, Belkziz SM, Dighe AS. A novel strategy for evaluating the effects of an electronic test ordering alert message: optimizing cardiac marker use. J Pathol Inform. 2012;3:3.
62. Vashitz G, Meyer J, Parmet Y, Liebermann N, Gilutz H. Factors affecting physicians compliance with enrollment suggestions into a clinical reminders intervention. Stud Health Technol Inform. 2010;160(Pt 2):796–800.

63. Payne TH, Hines LE, Chan RC, Hartman S, Kapusnik-Uner J, Russ AL, et al. Recommendations to improve the usability of drug-drug interaction clinical decision support alerts. J Am Med Inform Assoc. 2015;22(6):1243–50.
64. Middleton DB, Lin CJ, Smith KJ, Zimmerman RK, Nowalk MP, Roberts MS, et al. Economic evaluation of standing order programs for pneumococcal vaccination of hospitalized elderly patients. Infect Control Hosp Epidemiol. 2008;29(5):385–94.
65. Honeycutt AA, Coleman MS, Anderson WL, Wirth KE. Cost-effectiveness of hospital vaccination programs in North Carolina. Vaccine. 2007;25(8):1484–96.
66. Task Force on Community Preventive Services. Guide to community preventive services – vaccination: standing orders 2015. updated 5/26/2016. Available from: http://www.thecommunityguide.org/vaccines/standingorders.html
67. McKibben LJ, Stange PV, Sneller VP, Strikas RA, Rodewald LE, Advisory Committee on Immunization Practices. Use of standing orders programs to increase adult vaccination rates. MMWR Recommendations and reports: Morbidity and mortality weekly report Recommendations and reports / Centers for Disease Control. 2000;49(RR-1):15–6.
68. Eckrode C, Church N, English WJ, 3rd. Implementation and evaluation of a nursing assessment/standing orders-based inpatient pneumococcal vaccination program. Am J Infect Control 2007;35(8):508–515.
69. Dexter PR, Perkins SM, Maharry KS, Jones K, McDonald CJ. Inpatient computer-based standing orders vs physician reminders to increase influenza and pneumococcal vaccination rates: a randomized trial. JAMA. 2004;292(19):2366–71.
70. Goebel LJ, Neitch SM, Mufson MA. Standing orders in an ambulatory setting increases influenza vaccine usage in older people. J Am Geriatr Soc. 2005;53(6):1008–10.
71. Logue E, Dudley P, Imhoff T, Smucker W, Stapin J, DiSabato J, et al. An opt-out influenza vaccination policy improves immunization rates in primary care. J Health Care Poor Underserved. 2011;22(1):232–42.
72. Stewart AM, Cox MA, Rosenbaum SJ. The epidemiology of U.S. Immunization law: translating CDC immunization guidelines into practice: state Laws related to the use of standing orders covering immunization practice. 2005.
73. Gamble GR, Goldstein AO, Bearman RS. Implementing a standing order immunization policy: a minimalist intervention. J Am Board Fam Med JABFM. 2008;21(1):38–44.
74. Weiner BJ. A theory of organizational readiness for change. Implement Sci. 2009;4:67.
75. Bordley WC, Chelminski A, Margolis PA, Kraus R, Szilagyi PG, Vann JJ. The effect of audit and feedback on immunization delivery: a systematic review. Am J Prev Med. 2000;18(4):343–50.
76. Tomoaia-Cotisel A, Scammon DL, Waitzman NJ, Cronholm PF, Halladay JR, Driscoll DL, et al. Context matters: the experience of 14 research teams in systematically reporting contextual factors important for practice change. Ann Fam Mcd. 2013;11(Suppl 1):S115–23.
77. Mechanic D. Physician discontent: challenges and opportunities. JAMA. 2003;290(7):941–6.
78. Lahariya C. Vaccine epidemiology: a review. J Family Med Prim Care. 2016;5(1):7–15.
79. Hudsonmh U. Socio-ecological model: a framework for community based programs. In: Model.png S-E, editor.: Wikipedia; 2014.

Chapter 8
Sources and Resources in Determining Immunization Status of Your Patients

Donald B. Middleton

Every day practicing physicians must accomplish numerous goals during a patient's office visit. Taking care of the acute or chronic problems that brought the patient into the office is obviously first among these goals, but health maintenance, including determination of a patient's immunization status, is of competing importance. Immunization has repetitively been recognized as among our most important and proven effective individual and societal health maintenance stratagems, both nationally and worldwide. Centers for Disease Control and Prevention (CDC) states that between 1994 and 2013, immunization of children was responsible for preventing an estimated 322 million illnesses, 21 million hospitalizations, and 732,000 deaths [1]. The net savings from vaccination is estimated to be $295 billion in direct healthcare costs and $1.38 trillion in total society costs, not to mention the prevention of lifelong heartache following the death of a child or loved one. The Vaccines for Children (VFC) program, created in 1993 and providing immunization coverage for families who cannot pay for childhood vaccines, is one major contributor to this stunning achievement. Estimates are that through VFC vaccinations, for each dollar invested in vaccines, on average the return is $3 in indirect benefits and $10 in societal benefits. Adding in successes in adult vaccination, the overall net benefit of universal immunization for all children and adults is astounding. The National Vaccine Advisory Committee (NVAC) stated in 2014 that all healthcare providers in all settings have a fundamental responsibility to ensure that all patients are up to date with respect to recommended immunizations [2]. Regardless of specialty physicians who do not offer immunizations to their patients should routinely assess the immunization status of their patients and refer patients to immunizing providers when needed. Physicians who do not offer immunizations to their patients should also follow up on vaccine recommendations to confirm that their patients did in fact

D.B. Middleton, MD (✉)
University of Pittsburgh School of Medicine, UPMC St. Margaret, Department of Family
Medicine, Pittsburgh, PA, USA
e-mail: middletondb@upmc.edu

© Springer International Publishing AG 2017   273
P.G. Rockwell (ed.), *Vaccine Science and Immunization Guideline*,
DOI 10.1007/978-3-319-60471-8_8

Table 8.1 Adult vaccination rates in the United States

Vaccine	Year	Age group	National rate (%)	Healthy people 2020 goals (%)
Tdap	2013	≥19 years	17.2	80[a]
Zoster	2013	≥60 years	24.2	30
High-risk pneumococcal	2013	19–64 years	21.2	60
Pneumococcal	2013	≥65 years	59.7	90
Influenza	2013–14	≥19 years	42.2	70

Source: Flu: CDC National early season flu vaccination coverage, United States, November 2014. Online at http://www.cdc.gov/flu/fluvaxview/nifs-estimates-nov2014.htm
Other vaccines: Vaccination coverage among adults, excluding influenza vaccination—United States, 2013. Online at http://www.cdc.gov/mmwr/preview/mmwrhtml/mm6404a6.htm#Tab1
[a]Includes Td vaccine

receive recommended vaccines. Unfortunately, this goal of a shared responsibility to ensure adequate immunization for all patients has not as yet been achieved. In fact, immunization rates fall well below Healthy People 2020 goals set by the Office of Disease Prevention and Health Promotion at the United States Department of Health and Human Services, especially for adult patients (Table 8.1).

Accepting that a high vaccination rate is a laudable goal, the clinician is faced with the challenge of determining a patient's current vaccination status, determining which vaccines are due at the time of each visit and in some situations overcoming a lack of confidence in vaccine recommendations [3]. The first task requires some investigative skill; the second, maintaining an increasingly complex knowledge base and access to supportive immunization resources to confirm the accuracy of vaccine recommendations; and the third, a demonstration of sensitivity to concerns about vaccines while maintaining a firm commitment to Advisory Committee on Immunization Practices (ACIP) recommendations. Despite high vaccination rates among children, rates among adolescents and adults remain below desirable levels (Table 8.1). Adult vaccination rates are unlikely to change or will change slowly without additional interventions. The annual rates for influenza vaccination and pneumococcal vaccination (23-valent polysaccharide vaccine [PPSV23]) have not improved significantly in over a decade. Similarly, adolescent vaccination rates, particularly for human papillomavirus (HPV) vaccine, remain below desired levels. Effective measures of dealing with threats to confidence in vaccination are under constant review [3].

This chapter is devoted to helping physicians and other healthcare providers determine a patient's current vaccine status and to review the many resources designed to enhance the clinician's ability to improve patients' health through appropriate vaccination administration and vaccine record keeping. Of note, many of the resources mentioned in this chapter are online. Because of the constant updates to vaccine recommendations, checking resources online is of critical importance. A multitude of websites provide ready access to a wide range of materials to assist with clinical dilemmas and to bolster basic immunization knowledge.

Determination of Vaccine Status

One goal during any patient encounter, whether a health maintenance encounter (e.g., Medicare Annual Wellness Visit, annual physical, well-child exam) or routine checkup or acute-care visit, should be to determine the patient's immunization needs. Assessing the immunization status should be considered a routine part of the vital signs and intake information, investigated alongside the blood pressure and smoking history. Determination of a patient's vaccine status is not always easy and may take time. The steps toward determining a patient's vaccination status and requirements are (1) reviewing vaccination records and their veracity to uncover any vaccine deficits, a process which is normally based upon age, underlying disease, employment, lifestyle, and time of year, (2) overcoming any vaccine hesitancy either on the part of the patient or clinician, (3) supplying the patient with the vaccine information statement (VIS) and administering the appropriate vaccine, and (4) recording vaccine information in the patient's record and supplying the patient with proper documentation of vaccination plus plans for future vaccines.

For the family physician or other immunizing practitioner, the three major sources detailing vaccine status are the patient self-report, the electronic health record (EHR) or office chart, and the state immunization system (IIS). Sometimes the three sources are in agreement, but not always, so care in accepting recorded information is warranted. Other sources of vaccination history are often available for review: health department records, patient or prior physician-supplied documented vaccine records, links to other state IISs, records from places of employment or schools, and records of vaccinations given at pharmacies. Some or all of these sources may require review for completeness in documentation and determination of vaccine status.

Self-Report

Self-reported vaccination is often utilized to assess vaccination status but has variable reliability [4]. On a societal level, the validity of vaccination self-report is important in determining vaccine effectiveness (VE): high self-report of vaccination tends to increase VE estimates. Positive predictive values of self-reporting receipt of vaccines (the patient stating that he or she has had a particular vaccine when in fact the vaccine was received) are dependent upon the patient's age, underlying disease state, behavior, familiarity with the physician or practice, the detail of the report (specific date and place of vaccination), and the vaccine in question. Unfortunately, self-reporting of vaccine receipt is highly inaccurate for most patients and for most vaccine recall. In 2013 in a telephone survey, Rolnick et al. compared self-report of vaccination against electronic medical records for eight adult vaccines in 11,760 individuals [4]. These authors found that self-reported vaccination was overstated in those who were retired and those with household incomes less than $75,000. The sensitivity of self-report ranged from a low of 63% for hepatitis A vaccine to over 90% for tetanus, HPV, shingles, and flu vaccines. Self-report from adolescents is also often inaccurate. A 2013 article from Rhode Island by Oh et al. documented that by self-report 40% of girls and 60% of boys did not receive or were not certain of receipt of HPV vaccine, yet data from immunization records showed that 77% of girls and 69% of boys had had at least one dose of HPV vaccine [5]. A false-positive report of vaccination leaves the patient at risk of acquiring the disease. On the other hand, true-negative predictive values (the patient reports never being vaccinated or does not know when in fact the patient did not receive the vaccine in question) are generally high, meaning that administration of a vaccine dose is indicated, but a false-negative report can lead to an unnecessary additional dose of vaccine. Fortunately, with rare exception, CDC considers these "extra" doses to be safe. For example, an infant who receives a hepatitis B vaccine at birth and is given Pediarix® (contains DTaP, IPV, and hepatitis B vaccine) at times 2, 4, and 6 months receives four dose of hepatitis B vaccine in toto instead of the recommended three doses but has no increase in adverse effects following immunization [6].

Historically, the vaccination with the most accurate self-report which is valid in both sensitivity and specificity is the influenza vaccine [7]. A 2009 study from Wisconsin by Irving et al. confirms this fact. The sensitivity and specificity of self-reported influenza vaccination compared to immunization registry records were 95% and 90%, respectively. The positive predictive value was 89%, while the negative predictive value was 96% [8]. Misclassification with a variance of 10% was more commonly found among young children. Because flu vaccine is given annually, the proximity of vaccination to the query about vaccination status may in part explain these results. However, a study in 2015 by Lochner et al. found that self-report of influenza vaccination for 9378 Medicare beneficiaries was 69.4%, while Medicare claims for vaccination were only 48.3%. The positive predictive value of claiming to be vaccinated was 97.6%, while the negative predictive value was only 56.7% [9]. Some of those vaccinated might have received free flu vaccine in other venues which do not generate a Medicare charge accounting in part for the disparity. The rate of flu vaccine claims was lower for beneficiaries who were age <65 years, male, non-Hispanic black or Hispanic, and had less than a college education. Thus, the sources of discordance may be somewhat dependent on social factors. Self-reports of receiving pneumococcal PPSV23 vaccination as compared to medical record documentation showed interesting results: in a 2006 study from Pittsburgh, Nowalk et al. found that the PPSV23 self-reported vaccination rate was 45% compared to 55% by medical record review [10]. For this vaccine, the medical record documented a higher vaccination rate than did self-report, perhaps pointing out a failure to adequately educate patients about vaccine receipt. On the whole, clinicians can be fairly confident of positive and negative self-reported influenza vaccine and positive self-report for PPSV23 [11].

State Immunization Registry: Immunization Information System (IIS)

A good source to check on vaccination self-report and to determine which other vaccines are needed is the state IIS [12]. Fifty one of 53 state IIS programs are authorized to collect immunization records for all age groups [13]. CDC review of these information exchanges is online at immunization information systems (IIS): http://www.cdc.gov/vaccines/programs/iis/resources-refs/faq.html.

A 2015 systematic review of 240 articles and abstracts supported IIS capabilities as being effective in both the public and private sectors [14], but how often the IIS is consulted during an office visit is open to debate. In 25,866 girls and women who made 47,665 office visits during which each received at least one vaccine, review of the state IIS revealed that 43% could have also received the HPV vaccine but did not [15]. Unfortunately, some state registries do not record HPV vaccination so the immunizing provider must be familiar with their local state IIS [16].

Adopted and Immigrant Children

Immigration and adoption of foreign children pose a further problem to assessing vaccination status. Vaccine records may be incomplete and vaccine names can be confusing. Excellent sources to consult for patients who have received immunizations in countries other than our own include CDC Guidelines New Vaccination Criteria for US Immigration available online at http://www.cdc.gov/immigrantrefugeehealth/laws-regs/vaccination and immigration/revised-vaccination-immigration-faq.html.

The 2016 Yellow Book discusses international adoption online at http://wwwnc.cdc.gov/travel/yellowbook/2016/international-travel-with-infants-children/international-adoption.

Immunization Action Coalition (IAC) provides excellent international adoption information at http://www.immunize.org/adoption/ including an International Adoption Handout for physicians and their patients.

Pharmacy, Workplace, and School-Provided Immunizations

Each year, pharmacist-provided immunizations are helping improve immunization rates in the United States [17]. Individuals >65 years of age who lived in states where pharmacists could provide influenza vaccines had higher rates of immunization than individuals who lived in states where pharmacists could not provide vaccines [18]. Vaccination in a pharmacy is particularly important for adults over the age of 65 years who frequently receive zoster or Tdap/Td vaccine under Part D of Medicare. A 2015 investigation revealed that consumer demand and profitability of vaccine administration were the main motivators for retail clinics to administer vaccines, but in reality vaccinating anywhere is beneficial for both personal and public health [19]. In the 2010–2011 flu season, approximately 18% of adult influenza vaccine was given at a pharmacy and 17% in the workplace [20, 21]. CDC has information for businesses and employers to learn strategies for preventing the flu with sources on how to host a flu vaccination clinic in the workplace and promote flu vaccination in the community [22] found at http://www.cdc.gov/flu/business/index.htm.

Children can also be vaccinated in nontraditional places such as pharmacies and schools: in the 2014–2015 flu season, 4.5% of children were vaccinated in pharmacies and 4.7% in schools [21].

Recording Vaccinations and Vaccination Records

Given that so many vaccines may be administered outside the traditional doctor's office, one must be aware that proper documentation of these vaccines takes effort. Pharmacies, including pharmacies in supermarkets or other retail establishments, often fax reports of immunization records to physician offices, but many retail or travel clinics or employers providing vaccinations are not adequately linked to primary care physician offices or integrated into state IISs. Every attempt should be made to connect with pharmacies and retail clinics either online or through faxes to the physician's office. Patients vaccinated in the workplace or school, in pharmacies, or in other clinics need to be encouraged to send their physician proof of such vaccination, to ask that their records be faxed to their medical home and recorded in their state registry. The patient's medial home's office staff can then record the vaccination in the patient's personal health record and inform the state IIS if needed.

Vaccine administration in the office must be carefully noted including in particular the vaccine name, dose, and date of administration. Records patients brought in from elsewhere without this basic information are suspect. Often vaccine records that a new patient brings into the office are hand written or recorded in a vaccine booklet or on a card. These records should be checked against documentation in the patient's medical records from the patient's prior medical home. Realize, too, that EHRs and office charts can be inaccurate. Reasons for inaccuracies include the recording of a patient's verbal report into the immunization chart of the medical record as if that vaccine had truly been administered when in fact, it had not been. Additionally, failure to report past episodes of disease may prompt electronic health maintenance advisories that a vaccine is due when it is not. This issue is particularly common with a disease like varicella [23]. In 2015 in Arizona, Hendrickson et al. reviewed 2017 unique vaccination histories from a large community health provider for record completeness [24]. The state registry was 71.8% complete, the health provider EHR was 81.9% complete, and the personal health record was 87.8%

complete. Sixty five percent of vaccine histories were recorded in all three sources, but only 11% of patients had records in complete agreement across all three sources. Interestingly, findings for influenza vaccination documentation were flipped. The state registry had a higher percentage of influenza vaccinations documented in comparison to patients' personal records: only 64.4% were recorded in the personal record as opposed to 81.7% in the Arizona state IIS. Another study further corroborates this discrepancy in records. From Alberta in 2014, MacDonald et al. found 60 discrepancies in a review of 461 childhood vaccination records comparing parent self-report to the province registry [23]. Forty-two of these 60 discrepancies were due to the parent report that the child was up to date with immunizations. Primary reasons for the parental errors were missed doses or a refusal to allow administration of a particular vaccine, in this case varicella, but stating that the vaccine had already been given. In two cases, the parent thought the child was not up to date but in fact the child was. Clearly efforts to improve the interconnectedness of these administration records are needed. Of note, school entry laws requiring proof of vaccination prior to student registration and vigilant school nurses improve the accuracy of vaccination records. School administrations that promote programs to administer vaccines on site, particularly annual influenza vaccine, need to be connected to the state IIS and have in place a system to connect with the students' primary care physicians either through written or faxed reports or electronically. Among the areas of concern about IISs are questions of confidentiality and completeness. IISs are subject to a number of state and federal regulatory statutes some of which reduce the exchange of information between healthcare providers and the IISs [13]. Receipt of a vaccine such as influenza vaccine or Tdap given in the place of employment, especially during free vaccine drives, may not be recorded in an IIS. Some experts hold the view that the EHR incentive program from the federal government will improve immunization data management [25]. A national IIS would be a great solution to improve data discrepancies but is unlikely to be available soon. Clearly physicians who wish to support or to improve vaccination practices will need to consult their state IIS whenever vaccines are recommended, given, and documented.

In summary, a three-pronged approach to the documentation and storage of adequate, accurate vaccine records includes (1) maintenance of up-to-date office records and EHRs; the individual administering the vaccinations should be the one who is doing the recording into these records; (2) contacting other vaccine providers patients may have seen, office personnel should feel free to contact pharmacies, schools, and workplaces where vaccinations may have been given to confirm the dates and types of vaccines; (3) distribution of personal patient records, every vaccinated individual should be given a record of vaccines received. The record can be in the form of a vaccination booklet for a child, an immunization record card such as those available from IAC (Fig. 8.1) for roughly $0.05 to 0.20 apiece [26] or an iPhone or android immunization application. Examples of free vaccines apps are *My Immunizations* by Sunny Nagra, *Immunization Log* by Manu Gupta, and *Vaccines Tracker* by Asif Khalyani available from the app store. Of course patients can also simply keep a note on their personal electronic devices. Such vaccine

a

Vaccine	Type of vaccine	Date given mo/day/yr	Health care professional or clinic name	Date next dose due
Hepatitis B (HepB, HepA-HepB)				
Hepatitis A (HepA, HepA-HepB) If combo				
Measles, Mumps, Rubella (MMR)				
Varicella (chickenpox) (Var)				
Zoster (shingles)				
Tetanus, Diphtheria, Pertussis (whooping cough) (Tdap,Td)				

ADULT IMMUNIZATION RECORD
Always carry this record with you and have your health care professional or clinic keep it up to date.

Last name   First name   M.I.

Birthdate: (mo) – (day) – (yr)

Patient Number:

Immunization Action Coalition • Saint Paul, Minn. • www.immunize.org
To order additional record cards, visit www.immunize.org/shop Item #P2005 (9/15)

b

Vaccine	Type of vaccine	Date given mo/day/yr	Health care professional or clinic name	Date next dose due
Pneumococcal (PCV13, PPSV23)				
Influenza (IIV, LAIV)				
Human Papillomavirus (HPV2, HPV4, HPV9)				
Meningococcal (MCV4, MenB, MPSV4)				
Other				

To learn more about vaccines, visit www.vaccineinformation.org

Last name   First name   M.I.

Medical notes (e.g., allergies, vaccine reactions):

Health care provider: List the mo/day/yr for each vaccination given. Record the generic abbreviation (e.g., PPSV23) or the trade name. For combination vaccines (i.e., HepA-HepB), fill in a row for each separate antigen in the combination.

Fig. 8.1 (**a, b**) IAC adult immunization record cards (Reproduced with permission of Immunization Action Coalition)

recording may be especially helpful and desirable for adolescents and young adults. Physicians should also encourage individuals to take more responsibility in staying current with their own immunization requirements. Encouraging adolescents to do so may be particularly rewarding. Many practices now utilize secure EHR communication with patients. Email exchanges may also be helpful to increase accurate reporting of vaccination if individuals receive vaccination outside of the practice particularly when a vaccination is given at the place of employment, but security remains an issue [27].

Depending on one's EHR and one's state registry, the process of documenting vaccine administration is often not a two-way exchange of data between the two systems. Some EHRs send data automatically to the IIS but do not download data automatically from the IIS. Technology is continually improving to enhance communication, but barriers to a seamless exchange of information still remain. After vaccinating, the office staff should be supported in any efforts needed to accurately record data in the charts. Documentation processes unique to each office are required. Parents who do not have their child's immunization records and need information as to how to go about retrieving them or have questions on record keeping for immunizations can consult *For Parents: Vaccines for Your Children* at http://www.cdc.gov/vaccines/parents/records-requirements.html.

Resources to Help with Administration of Appropriate Vaccines

Once the vaccine history has been verified, the physician or other healthcare provider must decide which vaccines are necessary and administer those recommended vaccines. CDC's unified immunization schedules solve the issue of which vaccines are due at what age and for which underlying medical condition, travel plan, lifestyle, or field of employment and can be found at https://www.cdc.gov/vaccines/index.html.

Obviously at certain times of the year as with flu season, typically beginning in the fall and ending in the spring, the opportunity for this process of immunization assessment is made more convenient. Once flu vaccine is available in the office, it can be given to anyone who walks in including the office staff or who is over 6 months of age and carried through the door! As patients are already in the office and receptive to receipt of the flu vaccine, the clinician can then check the CDC schedule to look up which other vaccines may be due, based on the patient's age, medical condition, or employment. CDC "easy to read" schedules aimed for public use but helpful to healthcare providers as well are available at https://www.cdc.gov/vaccines/schedules/downloads/adult/adult-schedule-easy-read.pdf.

CDC has online tools to guide which vaccines are needed. CDC Screening Checklist for Contraindications for Vaccines for Children and Teens is available at http://www.immunize.org/catg.d/p4060.pdf. The adolescent and adult form to determine which vaccines are necessary or should have been given is online at https://www2.cdc.gov/nip/adultimmsched/. In addition, IAC has an excellent chart documenting Recommendations for Children and Adults by Age and/or Risk Factor at http://www.immunize.org/catg.d/p2019.pdf.

When a patient comes in for an office visit, many EHRs automatically notify their users as to which vaccines are required or overdue in the form of "alerts" which prompt the clinician to consider immunization updates. Vaccines can be given in general whenever a patient is seen for whatever reason.

Patient Education

A critical portion of maintaining good immunization practice is to educate the patient and family about vaccine preventable diseases (VPDs) and vaccination. Techniques to motivate patients to receive vaccines should be part of everyone's practice [28]. Most patients and parents understand that children are recommended to receive many childhood vaccines, but many patients are unaware of adult vaccine recommendations. Except for influenza vaccine, 19% of Americans think vaccination is generally not recommended for adults and 58% admit to a gap in awareness about which vaccines they need [29]. Vaccination rates for children are much better than those for adults as shown in a 2012 National Foundation for Infectious Diseases (NFID) publication Call to Action: *Adult Vaccinations Saves Lives*. A disappointing statistic cited in that publication was that 88% of consumers said they were likely to be vaccinated if their doctor recommended it, but only about half of patients say they recall having had a vaccination discussion with their physicians. However, when polled, almost all primary care physicians say they initiate vaccine discussions with their patients. This disconnect demonstrates the need for more clear communication from physicians and all healthcare providers to their patients and our community at large [29].

The best method to confirm that a patient or family has been given counseling about vaccines is to document the discussion in the chart and provide the appropriate Vaccine Information Statement (VIS) to the patient. VISs are information sheets produced by CDC that explain both benefits and risks of vaccines. In 1987, the National Vaccine Injury Compensation Program (VICP) mandated that a VIS be given out with every vaccine. VIS forms from CDC for all routine vaccines are available for resource and printing at http://www.cdc.gov/vaccines/hcp/vis/index. html. These forms may also be found on the IAC resource site at http://www.immu-nize.org/vis/. An internet search can also easily get one to these websites to print off the appropriate VIS, and many EHRs also provide printable VISs.

Up-to-date data on the use of the VIS in the office is minimal. Despite the mandate that a VIS be handed out with every corresponding vaccine administration, a 2001 study reported that only 69% of pediatricians and 72% of family physicians actually give parents or patients a VIS [29]. Only 70% of physicians in this study reported discussing vaccine side effects. Lack of time was the number one reason for these deficits. Perhaps the VIS is not uniformly given out because it adds little to the physician's ability to achieve vaccine compliance, especially for those who are vaccine hesitant. For some vaccines, the VIS mentions frightening side effects such as a chance of death following immunization. The risk of death is infinitesimally small (if it ever occurs) but, if noticed on the VIS, could potentially lead to vaccine refusal. Fortunately, the majority of patients and parents are committed to the process of vaccination. From the author's clinical practice is the case of the mother who expressed her disappointment upon learning that her child was not to receive any vaccination during the 9-month well-child visit. She was clearly a vaccine advocate!

During an office visit, in addition to receiving the VIS prior to vaccination, patients and parents should be given materials about the vaccines administered and the expected beneficial results [30, 31]. All patients should maintain records of administered vaccines and anticipate those that are to be given in the future. Unfortunately, physicians often fail to educate patients or parents about which vaccines will be needed at the next visit or fail to have patients' appointments made for future vaccination administration for series completion. Anticipatory guidance material is available through *Bright Futures* 4th edition 2017 [32] for pediatric patients and on CDC and IAC websites.

How Can a Patient or Family Get Supportive, Accurate Information on Vaccines?

Random internet searches for immunization materials can lead to unscientific anti-vaccine publications or to in-depth medical textbooks which the public are unlikely to buy. Ideally physicians should refer patients and parents to both the CDC and IAC websites which are geared toward the public. A reference section is also available in most EHRs. Vaccine information material written or produced for wide dissemination abounds on these sites: printouts on each vaccine, materials on underlying reasons for being vaccinated, videos detailing the vaccine process, videos detailing VPDs, and many other materials. CDC provides a list of materials that can be helpful in patient education entitled *Immunization Education & Training: Patient Education* at http://www.cdc.gov/vaccines/ed/patient-ed.html. Subheadings are *materials that can be used to educate patients, links to resources/websites providers can refer patients to for their own use, answers to parents' frequently asked questions*, and *printed materials for parents of infants and toddlers, parents of preteens and teens, pregnant women, and college students, young adults, and adults*. One particularly useful item on the CDC site for patients and parents is "How to evaluate materials on the web," which offers guidelines that could be given to every patient referred to the web. In 2016, CDC posted the 64-page "Parents Guide to Childhood Immunizations," a 2016 National Health Information Award winner, online at https://www.cdc.gov/vaccines/parents/tools/parents-guide/index.html. A potential approach to sorting through the myriad of materials available is to meet with one's office staff to decide which routine information will be given out with each visit or vaccination.

Additional patient-centered resources are available from the vaccine manufacturers, each with its own website. The United States government does not manufacture vaccines: vaccines are made by private industry which funds much vaccine research, perhaps raising worries about conflict of interest. However, vaccinating professionals must trust that the Food and Drug Administration and ACIP do the work required to assure vaccine safety and accurate information about effectiveness. Most of the materials which manufacturers provide are generic in their approach to improving vaccination rates because most practices will not disseminate branded information. Often private industry resources have good insight into the process of motivating individuals to be vaccinated and to help physicians be aware of vaccine requirements.

Resources for Clinicians

CDC Guidelines and Schedules CDC general recommendations on immunization are online at https://www.cdc.gov/mmwr/preview/mmwrhtml/rr6002a1.htm. In addition to general guidelines, this site advises on many special situations like vaccination of persons with latex allergy and bleeding disorders. Several basic principles apply in vaccinating according to CDC recommendations. Vaccine should always be given on time if possible. Delays in completing vaccinations lead to increased periods of being at risk for VPDs. Alteration of the ACIP universal vaccine schedules is not advisable. No scientific studies document side effects, effectiveness, or outcomes based on alternate vaccine delivery schedules. Notwithstanding, with rare exception such as for rabies vaccine, a vaccine series does not need to be restarted regardless of the interval between doses if that interval exceeds the minimum allowed interval between doses. Moreover, CDC recognizes a 4-day grace period if a vaccine is given too early. A vaccine given 5 or more days early must be repeated and not counted in completion of the overall vaccine series. The repeat dose should be given after the recommended minimal interval between doses has elapsed. As an example, a child given a dose of MMR on day 361 of life (the vaccine is due at 365 days of life) does not need to have that dose repeated. A child given a dose of MMR on day 360 of life needs to have a repeat dose given at a minimum of 28 days later. State or local policy may supersede the CDC 4-day grace period rule.

With the exception of MMR-V (ProQuad®) vaccine which is best used only for the 4–6-year dose to avoid febrile seizures in younger children, combination vaccines are preferred. In general, vaccines may be given simultaneously from different syringes at least 1 inch apart. An example of one exception to this rule is the simultaneous administration of Prevnar® (PCV 13) and Menactra® (MenACWY) in asplenic patients. These vaccines should be separated by at least 4 weeks. Killed and live vaccines may be given on the same day. However, if killed and live vaccines are not given on the same day, following a dose of a live vaccine all other vaccines should be delayed by at least 4 weeks. Two different killed vaccines or a live vaccine which is given following a dose of killed vaccine may be separated by any time interval. In a vaccine series administering the same vaccine product from a particular manufacturer is preferred. When the same product is not available, products covering the same VPD may be used interchangeably.

Catch-Up CDC Guidelines and Schedule The increasingly complicated but highly important ACIP vaccine schedule and the mobile American and international public make it extremely likely that some children can get behind on their vaccination schedules or present to your office with different vaccine histories unique to their home country. CDC catch-up vaccination schedule for children age 4 months through 6 years and 7 years through 18 years is online at http://www.cdc.gov/vaccines/schedules/hcp/imz/catchup.html or in the Society of Teachers of Family Medicine (STFM) app, *Shots Immunizations*, or CDC app. Copious footnotes about each specific vaccine are included in the online version or apps.

To keep up to date with immunization practices, physicians must have basic immunization knowledge either memorized or available through online sites or cell phone or handheld computer device applications; a well-trained office staff hopefully led by an office vaccine champion with additional training in immunization practices; access to journals, newsletters, and emails that inform the physician of immunization practice changes; and a reliable consultant from whom to ask specific questions [33]. In place of the latter, questions may be directed to the CDC staff at nipinfo@cdc.gov or the experts at IAC at www.immunize.org/askexperts. Prompt replies are the rule.

Apps

Apps serve as resources in several ways: they allow the patient to record administered immunizations, they provide a ready source for patient education, and they supplement the clinician's immunization knowledge base. As smartphones become universal accoutrements, apps have become useful to provide on-site, immediate access to information, not only for physicians but also for office staff and even for patients. IAC lists the multiple immunization apps available for iPhones and androids in alphabetical order at http://www.immunize.org/resources/apps.asp. This list is updated as new apps become available and is comprehensive. In 2015, Wilson et al. searched the Android app store and the Apple app store for immunization apps [34]. The Android store listed 225 apps and the Apple store 98 apps (some of which were for animals). These authors stated that paper records are missing 10–60% of important information or contained data errors. Unfortunately, smartphone apps are also subject to inaccurate data though recording errors, but they are portable so that they can be used on visits to the office, to emergency departments, to consultants, and during hospitalizations. Although the ownership of smartphones is almost universal, the acceptance of using the smartphone to record medical information is limited. Examples of free vaccines apps to record vaccine administration and to provide patient friendly information are noted above.

The Society of Teachers of Family Medicine (STFM) group on Immunization Education (GIE) produces an app called *Shots Immunizations* downloadable for free. In addition to the complete set of CDC vaccine schedules and footnotes, it includes graphics, images, and commentary about each vaccine. The drop-down list of headings includes the vaccine basics detailing all formulations of vaccine products, high-risk indications, adverse reactions, contraindications and precautions, catch-up advice, routine administration information, epidemiology about the disease being prevented with advice as to how to respond to vaccine hesitant individuals, vaccine brand names and ICD codes, educational information aimed at medical residents, and the excipients/additives in each vaccine. The app also presents immunization schedules containing brand names to reduce confusion about which product may be administered when a particular vaccine component is necessary. It contains a section on smallpox, references, and information about reporting adverse reaction to the Vaccine Adverse Event Reporting System (VAERS). *Shots* is automatically updated annually following changes to CDC unified immunization schedules which generally occurs in February of every new year and following any CDC change to vaccination recommendations throughout the year whenever the user accesses the app. It is also linked to the online STFM vaccine program, http://shotsonline.immunizationed.org/, which provides the same information for desktop or personal computers and to the STFM immunization website, Group on Immunization Education, http://www.immunizationed.org/.

CDC Vaccine Schedules app is widely recognized as the standard against which other apps are judged. It provides the same information found in CDC immunization schedules online. Basically the childhood, adolescent, and adult schedules, medical indications schedule for both children and for adults, catch-up schedule, and contraindications to vaccination are available with footnotes. One major advantage of this app is that it lists additional information and links to prior CDC website and publications which document the approaches to control specific VPDs. The app is automatically updated annually.

Other Apps Many specialties have produced immunization apps. The *AAFP mobile app* is downloadable at http://www.aafp.org/about/membership/services/app.html. The *AAP mobile app* is downloadable at https://www.aap.org/en-us/Pages/Get-the-AAP-Mobile-App.aspx. The *American College of Obstetrics and Gynecology (ACOG) mobile app* is downloadable at http://www.acog.org/ACOGapp. The *American College of Physicians (ACP) mobile app* is downloadable at https://www.acponline.org/acp-newsroom/american-college-of-physicians-immunization-advisor-app-makes-it-easier-for-doctors-to-identify and has a unique function in that it claims to be an "immunization advisor." All of these apps provide a great deal of information pertaining to that particular specialty but basically present the CDC unified immunization schedules with emphasis on the portions that are relevant to that specialty. All of these apps are automatically updated when opened.

Websites

Access to immunization websites is the best resource to maintain current knowledge, to answer questions that arise in practice, and to provide information for the patient, the patient's family, the office staff, and the clinician. Ideally, the reader should spend some time learning to navigate one or two sites (Table 8.2). Many excellent sites are available and each has advantages, but the two most clinically

Table 8.2 Immunization resource websites

Organization	Website
Centers for Disease Control and Prevention (CDC)	http://www.cdc.gov/
Immunization Action Coalition (IAC)	http://www.immunize.org/
Advisory Committee on Immunization Practices (ACIP)	https://www.cdc.gov/vaccines/acip/
Morbidity and Mortality Weekly Report (MMWR)	http://www.cdc.gov/mmwr
Society of Teachers of Family Medicine Group on Immunization Education (STFM GIE)	http://www.immunizationed.org/
National Foundation for Infectious Diseases (NFID)	http://www.nfid.org/
National Network for Immunization Information (NNii)	http://www.immunizationinfo.com/
Children's Hospital of Philadelphia (CHOP)	http://www.chop.edu
American Academy of Family Physicians (AAFP)	http://www.aafp.org/patient-care/public-health/immunizations.html
American Academy of Pediatrics (AAP)	http://www.aap.org/immunization/about/about.html
National Vaccine Advisory Committee (NVAC)	https://www.hhs.gov/nvpo/nvac/
Institute for Vaccine Safety at the Johns Hopkins University School of Public Health	http://www.vaccinesafety.edu/

useful sites are CDC and IAC because each has a mechanism through which the clinician can get a direct answer to a question. One can simply contact the CDC or send a question to IAC at *Ask the Experts (see above)*.

Centers for Disease Control and Prevention (CDC) CDC provides comprehensive information on its website, Vaccines & Immunizations, at https://www.cdc.gov/vaccines/index.html. Physicians and other healthcare providers can register for email updates from CDC at this site. A search engine allows entering the topic of interest which then leads to a list of articles published through the CDC. One difficulty with this approach is that the date for these articles is generally not evident in the resulting list so that the searcher has to open an article to see whether it is the most current. Information categories on the website include "Parents (birth-18 years)," "Adults (19 and older)," "Pregnancy and Vaccination," and "Healthcare workers." Subheadings are available to cover Travel, Refugees, and Immigrants and specific diseases or conditions. Information on pregnancy and vaccines is online at http://www.immunize.org/catg.d/p2019.pdf. An excellent video is available at this site to encourage pregnant women to stay current with pertussis vaccination. Parents can go to CDC Immunization Schedules to create a childhood immunization schedule for each child (http://www2a.cdc.gov/nip/kidstuff/newscheduler_le/). The schedule can then be printed out and kept with the vaccination record. Doing so gives a great deal of information to parents about what vaccines will be expected and might save some time in the office when the child comes in for a routine checkup. A member of the office staff may choose to go through this exercise with each parent during a well-child check. CDC provides advice as to how to deal with vaccine hesitancy. Many physicians and most of their patients have not seen or suffered through the diseases which immunizations are designed to prevent. Pictures of VPDs are available at http://www.cdc.gov/vaccines/vpd-vac/photo-all-vpd.htm and online in the STFM website. Review of the photos from CDC's website with the patient might encourage a reluctant individual to accept vaccination. CDC answers questions from physicians and other healthcare providers at https://wwwn.cdc.gov/dcs/ContactUs/Form. CDC telephone information line is at 800-CDC-INFO (800–232-4636).

Advisory Committee on Immunization Practices (ACIP) ACIP updates are available on the ACIP website or through the CDC home page by clicking on the ACIP link in the right-hand column. ACIP recommendations are published three times a year after each meeting and rarely when an ad hoc meeting is necessary. Clicking on the "Get email updates" on the website ensures automatic notification of every ACIP update.

Immunization Action Coalition (IAC) IAC is a nonprofit organization devoted to immunization education and communication and improving immunization rates. The outstanding staff is under the direction of Deborah L Wexler, M.D., a family physician. Virtually any clinically important immunization fact is available at this website. IAC provides information both for the public and for healthcare professionals. This website contains the following headings: Handouts for Patients and Staff, Vaccine Information Statements (in numerous languages), Ask the Experts, Package Inserts (for virtually every available US vaccine product), State Laws and Mandates (for all states and territories), Clinic Resources, Directory of Resources, Standing Orders (for all vaccines and in a large number of languages), Photos of vaccine preventable diseases, Videos, PowerPoint presentations, Food and Drug Administration (FDA) updates, relevant journal articles, CDC schedules, Unprotected People Reports, Technically Speaking, Billing and Coding information, and Shop IAC which offers countless vaccination aids for sale.

National Network for Immunization Information (NNii) A project of the Infectious Diseases Society of America (IDSA) and the Pediatric Infectious Diseases Society (PIDS) serves as a source of comprehensive information on vaccination and vaccination-related issues for parents, healthcare professionals, and the media. Online at http://www.path.org/vaccineresources/details.php?i=305.

Children's Hospital of Philadelphia (CHOP) The CHOP Vaccine Education Center (http://www.chop.edu/centers-programs/vaccine-education-center#.V9cW32VTHcs) provides up-to-date information and comprehensive reviews of vaccines and VPDs for both parents and for healthcare professionals. The director of the center is Dr. Paul A. Offit, M.D., whose career in vaccine development and promotion is extraordinary. Among his published books and an excellent read for all who vaccinate is *Deadly Choices* which details the fight against anti-vaccination forces [35].

American Academy of Pediatrics (AAP) The AAP website offers the immunization schedules, the latest news on immunizations, and a long list of immunization resources designed for parents and clinicians. A search engine is available, but the lack of production or publication dates on the responses to a search makes it somewhat difficult to utilize. The AAP produces a series of online courses in the PediaLink Online Learning Center accessible through the immunization site. One needs to create an AAP account to use this learning center. Some of these courses are free while others have a low cost like the $14.50 charge for the *Challenging Cases: Pertussis* course. The *Challenging Cases: Vaccine Hesitancy* online course is free. It is quite detailed so takes some time to complete but, once completed, arms the clinician with reasonable responses to almost every worry that could possibly trouble a patient or parent. Most of the materials are open to the general public, but a few require membership in the AAP. AAP members save on all purchases, so if materials on the site are used, the cost of membership is mitigated.

American Academy of Family Physicians (AAFP) The AAFP website offers a great deal of information, but the materials on immunizations are somewhat limited. The basic schedules and a search engine are provided. One distinct advantage to the search engine on this site is that the responses to a search include the dates of publication for articles. Additionally, on the Immunization Schedules page is a heading advising the user how to earn continuing medical education (CME) credit through watching webcasts.

Additional websites: Medscape (http://www.medscape.com/resource/vaccines) from WebMD provides health professionals with an extensive collection of publications on immunizations and links to other useful sites. Site access is free after registration. A complete list of vaccine manufacturers and their websites are available through IAC at http://www.immunize.org/resources/manufact_vax.asp. These websites only provide FDA-approved information about vaccine products. A change in any FDA information is generally made to the website immediately. Most manufacturers accept questions about vaccines and respond quickly with scientifically accurate information. A general internet search usually leads to excellent sources but can also lead to anti-vaccine sites listed prominently and looking professional and legitimate, so when advising patients to look online advise that they specifically look at the IAC, AAFP, STFM, CDC, or specialty society sites. CDC guidelines to help evaluate web information are at http://www.cdc.gov/vaccines/vac-gen/evalwebs.htm entitled *Finding Credible Vaccine Information*.

Books, Journals, and Newsletters

Books

Interestingly, books devoted to immunization are often referred to by color. Anyone wanting ready access to VPD information should be aware of CDC Epidemiology and Prevention of Vaccine-Preventable Diseases (The Pink Book) [36], The Vaccine

Handbook (The Purple Book) [37], CDC Health Information for International Travel 2016 (The Yellow Book) [38], AAP The Red Book [39], and, of course, the non-colored outlier, Vaccines (it's blue and gray) [40] . The IAC lists these reference books and some periodicals online at http://www.immunize.org/resources/books_refer.asp. These books provide everything one needs to know about vaccines. They can be read to enhance basic vaccine knowledge and to answer clinical queries. All are available online and all can be downloaded into handheld devices.

The CDC Pink Book is the best all-around reference for a particular vaccine or VPD. One can sign up on the Pink Book homepage for email notification whenever a change is made. A 2017 supplement is available online. In June 2016 CDC started a 15-part chapter-by-chapter webinar series of the 2015 13th edition of the Pink Book. This series of 1-h webinars is available online, and CME credit is available for up to a year after the date of the session first went live. Registration and more information are available on CDC's Pink Book Webinar Series web page at https://www.cdc.gov/vaccines/ed/webinar-epv/. CDC National Center for Immunization and Respiratory Diseases (NCIRD) periodically presents a 2-day comprehensive review of immunization principles, VPDs, and the recommended vaccines from material in the Pink Book (see http://www.cdc.gov/ncird/isd.html). The course is designed for physicians, nurses, medical assistants, pharmacists, immunization providers, program managers, and nursing and medical students seeking the most comprehensive knowledge about immunization.

The Yellow Book is an essential reference for all those who provide immunizations for travelers. In 2016, the full version costs $9.99 to download to an iPhone or android. A free download, Dr. Gary Marshall's Purple Book is a superlative, comprehensive report on vaccine development, safety, surveillance, and utilization and all VPDs. A perusal of this work will provide the reader with the information required to answer almost any worry from a vaccine-hesitant patient or parent and greatly enhance the reader's understanding of the intense scrutiny in place to ensure vaccine safety and effectiveness. A paperback copy with 560 pages of information may be purchased for $30.

Most pediatricians consider the Red Book as a required reference text. One feature that is particularly useful in the office is the ability to show pictures online of different diseases to patients or parents who may be unsure about the benefits of vaccination. In addition to providing general information about all major infectious diseases, the Red Book covers many special situations including day care and school health immunization advice. It costs $150 to download or purchase. Red Book Online at http://redbook.solutions.aap.org/ also sends periodic updates about disease management and vaccine recommendations like the flu alert sent on 9/16/16.

Vaccines is the most comprehensive textbook on vaccinations. The 2013 6th edition is 1550 pages long and costs $385. Because it is so complete, it is somewhat difficult to use to answer on-the-spot clinical questions. However, it is an unbeatable source if one wishes to understand vaccine science and the worldwide issues involving VPDs.

Journals

The Morbidity and Mortality Weekly Report (MMWR) is absolutely essential reading for anyone hoping to keep current. This publication is online every week and documents current outbreaks, updates in vaccine recommendations, and provides up-to-date numbers on VPDs. It also publishes occasional special reports and supplements covering topics such as annual influenza vaccination recommendations and general guidelines on immunizations. It is free on the MMWR Website at Free Electronic Subscription, http://www.cdc.gov/mmwr/mmwrsubscribe.html. It can be linked to through Twitter or Facebook. Podcasts are available as well.

Many major journals routinely print articles on vaccines and vaccine research, but the preeminent journal for those interested in vaccines and vaccination processes is *Vaccine* edited by Gregory Poland, M.D., and available at http://www.journals.elsevier.com/vaccine. A personal subscription is $520.

Newsletters

CDC Immunization Works is published monthly and available free online at http://www.cdc.gov/vaccines/news/newsltrs/imwrks/index.html. It presents top immunization stories such as information about the planned 47th National Immunization Conference, updates from MMWR, specifics about currently required vaccines like influenza vaccine, resources and information like scheduled ACIP meetings, and a calendar of events that includes local and national conferences or courses with an emphasis on immunization.

IAC produces a free, weekly, online immunization information bulletin, *IAC Express*, which is essential reading for anyone wanting to stay current. IAC Express has an interesting feature called *Ask the Experts*, designed to deal with dilemmas from practice and manned by top-notch experts. An example from *Ask the Experts* comes from a clinician who wrote in asking about the use of Twinrix®, the combination hepatitis A and hepatitis B vaccine that is recommended to be given at times 0, 1, and 6 months and the use of the hepatitis B monovalent vaccine. He knew that the traditional hepatitis B vaccination series was a three-injection series, given at times 0, 1, and 6 months. He knew that the traditional hepatitis A vaccination series was a two-shot series given 6 months apart. He chose to substitute the second, middle dose of the Twinrix® vaccine with hepatitis B monovalent vaccine thinking he was sparing his patients an "extra dose" of hepatitis A vaccine. He was informed, as were the readers of the feature, that Twinrix® contains only half as much hepatitis A antigen as the two available hepatitis A vaccines given at times 0 and 6 months. Therefore, the total antigen load of hepatitis A vaccine given to the clinician's patient was 1/2 of what it should have been. The advice from the IAC expert was that to be fully protected the patient required another single dose of monovalent hepatitis A vaccine 5 months after the last dose of Twinrix®.

The IAC also regularly publishes *Needle Tips* and *Vaccinate Adults*, both of which are written for healthcare professionals who provide immunization services and are available either in print or online. Every issue includes the *Ask the Experts* feature, the *Vaccine Highlights* section with news from ACIP and CDC, materials from IAC to photocopy for staff and patients, products you can purchase from IAC, and special views such as patient schedules for adults. In the guidelines section are single page printouts with titles such as *Vaccinations for Adults—You're Never Too Old to Get Immunized* and *Vaccinations for Man Who Have Sex with Men* as well as items for persons with HIV or hepatitis C infection, with diabetes, heart disease or lung disease, or for persons without a spleen. The publication is found at http://www.immunize.org/nslt.d/n67/patient_schedules_adult_high-risk.pdf.   These sheets can be photocopied and handed to patients and are frankly great reviews for the office staff as well.

The AAP also publishes a newsletter online at http://www.healthychildren.org. To disseminate information about the worldwide status of immunization, the World Health Organization (WHO) produces an online monthly newsletter at http://www.who.int/immunization/gin/en/. NCIRD also publishes a periodic newsletter at http://www.cdc.gov/ncird/div/dbd/newsletters/2016/summer/meetings-presentations.html. The FDA newsletter is at http://www.fdanews.com/newsletters. One can also sign on to get email from the FDA to stay current with changes in drug and vaccine indications and warnings. Physicians and other healthcare providers should also consult local vaccine organizations and government entities like the state or county health department, many of which produce their own newsletters that provide critical local information.

Vaccines for Special Circumstances

Routine vaccination should be fundamental for health maintenance in all circumstances. Special situations such as immunosuppression, postexposure to infectious diseases, pregnancy, prematurity, certain chronic diseases, and some lifestyles (smokers, men who have sex with men) increase the risk of diseases or adverse postvaccination events. In some situations, special vaccines or different vaccination schedules are indicated, and some vaccines ought to be postponed or even forbidden [41]. Vaccination rates for persons in these categories are notoriously poor. For example, only 18% of persons aged 19–49 years with a chronic liver condition have received hepatitis A vaccine [42]. Other targeted vaccines are equally low. CDC Adult Immunization Schedule by Medical and Other Conditions and Child and Adolescent Immunization Schedule by Medical and Other Conditions, new for 2017, can be found at http://www.cdc.gov/vaccines/schedules/. Frequent consultation with these CDC schedules could potentially improve low immunization rates particularly in individuals with diabetes, asthma, or renal failure and in smokers. Regardless of the underlying condition, all persons need to have annual flu vaccine and one lifetime dose of Tdap. Unfortunately, the CDC schedule does not cover all diagnoses clearly within a risk category. For example, heart disease is listed with the specific exclusion of hypertension as an indication; whether coronary artery disease is a risk factor is not mentioned. Similarly, the time since recovery from cancer does not appear to be a factor as to which vaccines are necessary. Clearly an individual being treated for breast cancer now is at high risk. If the breast cancer resolved 15 years ago, the individual may no longer be at increased risk. Many of the recommendations are left to interpretation, but questions about specific issues can be sent to CDC for clarification as mentioned above.

Immunocompromised

The Infectious Disease Society of America has published a clinical guideline for vaccination of the immunocompromised host [43]. In general, killed vaccines are safe in all circumstances, while live vaccines are generally contraindicated. Many immunocompromised individuals require special attention prior to receiving a vaccination.

Some potentially immunocompromising conditions are not included in the CDC chart. For example, persons with *rheumatoid arthritis* (RA) have an increased burden of infectious disease related morbidity and mortality that is roughly twice that of the general population [44]. RA patients are frequently on immunocompromising medications such as steroids or methotrexate or receiving monoclonal antibody therapy. Few studies have been done in this group to determine which vaccines are safe and effective. Clearly annual influenza vaccination is important in this group. A single lifetime dose of Tdap is also indicated. However, the safety of herpes zoster vaccine and the potential benefit of revaccination against pneumococcal disease both need to be studied. Similar issues arise when patients such as those with inflammatory bowel disease are on monoclonal antibody treatment. In general, in congruence with recommendations for other immunocompromised patients, live vaccines are avoided in this situation.

Vaccination post-solid organ *transplantation* or bone marrow replacement is still in need of study. Some researchers have worried that vaccination might trigger rejection, but to date no such rejection has been found for influenza vaccine in heart transplant recipients [45]. Some live vaccines seem to be safe in those with immunocompromising conditions. For example, varicella vaccine can be given to children with HIV if the CD4 is ≥15% [46]. The timing of vaccination is also of import. If possible, vaccine should be given at least 2 weeks prior to undergoing any immunocompromising therapies or 3–6 months afterward.

Adults who are *asplenic* or suffering from hemoglobinopathies such as sickle cell disease should be fully vaccinated including annual flu vaccination and at least one lifetime dose of Tdap [47]. The vaccination schedule for those needing immunization update after splenectomy can be quite complicated in regards to pneumococcal vaccinations. Full vaccination after the spleen is already gone means one dose of pneumococcal vaccination with PCV13 followed ≥8 weeks later by pneumococcal vaccination with PPSV23. Another dose of PPSV23 will be needed in

5 years if the patient is under 65 years old. No further doses are needed if this second dose was given at age ≥65 years. If the dose was given at age ≤64 years, then a third and final dose of PPSV23 will be needed after the patient turns age 65 years and at least 5 years after the second dose. The order of pneumococcal vaccination is also important: if PPSV23 was given first, then the individual must wait 1 year to receive PCV13 whereas if PCV13 was given first, as recommended, PPSV23 is given ≥8 weeks later. Evidence for the timing of all vaccinations post-splenectomy is not abundant, but vaccinating any time 14 days after splenectomy is reasonable. If postoperative vaccine administration is performed prior to postoperative day 14, it is reasonable to repeat the post-splenectomy vaccines 8 weeks after the initial doses.

This scenario is further complicated by the recommendation to vaccinate patients prior to a planned and scheduled elective splenectomy when possible. Whenever elective splenectomy is considered, patients should undergo immunization against *Streptococcus pneumoniae* (pneumococcus), *Neisseria meningitides* (meningococcus), and *Haemophilus influenzae* type b (Hib) at appropriately timed intervals. Asplenic patients need two doses of meningococcal quadrivalent conjugate vaccine (groups A, C, Y, W) separated by 8 weeks with a booster dose every 5 years, two or three doses of meningococcal B vaccine depending upon which manufacturer's product is used. Whenever possible, these vaccines should be administered at least 2 weeks prior to splenectomy. Multiple vaccines can be given concomitantly except for the two pneumococcal vaccines as discussed above and separation of PCV13 from the specific product Menactra® (MenACWY). In patient undergoing immunosuppressive chemotherapy or radiotherapy, immunization should be delayed for at least 3 months after completion of therapy [43].

Pregnancy

Pregnant women should receive a dose of Tdap with every pregnancy preferably between weeks 27 and 36 of gestation, assuming prior vaccination against tetanus. Vaccinating during the 27–36th week of pregnancy provides the newborn with the highest level of antibody to protect against pertussis during the first few months of life. Women who have NOT ever been vaccinated against tetanus should be given Td early in pregnancy with a second dose of Td or Tdap at least 4 weeks later and a third dose at least 6 months later [48]. Hopefully the Tdap dose which is acceptable at any time during the second or third trimester can be given in the 27–36 week window. The total number of doses tetanus (up to three) administered will depend upon prior tetanus vaccination records. Pregnant women should also receive influenza vaccine during any trimester of pregnancy. In fact, asking about pregnancy is not required prior to giving a woman of childbearing age influenza vaccine. Of course pregnant women should also have antibody evidence of immunity to rubella and preferably evidence of vaccination or immunity to measles, mumps, and chickenpox. Women who are not immune to one of these diseases should receive appropriate vaccination immediately postpartum.

Travelers

Vaccines for travelers are best assessed by consulting the 2016 Yellow Book and checking online at CDC Features, *Travel Smart: Get Vaccinated* online at http://www.cdc.gov/features/vaccines-travel/. The best vaccines for travel will depend upon the specifics including the countries of destination and whether one will be in urban vs. rural areas, time of year one is traveling, specific diseases for which the individual should be on alert, and the individual's underlying health status. Disease outbreaks vary from time to time, so consulting these online resources is critical to being certain that one is safe for travel. Some countries still require a yellow fever vaccine certificate. The list is available at the WHO Country List Yellow Fever vaccination requirements and recommendations, malaria situation, and other vaccination requirements (http://who.int/ith/ITH_country_list.pdf). Young babies who travel to a region with a reported measles outbreak are recommended to receive MMR earlier than usual, at age 6–12 months, but this vaccination dose is not counted in the required two doses of MMR to be ultimately protected [49].

Other Special Circumstances

Other special circumstances include certain occupations. Service in the military, working in a laboratory, or working as a healthcare provider are a few examples of occupations which may require additional vaccines. Several vaccines such as adenovirus vaccine are only approved for use in the military because infection can be widespread and spreads quickly. Members of the military receive vaccines when they enter basic training and before deployment to protect against disease threats specific to those environments in which they may serve [50]. Smallpox vaccination is only recommended for laboratory workers who handle orthopoxviruses and for smallpox epidemic response teams (*Shots Immunization* app). Workers at high risk of exposure to rabies, such as veterinarians, animal handlers, rabies laboratory workers, spelunkers, and rabies biologics production workers should be offered rabies vaccine as a preventive three dose series [51]. Healthcare workers, including physicians, nurses, clinical medical staff, emergency medical personnel, dental professionals and students, medical and nursing students, laboratory technicians, pharmacists, hospital volunteers, and administrative staff are at risk for both contracting VPDs because of constant exposure and spreading VPDs to others. Vaccine recommendations for healthcare workers include the hepatitis B series, MMR, varicella, Tdap, meningococcal (for some workers regularly exposed to *N. meningitidis*), and annual influenza vaccine [52]. Many healthcare employers have wisely and justly mandated that employees receive annual influenza vaccination. In general, employers will clarify which vaccines are required of their employees.

Postexposure Prophylaxis (PEP)

Some vaccines are recommended to be given as postexposure prophylaxis (PEP) soon after exposure to certain infectious diseases. For example, varicella vaccination is ideally given 3–5 days after exposure to the disease for an unvaccinated person but may be given any time after exposure [53]. Post-animal bite when the rabies status of the animal is unknown, four doses of rabies vaccine are recommended along with rabies immune globulin to be given at the same time as the first immunization dose. Dose 1 is given immediately as quickly as possible after the bite, along with the immune globulin, and additional doses on the 3rd, 7th, and 14th day later. If a previously vaccinated individual is bitten by a suspect animal, only two doses of rabies vaccine are indicated, on day 1 and day 3, and rabies immune globulin is not needed [51]. For unvaccinated persons exposed to blood or body fluids that are known to be hepatitis B (HBV) positive, PEP in the form of hepatitis B immune globulin (HBIG) is indicated along with one dose of hepatitis B vaccine to be administered as soon as possible after the exposure. The person should then complete the vaccination series according to the vaccination schedule. Infants born to HPV-infected mothers should receive hepatitis B vaccine and HBIG within 12 h of birth [54]. Hepatitis A (HAV) vaccine is preferred over immune globulin (IG) for PEP for people ages 12 months to 40 years who have recently been exposed to HAV. For those over 40 years of age, IG is preferred, although the vaccine can be used if IG is unavailable [55]. In the face of an outbreak of pertussis, DTaP vaccine can be given as early as 6 weeks of age. A third dose of MMR may be needed to control a mumps outbreak [56]. Schools and colleges may require that students at least be offered certain vaccines such as meningococcal B vaccine. Meningococcal vaccines are recommended during times of meningitis outbreaks which can occur in communities, schools, colleges, prisons, and other populations. During an outbreak caused by meningitis serogroup A, C, W, or Y, vaccination with a quadrivalent meningococcal conjugate vaccine covering those four strains is indicated and for those 2 months or older. Meningococcal vaccine covering serogroup B is to be used in the appropriate outbreak setting [57].

Men Who Have Sex with Men (MSM)

MSM are affected by higher rates of sexually transmitted diseases than other men and therefore are recommended to complete the MenACWY, hepatitis A, and hepatitis B vaccine series along with an annual seasonal flu vaccine. For those MSM up to age 26 years, they are recommended to also complete the HPV vaccination series [58].

Summary

Physicians and other healthcare workers who immunize patients must incorporate a structured approach to determination and documentation of a patient's vaccine status beyond self-reporting. Doing so requires review of the patient's immunization record as documented in their personal files or office medical record, review of electronic state registries, and review of written medical records from various other sources. The vaccine status should be assessed at each office visit to keep the patient and the patient's family up to date. Careful attention should be made to the recording and documentation of the vaccine administered both in the state registry and in the patient's personal medical record. Lastly, patients should receive record of their vaccinations. To keep current on immunization recommendations, the author favors regular perusal of the MMWR, IAC Express, and emails from CDC. For in-depth study of a vaccine or VPD, the CDC Pink Book is an excellent resource. Both IAC and CDC websites are top-notch resources to utilize in helping to solve clinical vaccination questions and problems as well as for downloading patient-friendly materials. This author's preference is for the STFM *Shots Immunization* app which provides all the information one needs in daily office practice, but the CDC and AAFP apps come in as close seconds. All are free and are useful to help identify which immunizations your patient needs on any given day. Patients with special circumstances such as certain chronic diseases, immunosuppression, certain occupations, postexposure, and MSM may require additional vaccines or recommendations and follow different vaccination guidelines.

References

1. CDC. Whitney CG, Zhou F, Singleton J, Schuchat A. Benefits from Immunization During the Vaccines for Children Program Era — United States 1994–2013. MMWR [Internet] April 25 2014;63(16):352–355. [cited 2017 June 21] Available from: http://www.cdc.gov/mmwr/preview/mmwrhtml/mm6316a4.htm.
2. National Vaccine Advisory Committee. Recommendations from the National Vaccine Advisory Committee: standards for adult immunization practice. Public Health Rep [Internet]. 2014;129(2):115–23. [cited 2016 Oct 8]. Available from: http://www.ncbi.nlm.nih.gov/pubmed/24587544.
3. Orenstein WA, Beigi RH, Lynfield R, Maldonado Y, Rothholz MC, Smith N, et al. Assessing the state of vaccine confidence in the United States: recommendations from the National Vaccine Advisory Committee. Public Health Rep [Internet] 2015 Nov-Dec;130(6):573-95. [cited 2017 june 21] Available from: https://www.ncbi.nlm.nih.gov/pubmed/26556929
4. Rolnick SJ, Parker ED, Nordin JD, Hedblom BD, Wei F, Kerby T, et al. Self-report compared to electronic medical record across eight adult vaccines: do results vary by demographic factors? Vaccine [Internet]. 2013;31(37):3928–35. [cited 2016 Oct 8]. Available from: http://www.ncbi.nlm.nih.gov/pubmed/23806243.
5. Oh J, Washburn T, Kim HH. Missed opportunity to provide HPV vaccine and educate adolescents: Rhode Island middle and high school students' self-reported HPV vaccination, 2013 RI YRBS. R I Med J (2013) [Internet]. 2014;97(12):35–8. [cited 2016 Oct 8]. Available from: http://www.ncbi.nlm.nih.gov/pubmed/25463626.
6. CDC. Hepatitis B FAQs for Health Professionals. Division of Viral Hepatitis. [Internet]. [cited 2017 June 21] Available from: http://www.cdc.gov/hepatitis/hbv/hbvfaq.htm.
7. MacDonald R, Baken L, Nelson A, Nichol KL, Fedson DS, McBean AM, et al. Validation of self-report of influenza and pneumococcal vaccination status in elderly outpatients. Am J Prev Med [Internet]. 1999;16(3):173–7. [cited 2016 Oct 2]. Available from: http://linkinghub.elsevier.com/retrieve/pii/S0749379798001597.

8. Irving SA, Donahue JG, Shay DK, Ellis-Coyle TL, Belongia EA. Evaluation of self-reported and registry-based influenza vaccination status in a Wisconsin cohort. Vaccine [Internet]. 2009;27(47):6546–9. [cited 2016 Oct 8]. Available from: http://www.ncbi.nlm.nih.gov/pubmed/19729083.
9. Lochner KA, Wynne MA, Wheatcroft GH, Worrall CM, Kelman JA. Medicare claims versus beneficiary self-report for influenza vaccination surveillance. Am J Prev Med [Internet]. 2015;48(4):384–91. [cited 2016 Oct 8]. Available from: http://www.ncbi.nlm.nih.gov/pubmed/25700653.
10. Nowalk MP, Zimmerman RK, Tabbarah M, Raymund M, Jewell IK. Determinants of adult vaccination at inner-city health centers: a descriptive study. BMC Fam Pract [Internet]. 2006;7:2. [cited 2016 Oct 8]. Available from: http://www.ncbi.nlm.nih.gov/pubmed/16403215.
11. Skull SA, Andrews RM, Byrnes GB, Kelly HA, Nolan TM, Brown GV, et al. Validity of self-reported influenza and pneumococcal vaccination status among a cohort of hospitalized elderly inpatients. Vaccine [Internet]. 2007;25(25):4775–83. [cited 2016 Oct 8]. Available from: http://www.ncbi.nlm.nih.gov/pubmed/17499402.
12. IIS | State Programmatic and Technical Contacts | Vaccines | CDC [Internet]. Available from: http://www.cdc.gov/vaccines/programs/iis/contacts-registry-staff.html.
13. Martin DW, Lowery NE, Brand B, Gold R, Horlick G. Immunization information systems: a decade of progress in law and policy. J Public Health Manag Pract [Internet]. 2015;21(3):296–303. [cited 2016 Oct 8]. Available from: http://www.ncbi.nlm.nih.gov/pubmed/24402434.
14. Groom H, Hopkins DP, Pabst LJ, Murphy Morgan J, Patel M, Calonge N, et al. Immunization information systems to increase vaccination rates: a community guide systematic review. J Public Health Manag Pract [Internet]. 2015;21(3):227–48. [cited 2016 Oct 8]. Available from: http://www.ncbi.nlm.nih.gov/pubmed/24912082.
15. Kepka D, Spigarelli MG, Warner EL, Yoneoka Y, McConnell N, Balch A. Statewide analysis of missed opportunities for human papillomavirus vaccination using vaccine registry data. Papillomavirus Res (Amsterdam, Netherlands) [Internet]. 2016;2:128–32. [cited 2016 Oct 8]. Available from: http://www.ncbi.nlm.nih.gov/pubmed/27540595.
16. Niccolai LM, McBride V, Julian PR, Connecticut HPV-IMPACT Working Group. Sources of information for assessing human papillomavirus vaccination history among young women. Vaccine [Internet]. 2014;32(25):2945–7. [cited 2016 Oct 8]. Available from: http://www.ncbi.nlm.nih.gov/pubmed/24713369.
17. Skelton JB, American Pharmacists Association, Academy of Managed Care Pharmacy. Pharmacist-provided immunization compensation and recognition: white paper summarizing APhA/AMCP stakeholder meeting. J Am Pharm Assoc (2003) [Internet]. 2011;51(6):704–12. [cited 2017 June 21]. Available from: http://www.ncbi.nlm.nih.gov/pubmed/22068191.
18. Steyer TE, Ragucci KR, Pearson WS, Mainous AG. The role of pharmacists in the delivery of influenza vaccinations. Vaccine. 2004;22(8):1001–6.
19. Arthur BC, Fisher AK, Shoemaker SJ, Pozniak A, Stokley S. Business models, vaccination services, and public health relationships of retail clinics: a qualitative study. J Healthc Manag [Internet]. 2015;60(6):429–40. [cited 2016 Oct 8]. Available from: http://www.ncbi.nlm.nih.gov/pubmed/26720987.
20. Williams WW, Lu P-J, O'Halloran A, Kim DK, Grohskopf LA, Pilishvili T, et al. Surveillance of vaccination coverage among adult populations — United States, 2014. MMWR Surveill Summ [Internet]. 2016;65(1):1–36. [cited 2016 Oct 8]. Available from: http://www.cdc.gov/mmwr/volumes/65/ss/ss6501a1.htm.
21. CDC. Place of influenza vaccination among adults – United States, 2010–11 influenza season. MMWR [Internet] 2011;60(23):781-85. [cited 2017 June 21] Available from: https://www.cdc.gov/mmwr/preview/mmwrhtml/mm6023a3.htm.
22. CDC. Information for Businesses & Employers. Seasonal Influenza (Flu). [Internet]. [cited 2017 June 21] Available from: http://www.cdc.gov/flu/business/index.htm.
23. MacDonald SE, Schopflocher DP, Golonka RP. The pot calling the kettle black: the extent and type of errors in a computerized immunization registry and by parent report. BMC Pediatr

[Internet]. 2014;14:1. Available from: http://www.ncbi.nlm.nih.gov/pubmed/24387002. [cited 2016 Oct 8].

24. Hendrickson BK, Panchanathan SS, Petitti D. Evaluation of immunization data completeness within a large community health care system exchanging data with a state immunization information system. J Public Health Manag Pract [Internet]. 2015;21(3):288–95. [cited 2016 Oct 8]. Available from: http://www.ncbi.nlm.nih.gov/pubmed/24378608.

25. Abramson E, Kaushal R, Vest J. Improving immunization data management: an editorial on the potential of Electronic Health Records. Expert Rev Vaccines [Internet]. 2014;13(2):189–91. [cited 2016 Oct 8]. Available from: http://www.ncbi.nlm.nih.gov/pubmed/24350664.

26. Shop IAC: Immunization Record Cards [Internet]. Available from: http://www.immunize.org/shop/record-cards.asp.

27. Wilson K, Atkinson KM, Deeks SL, Crowcroft NS. Improving vaccine registries through mobile technologies: a vision for mobile enhanced Immunization information systems. J Am Med Inform Assoc [Internet]. 2016;23(1):207–11. [cited 2016 Oct 8]. Available from: http://www.ncbi.nlm.nih.gov/pubmed/26078414.

28. Savoy M. How to Motivate Patients to Immunize. STFM Blog [Internet]. [cited 2017 June 21] Available from: https://blog.stfm.org/2015/07/20/how-to-motivate-patients-to-immunize/.

29. National Foundation for Infectious Diseases. Call To Action: Adult Vaccination Saves Lives. [Internet]. Bethesda, Md. 2012;1-6. [cited 2017 June 21] Available from: http://www.adultvaccination.org/resources/cta-adult.pdf

30. Murkoff H. What to Expect. Guide to Immunizations. [Internet]. [cited 2017 June 21] Available from: http://www.gethealthystayhealthy.com/sites/default/files/whattoexpect_immunization-guide.pdf.

31. Valuing Vaccinations Across Generations — Intergenerational Program — Penn State Extension [Internet]. May 3, 2016. [cited 2017 June 21] Available from: http://extension.psu.edu/youth/intergenerational/news/2016/valuing-vaccinations-across-generations.

32. Bright Futures Guidelines and Pocket Guide [Internet]. Available from: https://brightfutures.aap.org/materials-and-tools/guidelines-and-pocket-guide/Pages/default.aspx.

33. Middleton DB, Zimmerman RK, Troy JA, Wolfe RM. Keeping up-to-date with immunization practices. Prim Care [Internet]. 2011;38(4):747–61, ix. [cited 2016 Oct 8]. Available from: http://www.ncbi.nlm.nih.gov/pubmed/22094144.

34. Wilson K, Atkinson KM, Westeinde J. Apps for immunization: Leveraging mobile devices to place the individual at the center of care. Hum Vaccin Immunother [Internet]. 2015;11(10):2395–9. [cited 2016 Oct 8]. Available from: http://www.ncbi.nlm.nih.gov/pubmed/26110351.

35. Offit P. Deadly Choices. [Internet]. Basic Books, New York City, NY 2011. [cited 2017 June 21] Available from: http://pauloffit.com/booksby/deadly-choices/.

36. Hamborsky J, Kroger A, Wolfe C, eds. National Center for Immunization and Respiratory Diseases (U.S.). Communication and Education Branch. Epidemiology and prevention of vaccine-preventable diseases, 13th ed. 2015. 2017 supplement. {internet}. [cited 2017 June 21] Available from: http://www.cdc.gov/vaccine/pubs/pinkbook/index.html

37. Marshall G. Shop IAC: The Vaccine Handbook: A Practical Guide for Clinicians, 6th ed. 2017. [Internet]. [cited 2017 June 21] Available from: http://www.immunize.org/vaccine-handbook/.

38. CDC. CDC Yellow Book 2018 Health Information for International Travel. [Internet]. [cited 2017 June 21.] Available from: http://wwwnc.cdc.gov/travel/page/yellowbook-home.

39. AAP. Kimberlin DW, Brady MT, Jackson MA, Long SS, eds. Red Book 2015. Red Book Online. Point-of-Care Solutions. [Internet]. [cited 2017 June 21.] Available from: http://redbook.solutions.aap.org/book.aspx?bookid=1484.

40. Plotkin SA, Orenstein WA, Offit PA. Vaccines. 6th ed. Philadelphia: Elsevier Saunders, St. Louis, Mo; 2013.

41. Succi RC d M, Farhat CK. Vaccination in special situations. J Pediatr (Rio J) [Internet]. 2006;82(3 Suppl):S91–100. [cited 2016 Oct 8]. Available from: http://www.ncbi.nlm.nih.gov/pubmed/16683052.

42. Williams WW, Lu P-J, O'Halloran A, Kim DK, Grohskopf LA, Pilishvili T, et al. Surveillance of vaccination coverage among adult populations – United States, 2014. MMWR Surveill Summ [Internet]. 2016;65(1):1–36. [cited 2016 Aug 27]. Available from: http://www.ncbi.nlm.nih.gov/pubmed/26844596.

43. Rubin LG, Levin MJ, Ljungman P, Davies EG, Avery R, Tomblyn M, et al. 2013 IDSA clinical practice guideline for vaccination of the immunocompromised host. Clin Infect Dis [Internet]. 2014;58(3):309–18. [cited 2016 Oct 8]. Available from: http://www.ncbi.nlm.nih.gov/pubmed/24421306.

44. Perry LM, Winthrop KL, Curtis JR. Vaccinations for rheumatoid arthritis. Curr Rheumatol Rep [Internet]. 2014;16(8):431. [cited 2016 Oct 8] Available from: http://www.ncbi.nlm.nih.gov/pubmed/24925587.

45. White-Williams C, Brown R, Kirklin J, St. Clair K, Keck S, O'Donnell J, et al. Improving clinical practice: should we give influenza vaccinations to heart transplant patients? J Heart Lung Transp [Internet] 2006 March; 25 (3): 320-23. [cited 2017 June 21]

46. CDC. Routine varicella vaccination. [Internet]. [cited 2017 June 21] Available from: https://www.cdc.gov/vaccines/vpd/varicella/hcp/recommendations.html.

47. CDC. Asplenia and adult vaccination. [Internet]. [cited 2017 June 21] Available from: https://www.cdc.gov/vaccines/adults/rec-vac/health-conditions/asplenia.html.

48. Pregnancy and Vaccination I Guidelines and Recommendations by Vaccine I CDC [Internet]. Available from: http://www.cdc.gov/vaccines/pregnancy/hcp/guidelines.html#tdap

49. Measles I Home I Rubeola I CDC [Internet]. Available from: https://www.cdc.gov/measles/.

50. Vaccine Recommendations I Health.mil [Internet]. Available from: http://www.health.mil/Military-Health-Topics/Health-Readiness/Immunization-Healthcare/Vaccine-Recommendations.

51. Vaccine Information Statement I Rabies I VIS I CDC [Internet]. Available from: http://www.cdc.gov/vaccines/hcp/vis/visstatements/rabies.html.

52. Recommended vaccines for healthcare workers. [Internet]. Available from: http://www.cdc.gov/vaccines/adults/rec-vac/hcw.html.

53. Vaccines: VPD-VAC/Varicella/Post-exposure Vaccination [Internet]. Available from: http://www.cdc.gov/vaccines/vpdvac/varicella/hcp-post-exposure.htm.

54. CDC Guidance for evaluating health-care personnel for hepatitis B virus protection and for administering postexposure management. [Internet]. Available from: http://www.cdc.gov/mmwr/preview/mmwrhtml/rr6210a1.htm.

55. Ask the Experts about Hepatitis A Vaccines – CDC experts answer Q&As [Internet]. Available from: http://www.immunize.org/askexperts/experts_hepa.asp.

56. Albertson JP, Clegg WJ, Reid HD, Arbise BS, Pryde J, Vaid A, et al. Mumps outbreak at a university and recommendation for a third dose of measles-mumps-rubella vaccine — Illinois, 2015–2016. MMWR [Internet]. 2016;65(29):731–4. [cited 2016 Oct 8]. Available from: http://www.cdc.gov/mmwr/volumes/65/wr/mm6529a2.htm.

57. Meningococcal I Outbreaks I CDC [Internet]. Available from: http://www.cdc.gov/meningococcal/outbreaks/.

58. For Your Health I Gay and Bisexual Men's Health I CDC [Internet]. Available from: http://www.cdc.gov/msmhealth/for-your-health.htm.

Index

© Springer International Publishing AG 2017
P.G. Rockwell (ed.), *Vaccine Science and Immunization Guideline*,
DOI 10.1007/978-3-319-60471-8

Printed in the United States
By Bookmasters